DIABETES – DAMAGES AND TREATMENTS

Edited by **Everlon Cid Rigobelo**

Diabetes – Damages and Treatments
Edited by Everlon Cid Rigobelo

Published by InTech

Janeza Trdine 9, 51000 Rijeka, Croatia

Publishing Process Manager Alenka Urbancic

Technical Editor Teodora Smiljanic

Cover Designer InTech Design Team

Additional hard copies can be obtained from orders@intechopen.com

Diabetes – Damages and Treatments, Edited by Everlon Cid Rigobelo
p. cm.
ISBN 978-953-307-652-2

For EU product safety concerns:
IN TECH d.o.o., Prolaz Marije Krucifikse Kozulić 3, 51000 Rijeka, Croatia,
info@intechopen.com or visit our website at intechopen.com.

Meet the editor

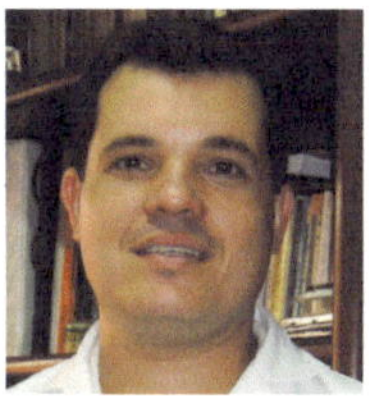

Dr. Everlon Cid Rigobelo graduated from Agronomy School Universidade Estadual Paulista, Brazil, in 2000. He received his M.S. degree in Animal Science Microbiology from the same University in 2002. He obtained his Ph.D from the same University. Rigobelo has experience in genetics, epidemiology and is active in the following subjects: microbial biotechnology, molecular genetics and bacterial genomics. He works with the probiotic strains against colonization caused by Escherichia coli STEC, Pasteurella multocida, Leptospirosis. He previously worked with physiological parameters caused by septicemia in pigs, among which is hypoglycemia.

Contents

Preface

Over the last few decades the prevalence of diabetes has dramatically grown in most regions of the world. In 2010, 285 million people were diagnosed with diabetes and it is estimated that the number will increase to 438 million in 2030.

Hypoglycemia is a disorder where the glucose serum concentration is usually low. The organism usually keeps the glucose serum concentration in a range of 70 to 110 mL/dL of blood. In hypoglycemia the glucose concentration remains normally lower than 50 mL/dL of blood. This book comprehensively reviews and compiles information on hypoglycemia in 18 chapters which cover occurrence, damages, treatments and preventions, and relevant discussions about the occurrence of hypoglycemia in neonates, drug-induced and caused by infections in animals.

This book is written by authors from America, Europe, Asia and Africa, yet, the editor has tried arrange the book chapters in a issue order to make it easier for the readers to find what they need. However, the reader can still find differ approaches on the same issue in same Section.

Section A, which includes chapters 1-2, mainly describes the management approach and Hypoglycemia in children. It includes some treatment methods and their applications.

Section B, which includes chapters 3-4, includes a contemporary review about Brittle Diabetes and Hypoglycemia in Critically Ill patients. It shows the great suffering of people that are affected by this specific disorder.

Section C, which includes chapters 5-8, covers the issues related with hypoglycemia's physiology.

Section D, which includes chapters 9 -12, deals with preventions of hypoglycemia and glucose homeostasis.

Section E, which includes chapters 13-14, covers hypoglycemia associated with tumors and with type B insulin resistant and also several neurologic manifestations.

Section F, which includes chapters 15-18, describes the role of incretin, zinc translocation, hyperinsulinaemic-hypoglycaemia and diabetes control.

Hopefully this book will be of help to many scientists, doctors, pharmacists, chemicals and other experts in variety of disciplines, both academic and industrial. In addition to supporting research and development, this book should also be suitable for teaching.

Finally, I would like to thank my daughter Maria Eduarda and my wife Fernanda for their patience. I extend my apologies for many hours spent on the preparation of my chapter and the editing of this book, which kept me away from them.

Prof. Dr. Everlon Cid Rigobelo
Laboratory of Microbiology & Hygiene,
Campus Experimental de Dracena
Animal Science Faculty
Dracena
Brazil

Part 1

Section A

1

Management Approach to Hypoglycemia

Miriam Ciljakova, Milos Jesenak,
Miroslava Brndiarova and Peter Banovcin
Pediatric Department of University Hospital and Jessenius Medical Faculty of Comenius University, Martin
Slovakia

1. Introduction

Management of hypoglycemia in children and adults depends on many factors. The most important point of view is the level of hypoglycemia and the relevance of clinical symptoms. In the case of severe hypoglycemia, all effort must be used to maintain euglycemia as soon as possible. However, the appropriate therapeutic approach relies on correct diagnostic evaluation. In relation to the age of onset, different causes of hypoglycemia should be considered in neonates, infants, children and adults.

The risk of hypoglycemia is declining during the life, low blood glucose level is the frequent problem, mainly in neonatal period. The majority of neonatal hypoglycemia are due to problems with the normal processes of metabolic adaptation after birth, and strategies enhance the physiologic transition should help prevent such episodes. Further investigation and specific intervention should be considered when hypoglycemia is unusual in severity, duration, or occurs in an otherwise low-risk infant (Desphande & Platt, 2005).

Important factor for diagnosis is timing of hypoglycemia in relation to fasting. If hypoglycemia occured in a short period after meal (2-3 hours) and after overnight fasting, hyperinsulinism would be assumed. Low blood glucose level within 4-6 hours after ingestion is typical for defect in glycogenolysis. If hypoglycemia occurs more than 6 hours after feeding, disorders of fatty acid oxidation or defect in gluconeogenenesis are supposed (de Leon et al, 2008). In older patients, the fasting period inducing hypoglycemia is usually longer.

Physical examination can also be helpful in diagnostic evaluation. The presence of central cleft lip (or palate), micropenis and undescended testes in male neonate strongly suggests the occurrence of hypoglycemia due to pituitary hormone deficiency. If TSH deficiency was associated, untreated infants would suffer from psychomotoric retardation, growth retardation is typical later at the age 2-3. Large for age newborns with recurrent hypoglycemia could be suspected of autosomal recessive form of hyperinsulinism, if mother did not suffer from diabetes in pregnancy. Short stature and hepatomegaly is a part of clinical picture of glycogen storage disease type 1 (Langdon et al, 2008).

Hypoglycemia is expected in a risk group of neonates (e.g. premature, small for age) and in diabetic patients. If etiopathogenesis of low blood glucose level is unknown and unexpected, the sampling of blood and urine at the time of hypoglycemia is crucial (critical sample). In diagnostic algorithm, it is necessary to measure plasma substrates: ketones (aminoacetate and hydroxybutyrate acids), lactate, free fatty acids, ammonia level, and hormones: insulin, C-peptide, cortisol, growth hormone at the time of low blood glucose level. Hypothyroidism ought to be excluded in all patients with low blood glucose level. If hypoglycemia was less than 2,8 mmol/l (50 mg/dl), repeated sampling and measurement of counter-regulatory hormones, such as cortisol and growth hormone, would be suggested 30 minutes after low blood glucose concentration. At the blood glucose level of 2,2 mmol/l and less, the peak values of cortisol and growth hormone are reached in half an hour, and are comparable to those in insulin stimulation test (Weintrob et al, 1998).

At the time of hypoglycemia, the lack of ketones makes pediatric frequent diagnosis of ketotic hypoglycemia nonprobable. Ketoacidosis is also common in cortisol deficiency, whereas lactic acidosis is part of disorders of gluconeogenenesis like as glucose 6-phosphatase deficiency. Ketones and lactate are the alternative fuel for brain, disorders with high plasma level of these substrates are linked with laboratory serious hypoglycemia without clinical symptoms of neuroglycopenia. Some patients may have only few symptoms at plasma glucose level as low as 1,1-1,7 mmol/l (20-30 mg/dl). On the other hand, in defects of ketogenesis, signs may begin to appear at plasma glucose level of 3,3 mmol/l (60 mg/dl) during fasting. The average cut point of plasma glucose level to provoke clinical adrenergic and neuroglycopenic symptoms is 2,8 mmol/l (De Leon et al, 2008).

High level of free fatty acids with hypoglycemia is a part of defects of fatty acid oxidation associated with coma, hepatocellular failure and hyperammonemia (Reye-like syndrome). Valproic acid can block β-oxidation, treatment of epilepsy may provoke Reye-like syndrome in some patients. Early supplementation with carnitine and riboflavin, avoidance of fasting and low-fat diet can be useful and lifesaving. Acyl-carnitine profile of blood spots in newborn screening is able to detect most fatty acid oxidation disorders. Free fatty acids do not pass blood-brain barrier and can not be used as a energy substrate in brain.

Hypoglycemic symptoms follow usually the same pattern for each patient. Especially in type 1 diabetes, it is important to teach patient and all family members how to recognize and treat hypoglycemia in a safe and effective manner as soon as possible. Coffee and cola caffeine may cause symptoms of hypoglycemia at a slightly higher blood glucose level than usually. The fact that caffeine enhances the intensity of symptoms warning hypoglycemia may be useful for patients with „hypoglycemia unawareness". On the other hand, treatment of high blood pressure with β-blockers may have opposite effect and makes symptoms of hypoglycemia less obvious. Patients with diabetes on β-blockers treatment should check blood glucose level in case of sweating without any reason. It may be the only sign of a very low blood glucose. Similarly, few symptoms are noticed in diabetics treating for depression with SSRIs, patients may suffer from hypoglycemia unawareness, too (Hanas, 2004).

The warning adrenergic symptoms precede typically neuroglycopenic ones and work as a brain protection. Diabetes mellitus may be associated with autonomic dysfunction, warning symptoms are being lost and hypoglycemia becomes unawareness. Frequent hypoglycemia may cause lowering of threshold for triggering adrenergic signs that start commonly at the blood glucose level 3,3-3,6 mmol/l (60-65 mg/dl) in diabetic patients. On the opposite side, if the average glycemia was 15 mmol/l within a week, the warning symptoms could start at the blood glucose level 4,5-5,5 mmol/l (80-100 mg/dl). Neuroglycopenic signs are mostly independent on the recent blood glucose values, observed in glycemia below 2,8 mmol/l (Hanas, 2004) .

For correct management of patients with hypoglycemia, two glucose thresholds must be distiguished. The first one is diagnostic glucose level, hypoglycemia is usually considered in

the case of plasma glucose value below 2,8 mmol/l. Such glucose concentration is helpful for immediate sampling of alternative fuels and hormones, and consequently for differential diagnosis of hypoglycemic patients. The second one is therapeutic glucose value, the goal of appropriate treatment of hypoglycemia is to maintain plasma glucose within normal range 3,9-5,5 mmol/l (70-100 ng/ml) (Langdon et al, 2008).
The glucose level can be measured as whole blood glucose or plasma glucose. Plasma glucose is approximately 11% higher than whole blood glucose. Methods of measuring glucose level with bedside glucose meters were originally designed for diabetes management. These monitors are adequate for management of hypoglycemia, but are not accurate enough for measurement of hypoglycemic level. Latest development in bedside monitoring has improved the technology, but is not sufficiently accurate and precise to establish a diagnosis of hypoglycaemia. As a screening test it may be useful, any meter blood glucose level less than 3,3 mmol/l should be confirmed by more precise laboratory measurement of whole blood or plasma glucose concentration (Gamma et al, 2000).
Blood samples that are not processed promptly can have errorneously low glucose levels, as a result of glycolysis by red and white blood cells. At room temperature, the decline of whole-blood glucose can be 0,3-0,4 mmol/l/hr (5 to 7 mg/dl/hr). The use of inhibitors, such as fluoride, in collection tubes prevents this problem. Falsely low (or high) glucose values may occur with samples drawn from indwelling lines without adequate flushing of the saline (or glucose) infusate (de Leon et al, 2008).

2. Management of hypoglycemia in neonates and infants

Traditionally, lower standards for hypoglycemia were accepted in neonates. The major reason was statistical, low blood glucose is so common in neonatal period that it must be taken as a normal. Recently, the same definition and the same targets for treatment of hypoglycemia have been recommended in neonates and in older patients (de Leon et al, 2008). Moreover, the consequences of delayed diagnosis or inadequate management may be more harmful to a developing brain in neonates and infants (Menni et al, 2001).
Previously, the blood glucose concentration at which clinical signs occured were used to define hypoglycemia. These signs, such as changes in level of alertness and tone, apnoe, tremors or seizures are not specific in neonates and infants. In the first few hours, after birth fuels apart from glucose are also relevant in providing brain energy. Therefore the presence or absence of clinical signs can not be used to differ between normal and abnormal glucose levels, although decreased level of consciousness or seizures should always suggest the possiblity of hypoglycemia (Desphande & Platt, 2005).
The cerebral fuel economy depends on blood glucose level, the avaliability of alternative fuels such as ketones and lactate, the local adaptation of microcirculation, the interaction with other brain cells and the concurent neonatal condition such as hypoxia and sepsis (Salhab et al, 2004). The immediate consequence of transition from fetal to neonatal life is the interruption of continuous glucose supplies. After birth, there is a rapid fall in blood glucose level, reaching a nadir between 1-2 hr in healthy term infants as well. Such low blood glucose level is usually accompanied by ketogenic response, particulary in breast-fed infants. Ketones provides alternative fuel for brain and prevents the neonate to become symptomatic. Even in the absence of any nutritional intake, the blood glucose rises significantly within 3 hrs due to counter-regulatory hormone response. Therefore, healthy asymptomatic neonates are proposed to avoid the blood glucose measurement during the

first 2-3 hrs after birth and only glycemia less than 2,0 mmol/l requires other intervention (Desphande & Platt, 2005). However, up to 10% of normal term neonates are not able to maintain plasma glucose concentrations above 1,7 mmol/l (30 mg/dl), if their first feeding is delayed for 6 hrs after birth (Lindley & Dunne, 2005). In case of this late first feeding, glycemia above 2,8 mmol/l (50 mg/dl) has been observed only in two thirds of healthy neonates. Promotion of first feeding soon after delivery is the basic approach to prevention of such blood glucose declining.

Some common maternal or neonatal problems expose a baby at risk of significant hypoglycemia (Table 1). Often measurements of blood glucose are helpful, even though in asymptomatic risk neonates. Severely intrauterine growth retarded (IUGR) neonates may have low cord blood glucose concentrations due to intrauterine hypoglycemia. On the other hand, hypoglycemia should be excluded in all clinically unwell infants. Clinical signs of common neonatal illnesses are shared by those with hypoglycemia. Moreower, many neonatal disorders can lead to hypoglycemia (Desphande & Platt, 2005).

Blood glucose concentrations show a cyclic response to an enteral feeding, reaching a peak approximately one hour after meal and a nadir just before the next feeding. In risk neonates, initial blood glucose measurement, immediately before the second feeding, may detect the most babies who can not manage adequately glucose homeostasis. Once or twice a day pre-feeding blood glucose determination may be sufficient in stable neonates, since the clinical condition has not been changed or the previous volume of milk has not been restricted. Laboratory standard blood glucose measurement is reliable and preferable to inaccurate reagent strip-based estimations (de Rooy & Hawdon, 2002).

Maternal conditions	• Diabetes (pregestational and gestational) • Drug treatment (β - blockers, oral hypoglycemic agents) • Intrapartum glucose administration
Neonatal problems	• Preterm • Intrauterine growth restriction • Perinatal hypoxia - ischemia • Hypothermia • Infection • Polycythemia • Infants on parenteral nutrition • Obvious syndromes (e.g. midline defects, Beckwith - Wiedemann syndrome)

Table 1. „At - risk" infants who require monitoring of blood glucose concentrations (Deshpande & Platt, 2005).

The most common neonatal hypoglycemia is due to delay of normal metabolic adaptation after birth. Occasionally, especially in IUGR neonates, a period of a week or more with high intravenous glucose infusion rate may be required. Blood glucose concentration often falls down in perinatal asphyxia, polycythemia, sepsis and with maternal use of β-blockers. Rarely, hypoglycemia is the presenting symptom of hormonal disorders or inborn errors of metabolism, such as hyperinsulinism (Yap et al, 2004), hypopituitarism and fatty acid oxidation disorder. Some clues can make hormonal or metabolic disorder very suspected:

- Family history of sudden infant death, Reye-like syndrome, or developmental delay
- Healthy, appropriate for gestational age, term infant with symptomatic hypoglycemia
- Hypoglycemia with midline defects, micropenis, exomphalos
- Hypoglycemia with seizures or abnormalities of conciousness
- Persistent or recurrent hypoglycemia
- Glucose infusion rate more than 10 mg/kg/min

Sample	Investigations
Blood	• Intermediary metabolites (glucose, lactate, pyruvate, alanine, free fatty acid, glycerol and ketone bodies) • Serum electrolytes, liver functions and acid - base status, C reactive protein • Ammonia • Amino acids • Total and free carnitine • Acylcarnitine profile • Insulin, C - peptide, growth hormone, IGF1, IGFBP3, cortisol and thyroid hormones • Galactosemia screen
Urine	• Ketones by dipstick • Organic acids and aminoacids • Reducing substances (galactose and fructose)
Others	• Ophthalmic examination • Cranial ultrasound scan and/ or MRI

Table 2. Suggested investigations in hypoglycemic patient with suspected metabolic/ endocrine disorder (Deshpande & Platt, 2005).

If neonate meets criteria for metabolic-hormonal disturbances, crucial point will be to obtain appropriate samples for examination of intermediary metabolites and hormones at the time of hypoglycemia. The second sample in a half an hour after episode may be useful to evaluate counter-regulatory response, mainly in newborns suspected of pituitary deficiency. If such samples are not obtained, the correct diagnosis may be delayed, furthermore, invasive testing and controlled fasting may be required. It can be helpful to prepare a hypoglycemia kit with suitable containers and instructions for instance of sudden hypoglycemic episode (Table 2). Further management should involve consultation with a specialist in pediatric endocrinology and metabolic medicine (Desphande & Platt, 2005).

2.1 Hormone deficiency

Some newborns with hypoglycemia are supposed to have pituitary deficiency, those suffering from midline defects (cleft lip or palate) and micropenis with undescended testes. At first, the basal sample of free thyroxine, TSH, cortisol, IGF-1, IGF BP-3, sex hormones should be recommended. Typically, lower concentrations of thyroxine, cortisol and IGF BP-3

are measured in infants with pituitary deficiency. Decreased IGF BP-3 level has greater value to diagnosis of growth hormone deficiency in infancy. Despite importance of evaluation IGF-1 levels in children, these are rarely helpful in neonates. In fact, serum IGF BP-3 should be performed as the test of choice in suspected neonatal growth hormone (GH) deficiency. The use of standard GH stimulation tests is not recommended in newborns, except for safe glucagon test 0,03–0,1 mg/kg. Cortisol and GH levels are measured in a basal sample, and furthermore in 5 consequent samples (0, 60, 90, 120, 150, 180 min). Cortisol and GH sampling half hour after clinically significant and laboratory proved low blood glucose level (≤ 2,2 mmol/l) can confirm GH deficiency, and protect child from prolonged redundant testing (Weintrob et al, 1998). Several mutation in genes involved in pituitary development (POUF1, PROP1, TPIT) has been reported in infants with hypoglycemia due to pituitary deficiency. Congenital hypopituitarism may not be diagnosed until a baby is several months old. Abnormal growth is usually noticed only after 1-2 years of life and recurrent hypoglycemia in infants with confirmed GH deficiency is an indication to start GH treatment, especially in those on thyroxine and hydrocortisone therapy (Randell et al, 2007).
Neonates with ambigous genitalia are always suspected of congenital adrenal hyperplasia, although presenting clinical signs of mineral disturbances rather than hypoglycamia may be apparent from 2 to 4 weeks of life. Treatment with hydrocortisone and fludrocortisone should be started immediatelly in such infants, after appropriate hormonal sampling. Chromosome analysis, hormone measurements (especially 17-hydroxyprogesteron, androstendion, cortisol and testosterone) are necessary in diagnostic approach, the most common cause is 21-hydroxylase deficiency. If enzyme defect is comfirmed by hormonal measurements, identification of mutation in genes (CYP 21, CYP 11β, and other) should folow in management. Wolman disease and congenital adrenal hypoplasia, two other rare causes of adrenal failure have been described in neonates and infants (Randell et al, 2007).

2.2 Metabolic inborn error

Hypoglycemia induced by first feeding, especially in combination with vomiting, diarrhoea and jaundice, should be suspected from galactosemia (galactose-1-phosphate uridyl transferase deficiency or UDP galactose-4-epimerase deficiency). Exposure to milk results in acute deterioration of multiple organ systems, including liver dysfunction, poor feeding, weight loss, renal tubular dysfunction, neutropenia, coagulopathy and Escherichia coli sepsis. Galactosemia should also be excluded in all neonates with these findings and concomitant E.coli sepsis. Some screening programs in newborns have included galactosemia routinely. A galactose restricted diet will reverse effectively multiorgan dysfunction, and will eliminate the risk of hypoglycemia during childhood. However, long-term effect on mental functions, speech and ovarian function may persist despite appropriate dietary therapy in individuals with galactosemia (Leslie, 2003).
Nonspecific symptoms occuring 3-6 months after birth, such as failure to thrive and vomiting, may be a part of clinical picture of hereditary fructose intolerance due to fructose 1-phosphate aldolase deficiency. Exclusively breast-fed and formula-fed infants are healthy unless fruits and juices are added into diet. The worsening of symptoms and hypoglycemia with feeding should rise clinical suspicion. Low chronic exposure to fructose causes failure to thrive and chronic liver disease. Biochemical findings of elevated fructose level may be

confirmed by enzyme assay of liver or small intestinal biopsy. Treatment consists of strict dietary avoidance of fructose, sucrose and sorbitol (Wong, 2005).
Disorders of gluconeogenesis should be considered in infants with fasting hypoglycemia during intercurrent illness, especially in the case of positive family history to unexplained sibling death. Pattern of characteristically abnormal organic acids in urine is usually present in infants with disruption of gluconeogenesis. Fructose 1,6-diphosphatase is a key regulatory enzyme of gluconeogenesis from all substrates (fructose, glycerol, lactate and amino acids). Deficiency of such enzyme leads to hepatomegaly, hypoglycemic seizures and hyperventilation due to lactic acidosis and ketoacidosis. Developmental delay and mental retardation may be the consequence of untreated infants. Unlike hereditary fructose intolerance, liver and renal tubular dysfunction are atypical. Infants with fasting hypoglycemia and lactic acidosis should be suspected of defects of gluconeogenesis, diagnosis is confirmed by enzyme assay in liver biopsy. Chronic treatment consists of avoidance of fasting and reduction of fructose in diet, correction of metabolic acidosis is necessary (Langdon et al, 2008). Continuous nasogastric infusion may be helpful overnigt and during intercurrent illness. Rarely, pyruvate carboxylase deficiency has been found. In addition to hypoglycemia, hyperalaninemia and lactic acidosis, elevated pyruvate is comfirmed. Some infants develop hyperammonemia, hypercitrulinemia, hyperlysinemia and hyperprolinemia. Diagnosis may be proven by measurement of enzyme activity in fibroblasts. In addition to metabolic acidosis correction, substitution of Krebs cycle substrates has been suggested, as well as supplementation with coenzymes of pyruvate dehydrogenase complex - thiamine and lipoic acid (Ahmad et al, 1999). Except such genetic enzymatic defects, alcohol ingestion and salicylate treatment may cause iatrogenic block of gluconeogenesis.
Medium-chain acyl-coenzyme A dehydrogenase deficiency (MCAD) is the most frequent disorder of fatty acid oxidation. Neonatal screening in Pensylvania has shown an incidence 1:9 000 live birth (Ziadeh et al, 1995). Although there is a significant heterogeneity in presentation of MCAD, the most common sign is intermittent hypoketotic hypoglycemia during intercurrent infection with decreased oral intake. Family history of sibling death rises suspicion. Severe form presents as a Reye-like syndrome with hyperammonemia, hepatocellular failure and coma. Affected patients could also be misdiagnosed with sudden infant death syndrome (Roe & Ding, 2001). Evaluation of suspected errors in fatty acid oxidation should first include the determination of plasma acylcarnitine profile by mass spectrometry and measurement of plasma total, esterified and free carnitine. Determination of urinary organic acids with assessment of dicarboxylic aciduria is also very useful. Patients, whose disorder cannot be confirmed by these tests, may require further evaluations, including assays of fatty acids oxidation and specific enzyme assays in cultured skin fibroblasts or lymphoblasts. Direct DNA mutational analysis can be performed, particularly in MCAD. Therapeutic approach consists of avoidance of fasting and high fat intake, although normal amounts of fats do not seem to be harmful. The use of cornstarch (1-2g/kg every 4 hours) and carnitine supplementation has been advocated (Rinaldo et al, 2002).

2.3 Neonates at risk of hypoglycemia

Prevention of low blood glucose concentrations is the goal of management in newborns at risk of hypoglycemia. In healthy appropriately grown term infants, facilitating normal feeding is all that is needed. Breast-fed neonates demonstrate lower blood glucose and higher ketone concentrations than formula-fed ones. This starvating, ketogenic response is typical for physiologic transition from fetal to neonatal metabolism, as in other mammals (de Rooy & Hawdon, 2002). For infants, who are able to tolerate enteral feeding, increasing amount of milk should be the first strategy. Although oral dextrose solution may be recommended, the milk contains approximately twice more energy as equivalent volume of 10% dextrose.

Severely IUGR neonates may be hypoglycemic in utero, delayed metabolic adaptation will be expected in those infants soon after birth. Cord blood glucose level determination may be helpful, the concentration less than 2,0 mmol/l can reveal IUGR infants at high risk of symptomatic hypoglycemia. In order to precede clinical consequences, appropriate intervention seems to be prophylactic intravenous glucose infusion as soon as possible (Desphande & Platt, 2005). In IUGR infants, early enteral feeding is recommended and breast-feeding is the approach of choice. If child remains hypoglycemic despite an adequate milk intake, intravenous glucose infusion at a rate equal to the hepatic glucose production 6-8 mg/kg/min (85-120 ml of 10% glucose/kg/24 hrs) is necessary. Due to functional hyperinsulinism in some IUGR infants, glucose intake may be increased (10 mg/kg/min or more) occasionally.

Preterm infants with respiratory distress (usually less than 32 weeks of gestation) require always intravenous glucose infusion, at least 6 mg glucose/kg/min. Near term infants are often able to suckle the breast or bottle but skillful support of nurse may be needed. Supplementation of milk with glucose polymers and energy supplements may increase the risk of necrotizing enterocolitis due to bowel osmolality (Desphande & Platt, 2005).

In infant of diabetic mother, the highest incidence of hypoglycemia occurs between 4-6 hr after birth, interval of onset may extend up to 48 hrs. Tighter metabolic control during pregnancy and delivery is associated with decreased frequency of neonatal hypoglycemia. In particular, maternal blood glucose more than 8 mmol/l during parturition is linked with higher risk of hypoglycemia in neonate. Insufficient metabolic compensation of pregnant diabetic woman is the reason of neonatal macrosomia due to prolonged fetal hyperinsulinism (Taylor et al, 2002). Management approach to neonate of diabetic mother consists of early enteral feeding and regular pre-fed glucose monitoring, unless the later blood glucose level is normal one. Excessive glucose infusion rate in baby is responsible only for another pancreatic stimulation and should be avoided. Similarly, administration of glucagon immediately after birth is not routinely recommended, otherwise rapid hepatic glucose release can further stimulate insulin secretion and augment the tendency to hypoglycemia.

The use of intravenous glucose bolus is inevitable in symptomatic infants with glycemia below the normal range. Recommended bolus therapy is 2 ml/kg of 10% glucose solution (200 mg glucose/kg). The dose has been efficacious in rapid release of clinical symptoms like as depressed alertness, hypotonia, apnoe or seizures, otherwise it usually restores normal blood glucose level without later hyperglycemia. Intravenous administration of bolus should be followed by an increase in the rate of glucose infusion. Treatment of neonatal hypoglycemia with intermittent boluses alone is not logical, the need for such boluses is an indication for rising continuous glucose infusion rate. Boluses of hypertonic (20% or 40%) glucose solutions should be avoided. In a similar way, gradual rather than large reduction in the rate of intravenous glucose infusion is helpful to maintain stable blood glucose concentration.

Glucagon promotes early neonatal glycogenolysis from liver and also stimulates gluconeogenesis and ketogenesis. Intravenous bolus dose of 200 μg/kg was used in previous studies, such administration may provoke further hypoglycemia due to hyperglycemia induced insulin secretion. Therefore, application of glucagon bolus should be followed by continuous glucose infusion. In a study of 55 neonates with hypoglycemia of various etiologies, continous infusion of glucagon (0,5-1,0 mg/day) increased blood glucose concentration significantly within 4 hrs after starting of infusion. The frequency of subsequent hypoglycemia has been decreased with continuous glucagon therapy (Mirales et al, 2002). The occurrence of severe hyponatremia has been reported in a preterm infant, but the relationship with glucagon infusion seems to be unlikely (Charsa et al, 2003, Coulthard & Hey, 2002).

3. Management of neonatal hyperinsulinism

Most infants with hyperinsulinism present within neonatal period, although infantile and childhood forms are also described. In general, excessive glucose requirement with infusion rate more than 10 mg/kg/min is suspected of hyperinsulinism. Traditionally, the diagnosis of hyperinsulinism is based on demonstrating inappropriately high insulin concentration at the time of hypoketotic hypoglycemia (Table 3). Diagnosis is confirmed by insulin level more than 2,0 mIU/l and glycemia below 2,8 mmol/l at the same time. Intravenous adminstration of glucagon is followed by glycemic response bigger than 1,7 mmol/l within 15- 30 minutes in infants with hyperinsulinism (de Leon et al, 2008).

Criteria for diagnosing hyperinsulinism based on critical sample
Critical sample must be drawn at time of hypoglycemia (plasma glucose < 50mg/dl) • Detecable insulin (>2 mIU/l) • Low free fatty acids (< 1,5 mmol/l) • Low ketones (plasma β hydroxybutyrate < 2,0 mmol/l) Inappropriate glycemic response to 1mg intravenous glucogen at time of hypoglycemia (glucose rise > 30mg/dl in 20 minutes)

Table 3. Criteria for diagnosing hyperinsulinism based on critical sample (Langdon et al, 2008).

The majority of neonatal hyperinsulinism is transient, these form has been observed in neonates with maternal diabetes, Beckwith - Wiedemann syndrome, Sotos syndrome, Perlman syndrome, birth asphyxia, polycythemia, rhesus incompatibility and severe intrauterine growth retardation (Baujat et al, 2004). Such perinatal stress-induced hyperinsulinism may persist for several days to several weeks, but not longer than 6 months (Hoe et al, 2006). Infants with prolonged stress hyperinsulinism are usually good responders to diazoxide therapy. Glucocorticoids are not effective in controlling of hyperinsulinism.

Hyperinsulinism is the most common cause of persistent or recurrent hypoglycemia in infancy. Generally, the persistent hyperinsulinism is relatively rare (1:30 000- 1:50 000) but may lead to neurological damage and lifelong handicap. Up to 20% of infants suffering from congenital hyperinsulinism exhibits neurological defect (Menni et al, 2001). Approximately 60% of patients with persistent hyperinsulinism present within the first week of life, the

most severe forms start earliest. However, all of the genetic causes of hyperinsuslinism may be initially diagnosed in older infants and children (Langdon et al, 2008).
Infants with congenital hyperinsulinism are usually born in term and macrosomic, similar as neonates of diabetic mothers. On the other hand, low birth weight or preterm birth does not exclude persistent hyperinsulinism (Aynsley-Green, 2000, Yap et al, 2004). Most infants are apparently macrosomic and plethoric and may have characteristic facial features with high forehead, large and bulbous nose, smooth philtrum and thin upper lip. Later in infancy, the only clinical sign may be unexplained developmental delay (de Lonlay et al, 2002 a).
Exomphalos in neonates with macrosomia and macroglossia enables to diagnose Beckwith-Wiedemann syndrome (BWS 1:10 000). Hyperinsulinemic hypoglycemia occurs approximately in 50% infants, and is usually mild and transient. Higher predisposition to childhood tumors has been described in BWS patients, analysis of chromosome 11p15 finding aberrant H19 and KCNQ1OT1 hypomethytalion may identify patients at increased risk of cancerogenesis (Bliek et al, 2001). Sotos syndrome (cerebral gigantism) involves also combination of somatic overgrowth and hyperinsulinism, the major cause is haploinsufficiency of NSD1 gene (Baujat et al, 2004).
The appropriate management of hyperinsulinemic infants is based on maintaining of blood glucose above 3,5 mmol/l. Even though of sufficient enteral feeding, the supplemental 10-15% glucose intravenous infusion is often needed, otherwise glucose requirement is usually 15-20 mg/kg/min. A secure central intravenous access should be obtained immediately after diagnostic evaluation. If intravenous cannula is resited, intramuscular glucagon administration 100 μg/kg is recommended. Hyperinsulinemic infants require intensive medical care monitoring at a centre specialized in management of hyperinsulinism. Once the infant is stabilized, a planned transport should take place. Delayed refferal to the centre may be the reason of neurologic consequences associated with disorder (Desphande & Platt, 2005).
The majority of transient forms of congenital hyperinsulinism will settle during the first month of life. This period can be spent evaluating of responsiveness to drugs therapies and attempting to introduce normal enteral feeding. After 4 weeks, as soon as diagnosis of congenital hyperinsulinism is confirmed, rapid genetic analysis of the affected child and parents using HPLC screening followed by sequencing of target genes should be recommended (Lindley & Dunne, 2005).
The most common and severe cause of persistent hyperinsulinism is due to loss of function mutation of the pancreatic β-cell K+ATP channel consisting of 2 subunits. K+ATP hyperinsulinism may be diffuse or focal. More than 100 mutations of ABCC8 (encoding SUR1 subunit) and 20 mutations of KCNJ11 (encoding Kir6.2 subunit) have been found so far. Neonates with recessive form present as a large for gestational age with very severe hypoglycemia immediately after birth, characteristic sign is usually poor responsiveness to diazoxide. Dominant form of K+ATP hyperinsulinism may occur in family members, the onset of milder hypoglycemic symptoms is often later in infancy and childhood. These patients reflect better responsiveness to diazoxide (Grimberg et al, 2001). In addition, defects in SUR1 subunit may be inherited in three different mechanism, loss of heterozygosity has been identified, except for recessive and dominant patterns. The association of recessive mutations with diffuse hyperinsulinism, as well as loss of heterozygosity with focal form, has been found in infants with SUR1 defects (Langdon et al, 2008).
The second most common form in infants is hyperinsulinism/hyperammonemia (HI/HA) syndrome caused by gain of function mutation of GLUD1 (encoding glutamate

dehydrogenase GDH). Most cases are sporadic due to de novo mutations. Approximately 20% of these disorders are familial with autosomal dominant inheritance. Typically, neonates suffering from HI/HA syndrome are appropriate for gestational age. Episodes of symptomatic hypoglycemia may not been recognized until 1-2 years of age. Patients with HI/HA syndrome have relatively mild fasting hypoglycemia. However, after ingestion of protein meal, severe protein-sensitive hypoglycemia can happen within 30-90 minutes. Diazoxide therapy is usually effective to control fasting and protein-induced hypoglycemia. Differential laboratory finding is slightly elevated ammonia level (60-150 μmol/l) without therapy requirement. The lack of clinical hyperammonemic symptoms may be explained by increased GDH enzyme activity in brain of affected individuals (Li et al, 2006). Less frequent form of congenital hyperinsulinism presenting with fasting hypoglycemia is due to activating mutations of GCK (glucokinase), sometimes showing autosomal dominant pattern. The age of onset and severity of symptoms varies markedly (Cuesta-Munoz et al, 2004). Rarely, mutation of HADHSC gene (encoding short chain L-3-hydroxyacyl-CoA dehydrogenase SCHAD) with autosomal recessive inheritance may be identified as a cause of hyperinsulinism in infants (Hussain et al, 2006).

Occasionally, congenital carbohydrate-deficient glycoprotein syndrome, also known as congenital disorders of glycosylation (CDG), has been identified as a cause of neonatal hyperinsulinism. Unlike other forms of hyperinsulinism, CDG often leads to involvment of other systems, especially the brain, liver, gut and skeleton. The diagnosis is usually confirmed by identification of hyposialylated serum transferrin by isoelectric focusing (Fang et al, 2004).

Less than 20% of neonates with persistent congenital hyperinsulinism will respond to diazoxide therapy, a K+ATP channel opener (De Lonlay et al, 2002 b). Diazoxide binds to the SUR1 subunit of the K+ATP channel. Infants with no functional K+ATP channels at the β-cell membrane are not expected to respond to diazoxide therapy. On the other hand, patients suffering from hyperinsulinism-hyperammonemia syndrome with normal K+ATP channel are more likely better responders than those with ABCC8 loss of function mutation. So genetic analysis of congenital hyperinsulinism is useful in predicting of drug responsiveness. The daily requirement of diazoxide varies between 5-25 mg/kg divided in several doses. Otherwise, diazoxide as a channel opener retains sodium and water, chlorothiazide has been successfully added to counteract this side event. Appart from acting as a diuretic, chlorothiazide has also direct β-cell pottasium channel opening activity. In a purpose to supply sufficient glucose, large volumes of intravenous fluids are infused to hyperinsulinemic infants and enhance the danger of severe water retention (Silvani et al, 2004).

Somatostatin analogues are able to inhibit insulin secretion in various manners by inducing hyperpolarisation of β-cells, direct inhibition of the voltage-gated calcium channel and more distal insulin secretory pathways. Recommended dose of somatostatin analogues is 5-20 mg/kg/24 hrs intravenously or subcutaneously, usually in combination with diazoxide. If diazoxide is contraindicated and intravenous glucose requirement is too high, somatostatin therapy may be used as a first line treatment. Safety and efficacy of long term treatment in infants and children has been discussed (Dunne et al, 2004).

The intravenous administration of glucagon (1-10 μg/kg/hr) may be helpful in acute management of infants with hyperinsulinism, rising glycemia reflects the changes in gluconeogenesis and glycogenolysis. For long-term therapy, glucagon works like as insulin secretagogue and is recommended usually in combination with other treatment lowering insulin secretion (Aynsley-Green, 2000). Considerable distinction has been reported on glycemic effect of Ca 2+ channel blockers. According to reports of few centres, some hyperinsulinemic infants may profit from nifedipine chronic therapy (Lindley et al, 1996).

Seletctive drugs for hypoglycemic disorders

1. **Intravenous glucose rescue doses**
   - Dextrose emergency bolus: IV push 0,2g/kg bolus (2ml/kg of dextrose 10%), followed by D 10% continuous infusion of 5ml/kg/hr
   - If plasma glucose not corrected after 15 minutes, bolus 2ml/kg of 10% dextrose and increase continuous infusion by 25% to 50%
2. **Glucagon (emergency treatment only in case of insulin-induced hypoglycemia)**
   - 1 mg intramusculary or intravenously (0,03-0,1 mg/kg)
   - Side effects: vomiting and rebound hypoglycemia
3. **Diazoxide (use in hyperinsulinism or sulfonylurea overdose)**
   - 5 - 15mg/kg/day divided into two or tree doses (if given by IV route, must be given over 15 minutes to avoid hypotension)
   - Start with maximum dose (15mg/kg to test), then lower as possible (responders usually require 10mg/kg or less)
   - Side effect: fluid and sodium retention, hypertrichosis
4. **Octreotide**
   - Start at 2 to 5 mg/kg/day and increase to 20 mg/kg/day SC divided into 3 or 4 doses
   - Side effect: transient diarrhoea, abdominal discomfort, gallstones, transient growth impairment
5. **Cornstarch (for glycogen storage disease)**
   - 1 - 2g/kg/dose (freshly prepare each dose by suspending in cold sugar - containing liquid)
   - Effect last 4 to 6 hrs
   - Not well absorbed in infancy
   - Side effect: diarrhoea
6. **Carnitine (for free fatty oxidation disorder)**
   - 100mg/kg/day divided into three or four doses
   - Side effects: diarrhoea and fishy body odour

Table 4. Therapy of hypoglycemia (IV intravenous and SC subcutaneous) (Langdon et al, 2008)

Neonates with severe forms of cogenital hyperinsulinism can usually be stabilised using the measures mentioned above (Table 4). After clinical improvement and stable glucose infusion rate, the oral feeding can start substantially. The response to enteral feedings, as well as protein load, may result in further stimulation of insulin secretion and recurrent hypoglycemia. In such infants, the appropriate management seems to be parenteral

nutrition, although this approach may also augment insulin release from β-cells (Magge et al, 2004).
Clinically, infants with focal lesions are indistinguishable from those with diffuse hyperinsulinism. The focal lesions are potentially curable by surgery, whereas the outcome of diffuse K+ATP hyperinsulinism is worse. Furthermore, near total pancreatectomy (95-98% of pancreas), invasive treatment of severe diffuse hyperinsulinism, is associated with a high risk of later development of diabetes mellitus. Focal lesions (usually less than 10 mm in diameter) are frequently not visible at laparotomy, the determination of appropriate diagnostic methods is necessary to differentiate focal hyperinsulinism from diffuse one. Significant different surgerical approach depends on reliable and accurate diagnostic evaluation. Conventional imaging methods including ultrasound, ocreotid scintigraphy, and magnetic resonance imaging are usually meaningless (Lindley & Dune, 2005).
Interventional radiology methods, such as transhepatic portal venous insulin sampling and selective pancreatic arterial calcium stimulation have only modest success and are technically difficult and highly invasive, predominantly in small infants. During sampling procedure, the blood glucose concentrations should be kept below 3,0 mmol/l to demonstrate insulin hypersecretion in all or in isolated samples. Such glycemia without ketones may provoke clinical signs, especially in hyperinsulinism. Recently, positron emission tomography (PET) scans with fluorine-18, L-3, 4-dihydroxyphenylalanine (18F-fluoro-L-DOPA) have been found to accurately discriminate focal form from diffuse hyperinsulinism. In infants with focal hyperinsulinism, there is a local accumulation of 18F-fluoro-L-DOPA. Combined PET and computed tomography (CT) images make lesion possible to be localized (Ericson et al, 1997).

4. Management of hypoglycemia in children and adults

Comparing to adults, children have very limited glucose homeostasis because of smaller reserves of liver glycogen and muscle protein. Moreover, glucose consumption is relatively high due to larger brain-to-body-mass ratio in children. For example, the fuel stores of a 10 kg infant are only 15% of those of an adult. The real consequence of mentioned differences is varios approach to fasting in children and adults. Exposing infants to fasting is not without risk, particularly if fatty acid oxidation disorders or adrenal insufficiency are present (de Leone et al, 2008).
Infants younger than 1 year should not be fasted more than 24 hrs, while in older children the maximum fasting is 36 hrs. Adults usually require to decrease plasma glucose level below diagnostic threshold more than 48 hrs (maximally 72 hrs). The fasting test is interrupted, when the plasma glucose falls below 2,8 mmol/l. This starving may be ended sooner, if plasma β-hydroxybutyrate rises above 2,0 mmol/l or in the case of any clinical signs suggesting hypoglycemia. At the time of hypoglycemia, critical sampling of alternative fuels (ketones, lactate and free fatty acids), insulin and counter-regulatory hormones (mainly cortisol and growth hormone) is crucial (Table 5). The result of fasting test may be affected by β-blockers treatment and unrecognized hypothyroidism, these two possibilities should be excluded before fasting. Especially in suspicion of hyperinsulinism, the fasting test may be ended with intravenous glucagon admininstration to evaluate the glycemic response (de Leon et al, 2008).

	Fasting			
	Hypoglycemia			
	Acidosis		No Acidosis	
Fuel Response	Lactic acidosis	Ketoacidosis	Free fatty acids > 1,5 mmol/l	Free fatty acids < 1,5 mmol/l
Possible Disorders	G - 6 - Phosphatase deficiency Fructose 1,6 - diphosphatase deficiency Pyruvate carboxylase deficiency Normal neonates	Normal Ketotic hypoglycemic Glycogen storage disorder Growth hormone deficiency Cortisol deficiency	Fatty acid oxidation disorders Normal neonates	Hyperinsulinism Panhypopituitarism Small for gastational age, birth asphyxia
Further Test	Gluconeogenic precursors Glucagon stimulation test	Tests of pituitary & adrenal function Glucagon stimulation test	Acyl - carnitine profile	Glucagon stimulation test Tests of pituitary, adrenal, thyroid function Insulin assay Other tests for hyperinsulinism

Table 5. An algorithmic approach to hypoglycemia (de Leon et al, 2008).

4.1 Ketotic hypoglycemia

Ketotic hypoglycemia is the most common cause of low blood glucose level in chilhood. Usually, ketotic hypoglycemia begins as recurrent morning episodes of fasting hypoglycemia at the age of 2 or 3. The most of cases disappear spontaneously at the age of 8 to 9. Typically, partial or complete vomiting of evening meal is reported by parents in history. Especially, hypoglycemic episodes are likely to occur during periods of intercurrent illness with limited food intake. At the time of documented hypoglycemia, high level of ketones are measured in blood and urine, the plasma insulin concentration is typically low (< 2 mIU/l). Plasma alanine values are markedly reduced in children with ketotic hypoglycemia after ovenight fasting. Infusions of alanine produce a rapid rise in plasma glucose concentration without significant changes in lactate or pyruvate levels. This suggests that a deficiency of substrate, rather than defect in gluconeogenesis, plays a role in etiopathogenesis. Alanine, as a major gluconeogenetic amino acid precursor, is released from muscle during periods of caloric reduction. Children suffering from ketotic hypoglycemia are usually smaller than those of same age, reduced muscle mass in such patients may partially explain decreased supplies of gluconeogenic substrates (Stanley, 2006).

The diagnosis of ketotic hypoglycemia can be claimed only after exclusion of the others. Recurrent hypoglycemia with ketosis may occur in the case of hormone deficiencies, defects in gluconeogenesis and glycogen metabolism. Sometimes, the diagnosis demands the confirmation gained by supervised fasting. Low blood glucose level in combination with elevated ketones and free fatty acids develops within 14 to 24 hrs in most children with ketotic hypoglycemia. Prevention of ketotic hypoglycemia involves frequent high-carbohydrate feedings, as well as overnight fasting should be shortened. The child with ketotic hypoglycemia should not fast more than 12 hrs. During intercurrent illness, parents ought to test the urine of child, the presence of ketones precedes hypoglycemia by several hours, and such ketones in urine may be the indicator of subsequent low blood glucose. In the presence of ketonuria, high-carbohydrate liquids should be offered to child. Vomiting child with ketotic hypoglycemia should be reffered to the hospital for intravenous glucose administration (Langdon et al, 2008).

4.2 Hyperinsulinism

All genetic causes of hyperinsulinism may be diagnosed later in childhood, these are usually not so severe as persistent neonatal forms. In adolescence and adulthood, insulinoma appears more frequent cause of hyperinsulinism comparing to genetic ones. Insulin-secreting adenomas (insulinoma) of pancreas are extremely rare in young children, at this age diffuse or focal hyperinsulinism is more common. Insulinomas may occur sporadically, but familial form as a part of MEN 1 should be considered. Exclusion of parathyroid, pituitary and pancreatic hormone overproduction should be done in insulinoma patient and in family. MEN 1 may be confirmed by analysis of mutations of gene, encoding menin (Greenberg et al, 2000). Routine imaging of the pancreas (abdominal ultrasound, CT, MRI) often fails to reveal the tumor, unless it is bigger than 2 cm. Insulinomas are usually unvisible on octreotid scan. Elaborating noninvasive diagnostic methods, the endoscopic ultrasonography seems to be the most helpful before surgery, higher sensitivity (90%) is described only in intraoperative ultrasonographic investigation. In adolescents and adults, invasive pancreatic arterial stimulation with calcium and subsequent venous sampling of insulin levels may localize the insulinoma to a region of pancreas, method is technically difficult in small children. Accurate diagnosis of hyperinsulinism must precede all invasive examinations and surgery (Hirshberg et al, 2000). Factitious hyperinsulinism ought to be strictly excluded, especially in puberty and adolescence. Inspite of true hyperinsulinism, C-peptide level is low in the case of intoxication with human insulin. However, both true hyperinsulinism and sulfonylurea poisoning show high C-peptide concentration. If iatrogenic hyperinsulinism is suspected, the concentration of sulfonylurea drugs should be measured by specific toxicologic examination (Marks & Teale, 1999). Small number of children and adults may suffer from hypoglycemic seizures or syncope due to hyperinsulinism occurring with anaerobic exercise. The condition is inherited in an autosomal dominant pattern (Meissner et al, 2001).

4.3 Counter-regulatory hormone deficiency

Four hormones are involved in maintaining blood glucose level, but only cortisol and growth hormone deficiency are usually examined as a cause of hypoglycemia. Although all forms of hypocorticism may present by hypoglycemia, ACTH deficiency or unresponsiveness is more likely reflected in clinical sign of hypoglycemia than primary adrenal failure. Iatrogenic suppression of adrenal function is one of the most common causes of ACTH deficiency, but may be underdiagnosed due to absence of typical electrolyte abnormalities. Vomiting, hypotension and hypoglycemia can be provoked by a stressful event in a child who weaned high-dose glucocorticoid therapy. Milder clinical manifestation may be caused by topical, inhaled or intranasal glucocorticoid preparations. Such treatment is advocated for many persons, and combination of these forms may lead to episodic hypoglycemia and can have possible impact to growth in childhood (Pinney et al, 2007). ACTH deficiency should be excluded in obese patient with red hair, especially before planned surgery. POMC mutations has been indentified as a cause of hypocorticism in this atypical clinical presentation (Krude et al, 1998). Idiopathic ACTH deficiency can be acquired in childhood, adolescence and also later in life. An association with autoimmune thyroiditis or celiac disease suggests autoimmune hypophysitis. Detailed history and examination are recommended to exclude pituitary damage, e.g. head trauma, pituitary infarction, infection, cranial radiation and tumors.

Patients with primary adrenal insufficiency are hyperpigmented due to oversecretion of proopiomelanocortin (POMC) and subsequently high ACTH and MSH levels, hypoglycemia is usually associated with typical mineral disturbances. In adolescence and adulthood, the common cause is autoimmune adrenalitis. Other autoimmune disorders should be considered (as a part of APS1 or APS2a), the positivity of organ-specific antibodies (ACA, anti-21-hydroxylase) is helpful in diagnostic approach. Typically, hypoparathyroidism and mucocutaneous candidosis precede adrenal failure in child with autoimmune polyglandular syndrome type 1 (APS1), defect in autoimmune regulator gene (AIRE) has been determined with recessive inheritance. In boys with proven adrenal failure, adrenoleukodystrophy should be excluded. This X-linked recessive disorder is detected by high levels of very long-chain fatty acids in urine. Milder form - adrenomyelopathy develops in childhood and adolescence, and neurological disease follows 10-15 years later. Severe form is much rare and starts in infancy. Hyperpigmentation and high ACTH level are also found in ACTH resistance (Allgrove syndrome - tripple A), inherited autosomal dominantly. Main features are achalasia, alacrimia and adrenal failure, patients suffer from autonomic dysfunction and progressive neurological symptoms. Mutation in ALADIN gene has been found in patients with tripple A syndrome (Randell et al, 2007).

GH deficiency may be either isolated, or as a part of panhypopituitarism. Two stimulation tests (GH<10 ng/ml) are required for diagnosis in children with growth retardation (SDS<-2), hypothyroidism and celiac disease should be excluded before testing. One test may be sufficient in the case of positive history to cranial radiation, or MRI imaging of empty sella, septooptic dysplasia or corporus callosum agenesis. After head surgery due to craniopharyngeoma, observing period without GH therapy is 2 years at least. In the case of complete pituitary insufficiency, the significant growth rate slowing, low IGF1 level and previously claimed three hormone deficiencies, any testing is not necessary. Moreover, provocation of hypoglycemia may be harmful and dangerous due to lack of two counter-regulatory hormones in panhypopituitaric child. Imaging findings, such as agenesis of corpus callosum, septooptic dysplasia or empty sella must increase clinical suspicion (Rosenfeld & Cohen, 2008).

Thirty minutes after hypoglycemia, sampling of hormones may reveal counter-regulatory deficiency more sensitively than measurement of critical sample. At the time of low blood glucose level, higher concentrations of cortisol (>500 nmol/l) and GH (>10 ng/ml) exclude substantial lack of these hormones. However, decreased counter-regulatory hormones in critical sample are not diagnostic for hormonal deficiencies. The peak of these hormones is present approximately 30 minutes after hypoglycemic episode confirmed by laboratory blood glucose measurement below diagnostic threshold (<2,8 mmol/l). Such information about duration of hypoglycemia can not be usually obtained at the time of critical sampling. On the other hand, measurement of insulin and C-peptide levels at the time of low blood glucose level remains crucial for diagnosis of hyperinsulinism.

Teoretically, epinephrine deficiency may contribute to hypoglycemia of adrenal failure. However, hypoglycemia is rare in patients with bilateral adrenalectomy on adequate glucocorticoid replacement. Similarly, diabetic patients exhibit diminished epinephrine secretion more probably due to repeated hypoglycemia. Reduction of insulin-induced hypoglycemia can usually restore normal catecholamine response. Impaired glucagon secretion also increases the risk of hypoglycemia in patients with type 1 diabetes (Langdon et al, 2008).

4.4 Glycogen storage disease

Glucose is stored as a glycogen in the liver, muscles, and kidneys. If there is defect in formation or breakdown of glycogen, hypoglycamia may take part. In such group of metabolic inborn errors, glycogen storage disease (GSD) type 1 (glucose-6-phosphatase deficiency) is the most common cause of hypoglycemia. Appart from defect in glycogen metabolism, glucose-6-phosphatase deficiency is also essential enzyme for gluconeogenesis. Disruption of two metabolic pathways in GSD type 1 leads to significant persistent or recurrent hypoglycemia. Fortunately, glucose values within the range 30-50 mg/dl (1,7-2,8 mmol/l) are usually well tolerated, reflecting the adaptation of the brain to alternative fuel sources (lactate). Despite subtle clinical picture at the time of marked hypoglycemia, counter-regulatory hormones are elevated appropriately. Consequent promotion of glycogenolysis, gluconeogenesis and lipolysis increases lactate, triglycerides and ketones level. Clinically, glucose-6-phosphatase deficiency leads to massive glycogen stores and progressive hepatomegaly, renal tubular disease and malabsorbtion, later growth retardation is common. In addition to recurrent hypoglycemia, there is also lactic acidosis, elevated lipid levels and hyperuricemia in children with GSD type 1. Most cases are diagnosed in childhood, although sometimes GSD presents as a neonatal hypoglycemia Diagnosis is made by enzymatic studies of liver, kidney or intestine biopsy tissue or by elaborating specific gene mutations. Availability of mutation analysis has made the need for liver biopsy obsolete. Management approach involves continuous nasogastric or gastrostomy nocturnal feeding (6-8 mg/kg/min of glucose) and cornstarch supplementation (1-2g/kg every 4 hrs). Patients are fed every 2 hrs during the day, and glucose should be continuously provided overnight.

GSD type 3 (amylo-1,6-glucosidase deficiency) exhibits similar laboratory and clinical findings, such as hepatomegaly and growth failure, occasionally progressive muscle weakness and cardiomyopathy has been recorded. GSD type 6 and 9 (liver phosphorylase deficiency) has a comparatively benign course, mild episodes of hypoglycemia are not usually associated with lactic acidemia and hyperuricemia. Furthermore, elevated transaminase and hyperlipidemia are measured, affected children are investigated for hepatomegaly, hypotonia and muscle weakness. Most of these clinical features resolve by puberty, although some individuals may have a problem with cardiomyopathy, myopathy and renal tubular acidosis. In patient with concomitant liver and muscle involvment, the use of low-carbohydrate high-protein diet has been suggested to protect muscle from lack of alanin. Biochemical studies of leucocytes may confirm the diagnosis of GSD, except type 1 and 0. Glycogen synthase deficiency (GSD 0) is a rare but probably under-diagnosed cause of hypoglycemia. Fasting hypoglycemia is ketotic and unlike of other GSD, hepatomegaly is not observed. Diagnosis of GSD 0 can be determined by liver biopsy, recently mutation analysis of glycogen synthase gene has been available (Weinstein et al, 2006).

Glycogen accumulation in liver and kidney may be caused by GLUT2 deficiency (also known as Fanconi-Bickel syndrome). GLUT2 allows glucose transport across cell membrane of β-cells, renal tubule cells and hepatocytes. Except postprandial hyperglycemia due to reduced glucose transport on β-cell, clinical and laboratory findings are similar to Gierke disease (GSD type 1). Children suffer from fasting hypoglycemia, postprandial hyperglycemia, glucosuria, phosphaturia, aminoaciduria and metabolic acidosis. Furthermore, hepatomegaly, hypophosphatemic rickets and severe growth retardation can be present (Santer et al, 2002). Unlike GULT2 deficiency, GLUT1 is responsible for glucose transport across blood-brain barrier. The clinical consequence varies from classic picture of developmental encephalopathy with seizures to atypic presentations, e.g. mental retardation, intermittent ataxia, choreoatetosis, dystonia and dysartric speech. The diagnosis is confirmed by hypoglycorrhachia in cerebrospinal fluid despite normal plasma glucose concentration. Recent discovery of this condition may explain previously longtime reported positive effect of ketogenic diet in some patients with neurologic defect. The ketogenic diet successfully controls the seizures in patients with GLUT1 deficiency, but has smaller effect on the cognitive function (Wang et al, 2005).

4.5 Autoimmune hypoglycemia

Autoimmune hypoglycemia can result from antibodies directed either against insulin or insulin receptor, and may occur in all ages. The hypoglycemia is most often postprandial, but may be fasting. Laboratory findings are usually similar to exogeneous hyperinsulinism (high insulin and low C-peptide) in patients with anti-insulin antibodies positivity, whereas autoimmune hypoglycemia due to anti-insulin receptor antibodies shows typically undetectable insulin and C-peptide level. Rarely, antibodies directed against surface antigens on β-cells has been reported as a cause of autoimmune hypoglycemia (Redmon & Nutal, 1999).

4.6 Reactive hypoglycemia

The term of idiopathic postprandial syndrome, also known as reactive hypoglycemia, has been used for any clinical symptoms suggesting hypoglycemia that occur 2-4 hours after meal. Many healthy children and adults may have glycemia less than 60 mg/dl (3,3 mmol/l) without clinical presentation postpradially, consequently the oral glucose tolerance test has as a little diagnostic value in this syndrome. Most patients are adolescent girls with positive family history of similar symptoms in mother. At first, diagnosis such as panic attack, hyperventilation, vasovagal syncope and orthostatic hypotension should be excluded. Diagnosis of reactive hypoglycemia requires confirmation of low blood glucose level at the time of clinical symptoms suggesting hypoglycemia, and exclusion of other pathologic conditions (e.g. hyperinsulinism).

4.7 Alimentary hypoglycemia

All patients with Nissen fundoplication and gastrostomy tube are at risk of alimentary hypoglycemia. After surgery, rapid absorbtion of high-glucose fluids causes hyperinsulinism, responsible for hypoglycemia in 1-2 hours later. This condition, known as a late (glucose) dumping may occur in one third of patients with fundoplication and gastric tube. In long-term management, an avoidance high load of rapid carbohydrates, a supplementation of acarbose of 12-75 mg per dose, and a complex carbohydrate formula may be successful (Ng et al, 2002).

4.8 Hypoglycemia induced by exogenous agents

Many medicaments may cause hypoglycemia as a side effect, directly or indirectly. Unlike to direct effect of β-blockers, discontinuation of chronic high-dose inhaled corticosteroid treatment and subsequent adrenal suppression might cause hypoglycemia indirectly. The correct attitude to any person presenting with hypoglycemia is awareness of detailed drug history concerning all family members. Common causes of low blood glucose level due to poisoning are paracetamol or salicylate overdoses, sulfonylurea ingestion and insulin administration. Especially, insulin overdoses should be considered, if insulin concentration is too high despite of supressed C-peptide level. In such patients, family history is usually positive for type 1 diabetes treated by human insulins. Administration of insulin analogues may not be detected by immunoassay, the serum insulin concentration may be falsely low. Recommended treatment is glucose ingestion or infusion, in case of insufficiency of these procedures, the successful use of diazoxide and ocreotid has been reported (Lheurex et al, 2005). Sometimes, antidotes are necessary, for example, paracetamol poisoning requires addition of N-acetylcysteine. Similarly, salicylate intoxication may initiate changes in glucose metabolism, hyper- and hypoglycemia have been reported. Alcohol consumption reduces gluconeogenesis, hypoglycemia may occur in a several hours after acute intoxication. Ingestion of plants such as cocklebur (Xanthium strumarium) can cause hypoglycemia, kidney or liver dysfunction, and large amount may lead to multi-organ failure (Randell, 2007).

4.9 Hypoglycemia in non-insulin secreting tumors

Hypoglycemia has been reported in patients with non-insulin secreting tumors, predominantly large retroperitoneal ones. The serum evaluation of such patients shows elevated insulin–like growth factor 2 (IGF2). IGF-2 activates IGF-1 receptor and cross activates insulin receptor, causing hypoglycemia. In management approach, the method of choice is surgical removal of tumor. Some authors reffers to success with growth hormone treatment up to the time of definitive surgery (Agus et al, 1995). However, this approach may be contradictory and needs other evidence.

4.10 Hypoglycemia in critical illness and organ failure

Approximately 30% of patients with severe malaria suffer from hypoglycemia, and the presence of low blood glucose seems to be associated with increased mortality in malaric patients. In addition, the therapy for malaria can contribute to hypoglycemia, in particular, quinine stimulates insulin secretion. Hypoglycemia is also common in other critically ill patients and has been reported in organ failure or severe disease, such as sepsis, head injury, heart failure, chronic renal failure, acute hepatic necrosis, pancreatitis, severe enteritis and multiple organ failure. Etiopathogenesis of hypoglycemia in these patients is often multifactorial: lack of substrate, undernutrition, accelerated glucose consumption, impaired gluconeogenesis, misplaced infusion line, cytokine and drug effect (Langdon et al, 2008). On the other hand, an acute illness may reveal latent disorder of glucose metabolism (Weinstein et al, 2001).

4.11 Hypoglycemia in diabetes mellitus

In diabetic patients, clinical symptoms suggesting hypoglycemia should be promptly treated by rapid carbohydrate intake, 15 g of carbohydrates are recommended to 50 kg patient as usual. If signs last in 15 minutes, the same dose of carbohydrates should be taken. Clinical presentation of severe hypoglycemia, such as seizures and unconsciousness, must be cured by intramuscular or subcutaneous administration of glucagon with assistance of another person. The incidence of hypoglycemia induced by insulin therapy is higher than those caused by sulfonylureas. However, pre-existing renal failure may increase the risk of hypoglycemia in patients on sulfonyurea therapy. Measurements of ả particularly low HbA1c level should be suspected of unknown hypoglycemic episodes in past.

The frequency of severe hypoglycemia is declining due to improvement of techniques, therapeutic strategies and insulin structure (Baunduceau et al, 2010). Hypoglycemia may be harmful in patients with history of ischemic heart disease, association between severe hypoglycemia and sudden death has been described. Prolonged duration of type 1 diabetes is linked to higher risk of severe hypoglycemia due to profound lack of insulin, furthermore, protective hormone response may be diminished (Heller, 2010). In ADVANCE study, an increase in the frequency of severe hypoglycemia was found in elderly diabetics presenting with substantial cognitive disorders. However, dementia alone is a significant risk factor for occurrence of severe hypoglycemic episodes due to mistakes in diabetes management (Bauduceau, 2010). Similarly, infants and small children are not able to manage own diabetes, hypoglycemia must be resolved by help of another person, so all hypoglycemia in such patients should be considered as a serious.

During exercise, diabetic patients are usually at risk of glucose declining, sometimes falling to hypoglycemic levels. Adequate carbohydrate replacement during and after exercise seems to be the most important measure to prevent hypoglycemia, an insulin reduction from 20 to 30% can be reasonable only for exercise lasting more than one hour (Grimm et al, 2004). Repeated unexpected low blood glucose levels in type 1 diabetes (DM 1) may be the indicator of associated disorders. All patients with DM 1 requiring significant reduction of insulin dose, should be testing for autoimmune hypothyroidism, hypocorticism and celiac disease.

5. Conclusion

Diagnostic approach to hypoglycemia should be based on critical sample of intermediate metabolites and hormones at the time of laboratory proven low blood glucose level as well as 30 minutes after hypoglycemic episode. Authors suggest that repeating second sampling may be more helpful for determination of deficiency of counter-regulatory hormones. All management effort should be done to obtain such measurement as soon as possible, with consequent quick and appropriate treatment. Delayed or incorrect diagnosis of hypoglycemic symptoms may lead to many different irreversibile neurologic disturbances, especially in infants and small children.

6. References

Agus M.S., Katz L.E., Satin-Smith M., Meadows A.T., Hinth R.L., Cohen P. (1995) Non-islet-cell tumor associated with hypoglycemia in a child. Successful long-term therapy with growth hormone. J Pediatr, 127 (3), 403-407

Ahmad A., Kahler S.G, Kishanani P.S., Artigas-Lopez M. Pappu A.S., Steiner R., Millington D.S., Van Hove J.L. (1999) Treatment of pyruvate carboxylase deficiency with high dose citrate and aspartate. Am J Med Genet, 87, 331- 338

Aynsley-Green A., Hussain K., Hall J., Saudubray J.M., Nihoul-Fekete C., De Lonlay-Debeney P.(2000) Practical management of hyperinsulinism in infancy. Arch Dis Child Fetal Neonatal Ed, 82, 98-107

Bauduceau B., Doucet J., Bordier L., Garcia C, Dupuy O. Mayauduon H.: Hypoglycaemia nad dementia in diabetic patients.Diab Metab, 36, 106-110

Baujat G., Rio M., Rossignol S., Sanlaville D., Lyonnet S., Le Merrer M. (2004) Paradoxical NSD1 mutations in Beckwith -Wiedemann syndrome and 11p15 anomalies in Sotos syndrome. Am J Hum Genet, 74, 715-720

Bliek J., Maas S.M., Ruijter J.M., Hennekam F.E., Alders M. Westerveld A. (2001) Incresed tumour risk for BWS patients correlates with aberrant H19 and not KCNQ1OT1 methylation, occurrence of KCNQ1OT1 hypomethylation in familial cases of BWS. Hum Mol Genet, 10, 467-476

Charsa D.S., McKinley P.S., Whitfield J.M. (2003) Glucagon infusion for the treatment of hypoglycaemia, efficacy and safety in sick, preterm infants. Pediatrics, 111, 220-221

Coulthard M.G., Hey E.N. (2002) Glucagon is very unlikely to have caused hyponatremia. Pediatrics, 109 (5), 985

Cuesta-Munoz A.I., Huopio H., Otonkoski T. (2004) Severe persistent hyperinsulinemic hypoglycemia due to de novo glucokinase mutation. Diabetes, 53, 2164 - 2168

de Lonlay P., Cormier-Daire V., Amiel J., Touati G., Goldenberg J.C., Fournet J.C.: (2002) Facial appearence in persistent hyperinsulinemic hypoglycemia. Am J Med Genet, 111, 130-133 a

de Lonlay P., Fournet J.C., Touati G., Gross M.S., Martin D., Sevin C. (2002) Heterogeneity of persistent hyperinsulinaemic hypoglycaemia. A series of 175 cases. Eur J Pediatr, 161, 37-48 b

de Leon D.D., Stanely C.A., Sperling M.A (2008) Hypoglycaemia in neonates and infants. In Sperling M.A.: Pediatric endocrinology, third edition, Saunders Elsevier, 2008, 889, 165-197 ISBN 978-1-4160-4090-3

de Rooy L., Hawdon J.M. (2002) Nutritional factors that affect the postnatal metabolic adaptation of full-term small and large-for-gestational-age-infants. 109, e42

Desphade S., Platt M.,W. (2005) The investigation and management of neonatal hypoglycaemia. Seminars in Fetal and Neonatal Medicine, 10, 351-361

Dunne M.J., Cosgrove K.E., Shepherd R.M., Aynsley-Green A., Lindley K.J. (2004) Hyperinsulinism in infancy, from basic science to clinical disease. Physiol Rev, 84, 239-275

Ericson L.E., Hakanson R., Lundkiust I. (1997) Accumulation of dopamine in mouse pancreatic β cells following injection of L-DOPA. Localisation to secretory granules and inhibition of infusion solution. Diabetologia 13 (2), 117 - 124

Fang J., Peters V., Assmann B., Korner C., Hoffmann G.F. (2004) Improvement of CDG diagnosis by combined examination of several glycoproteins. J Inherit Metab Dis 24 (8), 858-862

Gamma R., Anderson N.R., Marks V. (2000). Glucose meter hypoglycaemia: Often a non-disease. Ann Clin Biochem 37(5), 731-735

Greenberg L.W., Badosa F., Niakosari A., Schneider A., Zaeri N., Schindler A.M. (2000) Clinopathologic exercise: Hypoglycaemia in a young women with amenorrhea. J Pediatr, 136(6), 818-822

Grimberg A., Ferry R.J.Jr., Kelly A. (2001) Dysregulation of insulin secretion in children with congenital hyperinsulinism due to sulfonylurea receptor mutations. Diabetes, 50, 322 - 328

Grimm J.J., Ybarra J., Berné C., Muchnick S., Golay A. (2004) A new table for prevention of hypoglycaemia during physical activity in type 1 diabetic patients. Diabetes Metab, 30, 465-470

Hanas R. (2004) Type I diabetes in children, adolescents and young adults. Second edition, Class Publishing, London, ISBN 185959 – 078 - 0, 385

Heller S (2010) Hypoglycemia in diabetes. Medicine v38 (12), 671-675

Hirshberg B, Livi A., Bartlett D.L., Libutti S.K., Alexander H.R., Doppman J.L (2000) Forty-eight-hour fast: The diagnostic test for insulinoma. J Clin Endocrino Metab, 85(9), 3222-3226

Hussain K., Clayton P.T., Krywawych S. (2005) Hyperinsulinism of infancy associated with a novel splice site mutation in the SCHAD gene. J Pediatr 146, 706 - 708

Krude H., Biebermann H., Luck W., Horn R., Brabant G., Gruters A.(1998) Severe early onset obesity, adrenal insufficiency and red hair pigmentation caused by POMC mutations in human. Nat Genet 19(2), 155-157

Langdon D.R., Stanley C.A., Sperling M.A. (2008) Hypoglycemia in the infant and child. In: Sperling M.A.: Pediatric endocrinology, Philadelphia, Saunders Elsevier, third edition, 889, 422-443, ISBN 978–1–4160-4090-3

Leslie N.D. (2003) Insights into the pathogenesis of galactosemia. Annu Rev Nutr, 23, 59 - 80

Lheureux P.E., Zahir S., Penaloza A. (2005) Bech –to-bedside review. Antidotal treatment of sulfonylurea-induced hypoglycaemia with ocreotide. Crit Care, 9, 543-549

Li C., Matter A., Kelly A. et al (2006) Effects of a GTP-insensitive mutation of glutamate dehydrogenase on insulin secretion in transgenic mice. J Biol Chem, 281, 15064 - 15072

Lindley K.J., Dunne M.J., Kane C., Shepherd R.M., Squires P.E., James R.F. (1996) Control of beta cell function in nesidioblastosis. A possible therapeutic role for calcium channel blockade. Arch Dis Child 74, 373-378

Lindley K.J., Dunne M.J. (2005) Contemporary strategies in the diagnosis and management of neonatal hyperinsulinaemic hypoglycaemia. Early Human Development, 81, 61-72

Magge S.N., Shyng S.L., McMullen C., Steinkrauss L., Ganguly A., Katz L.E. (2004) Familial leucine sensitive hypoglycemia of infancy due to a dominant mutation of the beta – cell sulfonylurea receptor. J Clin Endocrinol Metab, 89, 4450-4456

Marks V., Teale J.D (1999) Drug-induced hypoglycemia. Endocrinol Metab Clin North Am, 28 (3), 555-577

Menni F. de Lonlay P., Sevin C., Touati G., Peigne C., Barbier V. (2001) Neurologic outcomes of 90 neonates and infants with persistent hyperinsulinemic hypoglycemia . Paediatrics 107 (3), 476-479

Meissner T, Otonkoski T., Feneberg R, Beinbrech B., Apostolidou S., Sipila I. (2001) Exercise induced hypoglycaemic hyperinsulinism. Arch Dis Child 84 (3), 254-257

Miralles R.E., Lodha A., Perlman M., Moore A.N. (2002) Experience with intravenous glucagon infusions as a treatment for resistant neonatal hypoglycaemia. Arch Pediatr Adolesc Med, 156, 999-1004

Ng D., Ferry R.J., Weinzimer S.A. Stanley C.A., Levitt Katz L.E. (2002) Acarbose treatment of postprandial hypoglycemia in children after Nissen fundoplication. J Pediatr, 139, 877-879

Pinney S.H., Heltzer M., Brown-Whitehorn T., Langdon D.R.(2007) Hypoglycemia and growth failure due to inhaled corticosteroids. The Endocrine Society 89 th annual Meeting, Toronto

Randell T.L. (2007) Diagnosis and management of hypoglycaemia beyond the neonatal period. Paed Child Health 17, 7, 266-272

Redmon J.B., Nutall F.Q. (1999) Autoimmune hypoglycemia. Endocrinol Clin Metab North Am 28 (3), 603-618

Rinaldo P., Matern D., Bennett M.J. (2002) Fatty acid oxidation disorders-. Annu Rev Physiol 64, 477 - 502

Roe C.R., Ding J.H. (2001) Mitochondrial fatty acid oxidation disorders. In CRS Scriver: The metabolic and molecular bases of inherited disease, Eight edition, New York, Mc Graw-Hill, 2297-2326

Rosenfeld R.G., Cohen P, (2008) Disordes of growth hormone/insulin-like growth factor secretion and action. In: Sperling M.A.: Pediatric endocrinology. Philadelphia, Sauders Elsevier, 889, 254-334

Salhab W.A., Wyckoff M.H., Laptook A.R., Perlman J.M. (2004) Initial hypoglycemia and neonatal brain injury in term infants with severe fetal acidaemia. Pediatrics, 114, 361-366

Santer R., Groth S., Kinner M., Dombrowski A., Berry G.T., Brodhel J. (2002) The mutation spectrum of the facilitative glucose transporter gene SLC2A2 (GLUT2) in patients with Fanconi-Bickel syndrome. Hum Genct, 110(1), 21-29

Silvani P., Camporesi A., Mandelli A., Wolfler A., Salvo I. (2004) A case of severe diazoxide toxicity. Paediatr Anaesth, 14, 607-609

Stanley C.A. (2006) Parsing ketotic hypoglycaemia. Arch Dis Child, 91(6) 460-461

Taylor R., Lee C., Kyne-Grzebalski D., Marshall S.M., Davison J.M. (2002) Clinical outcome of pregnancy in women with type 1 diabetes. Obstet Gynecol, 99, 537-541

Wang D., Pascual J.M., Yang H. (2005) Glut-1 deficiency syndrome: clinical, genetic and therapuetic aspects. Ann Neurol, 57, 111 - 118

Weinstein D.A., Correia C.E., Saunders A.C. (2006) Hepatic glycogen synthase deficiency: an infrequently recognised cause of ketotic hypoglycemia. Mol Genet Metab, 87, 284-288

Weinstein D.A., Raymond K., Korson M.S., Weiner D.L., Wolfsdorf J.I.: (2001) High incidence of unrecognized metabolic and endocrinologic disorders in acutely ill children with previously unrecognized hypoglycemia. Pediatr Res 49, S 2, 88

Weintrob N., Sprecher E., Josefsberg Z., Weininger C., Aurbach - Klipper Y. (1998) Standard and Low-Dose Short Adrenocorticotropin Test Compared with Insulin-Induced Hypoglycemia for Assessment of the Hypothalamic-Pituitary-Adrenal Axis in Children with Idiopathic Multiple Pituitary Hormone Deficiencies. J. Clin. Endocrinol. Metab. 1998 83: 88-92

Wong D. (2005) Hereditary fructose intolerance. Mol Genet Metab, 85, 165 - 167

Yap F., Hogler W., Vora A., Halliday R., Ambler G (2004) Severe transient hyperinsulinaemic hypoglycaemia: two neonates without predisposing factor and a review of the literature. Eur J Pediatr , 163, 38-41

2

Hypoglycemia in Children Attending the Critical Care Medicine in Developing Countries

Mohammod Jobayer Chisti, Tahmeed Ahmed,
Hasan Ashraf, Abu Syeed Golam Faruque,
Sayeeda Huq and Md Iqbal Hossain
International Centre for Diarrhoeal Disease Research, Bangladesh
Bangladesh

1. Introduction

Hypoglycemia is a biochemical symptom, which refers to the presence of an underlying cause. As glucose is the fundamental energy currency of the cell, disorders that affect its availability or its use can cause hypoglycemia (DePuy et al., 2009, Schaefer-Graf et al., 2002). Glucose is a source of energy storage in the form of glycogen, fat, and protein and hypoglycemia is the most common metabolic problem among pediatric patients in the critical care medicine (DePuy et al., 2009, Tita et al., 2009, Adamson et al., 1995, Alkalay et al., 2006). The lower limit of the accepted normal value of blood glucose level in newborn infants with associated illness especially in presence of hypoxemia and ischemia that already impairs the cerebral metabolism has not been determined (Sperling et al., 2008, Alkalay et al., 2006). Moreover, there are controversies regarding the definition of hypoglycemia (Cornblath et al., 2000). However, some reasonably accepted definitions of hypoglycemia for the purpose of the clinical management of the entity are in practice. In children, a blood glucose value of less than 40 mg/dL (2.2 mmol/L) represents hypoglycemia (Tita et al., 2009, Guideline, 2004, Jain et al., 2008). A plasma glucose level of less than 30 mg/dL (1.65 mmol/L) in the first 24 hours of life and less than 45 mg/dL (2.5 mmol/L) thereafter constitutes hypoglycemia in the newborn (DePuy et al., 2009, Tita et al., 2009, Daly et al., 2003, Guideline, 2004, Cornblath et al., 2000). However, in children with severe acute malnutrition (SAM) the cutoff value is a bit high, and, a blood glucose value of less than 54 mg/dL (3.0 mmol/L) represents hypoglycemia (WHO, 1999, Ahmed et al., 1999).

2. Incidence of hypoglycemia

Incidence of hypoglycemia varies with the definition, population, method and timing of feeding, and the type of glucose assay (Guideline, 2004). The age is also helpful in assessing the probable diagnosis of hypoglycemia. The incidence is highest in the immediate post neonatal period (Halamek et al., 1997a, Cornblath and Ichord, 2000). The incidence decreases with increasing age (Halamek et al., 1997a, DePuy et al., 2009).

The overall incidence of symptomatic hypoglycemia in newborns varies from 1.3-3 per 1000 live births (Cranmer, 2009, Guideline, 2004). Serum glucose levels are higher than whole blood values (Cowett and Loughead, 2002, Deshpande and Ward Platt, 2005). The incidence of hypoglycemia is greater in high-risk neonatal groups (DePuy et al., 2009, Guideline, 2004, Cornblath and Ichord, 2000). Hypoglycemia is more common in premature neonates especially born at less than 37 weeks of gestation and in those especially born at more than 40 weeks gestation, with incidence rates of 2.4% in neonates born at 37 weeks' gestation, 0.7-1.8% in neonates born at 38-42 weeks of gestation (Tita et al., 2009, Narchi and Skinner, 2009, Cornblath and Ichord, 2000). The incidence of hypoglycemia in children older than 6 months in a large urban critical care department was 0.034% (Daly et al., 2003). In a recent Japanese study, more than 80% of admissions from the nursery to the neonatal ICU after birth were due to apnea or hypoglycemia in neonates born at 35-36 weeks' gestation (Ishiguro et al., 2009). Incidence of hypoglycemia among 1-5 years old children with acute gastroenteritis and dehydration was found 9.2% (Reid and Losek, 2005). However, study conducted among the hospitalized malnourished children in the critical care medical units of the developing countries, 16-39% were found to be hypoglycemic on admission (Bennish et al., 1990, Huq et al., 2007, Chisti et al., 2010).

Early feeding decreases the incidence of hypoglycemia (Wight, 2006, Meier et al., 2007, Chertok et al., 2009). The incidence of inborn errors of metabolism that lead to neonatal hypoglycemia are rare but can be screened in infancy (Schwartz, 1997b, Guideline, 2004, Cranmer, 2009):

Common inborn errors of metabolism:

- Carbohydrate metabolism disorders (>1:10,000)
- Fatty acid oxidation disorders (1:10,000)
- Hereditary fructose intolerance (1:20,000 to 1:50,000)
- Glycogen storage diseases (1:25,000)
- Galactosemia (1:40,000)
- Organic acidemias (1:50,000)

Uncommon inborn errors of metabolism:

- Phosphoenolpyruvate carboxykinase deficiency
- Primary lactic acidosis

3. Objectives

- To develop a guideline for the physicians and nurses working at the critical care medicine in the developing countries for the bed side diagnosis and prompt management of hypoglycemia and
- To evaluate its role as a predictor of fatal outcome in children with SAM.

4. Options

- Clinical assessment
- Bed side testing
- Prompt bed side management
- Empirical antimicrobial therapy according to cause

5. Benefits of this chapter

- Increase awareness for the rapid diagnosis of hypoglycemia in children with SAM, and those with dehydrating diarrhea
- Better utilization of the available diagnostic equipments
- Understanding the value of rapid management of hypoglycemia in children with SAM
- Understanding the need for antimicrobial therapy according to cause
- Decreased morbidity and mortality due to hypoglycemia
- Increase the awareness of the causes of pediatric hypoglycemia
- Immediate diagnosis
- Prompt treatment
- Reduced cost associated with unnecessary investigations and complications due to inappropriate treatment

6. Importance of the chapter

Health professionals in developing countries often rely on clinical signs to predict the severity of disease in hospitals with limited facilities, which is often reliable in children with better nutritional status (WHO, 2005, Chisti et al., 2009c) but severely malnourished children often have severe infection (Chisti et al., 2010) and die without any prior overt clinical signs, which may prevent their appropriate and timely management (Suskind and Suskind, 1990, Morgan, 1997). Laboratory investigation, an essential alternative measure of suppressed clinical signs, often involves many efforts, time and cost, as in blood culture. Availability of pertinent laboratory investigations in resource poor settings is very limited. Furthermore, data on simple, less time-consuming and inexpensive laboratory diagnostic tool(s) that can predict the outcome of such infants are scarce. However, limited data for predicting factors of fatal outcome in severely malnourished children in pediatric critical care medicine revealed that hypoglycemia, measured by a simple portable bedside glucose test, is significantly associated with fatal outcome especially in children presenting with SAM (Chisti et al., 2010, Huq et al., 2007). It may be a useful rapid diagnostic test, allowing prompt comprehensive management of such children following WHO guidelines (WHO, 2005), thus reducing deaths even in resource poor settings.

7. Associated factors of hypoglycemia

Hypoglycemia is common in critically ill children and is associated with increased mortality rates in critically ill nondiabetic children (Faustino and Bogue, Cornblath and Ichord, 2000, Reid and Losek, 2005). A recent study by Faustino et al. showed that hypoglycemia was associated with worsening organ function (Faustino and Bogue) and concluded that it may be a marker of severity of illness. He also suggested that further investigations are needed to establish the mortality risk with hypoglycemia due to the effect of insulin compared to spontaneous hypoglycemia (Faustino and Bogue). One recent study revealed that infants with serious illness such as sclerema requiring admission to critical care medicine in an urban diarrhea hospital were significantly associated with hypoglycemia (Chisti et al., 2009a). Another study from the same center revealed that patients with enteric encephalopathy having fatal outcome more often presented with hypoglycemia compared to those who survived (Chisti et al., 2009b).

A most recent study from the critical care ward of Dhaka hospital of ICDDR,B revealed that among all relatively rapid laboratory investigations in neonates, hypoglycemia was the independent predictor of fatal outcome (Table 1). The study revealed that to predict death, the sensitivity, specificity, and positive predictive value of hypoglycemia with their 95% confidence intervals were 40% (14–73%), 88% (75– 95%), and 40% (14–73%), respectively (Chisti et al., 2010). The study concluded that most of the laboratory markers used to predict fatal outcome in diarrheal infants with SAM take several hours to become available, except a bedside glucose test, which takes less than a minute but is inexpensive. The study suggested that presence of hypoglycemia, measured by a portable bedside glucose test, is significantly associated with fatal outcome with high specificity in infants presenting with diarrhea and SAM (Chisti et al., 2010). It may be a useful rapid diagnostic test allowing prompt detection followed by comprehensive management of such infants according to WHO guidelines, which would help in reducing deaths even in resource poor settings (WHO, 2005). The findings of the study was also supported by another previous study from the same country where children with hypoglycemia more often had bacteremia (Huq et al., 2007).

Variable	Death N = 10 (%)	Survivor N = 51 (%)	Non-adjusted OR (95% CI)	p value	Adjusted OR (95% CI)	p value
Hypoglycemia	4 (40)	6 (12)	5.0 (1.01 - 29.8)	0.027	5.0 (1.1 - 23.0)	0.039
Abnormal WBC count	6 (60)	36 (71)	0.6 (0.1 - 3.1)	0.710	0.5 (0.1 – 2.5)	0.438
Higher S. CRP level	9 (90)	33 (65)	4.9 (0.6 - 111.7)	0.151	4.5 (0.5 - 39.5)	0.179
Hyponatremia	3 (30)	14 (28)	1.1 (0.2 - 6.0+)	1.00	0.8 (0.2 - 4.2)	0.813
Hypokalemia	4 (40)	25 (49)	0.7 (0.1 - 3.3)	0.735	2.2 (0.3 - 14.4)	0.409
Hypocalcemia	4 (40)	11 (22)	2.4 (0.5 - 12.4)	0.243	1.8 (0.3 - 10.2)	0.529
Hypomagnesemia	0 (00)	2 (4)	0.0 (0.0 - 23.5)	1.00	0.0 (0.0 - unidentified)	1.0

OR: odds ratio, CI: confidence interval, S: serum, CRP: C-reactive protein.
Illustrated from the Tropical Medicine and International Health by Chisti et. al. (2010)

Table 1. Comparison of the characteristics of severely malnourished infants with fatal outcome and those who survived

8. Hypoglycemia and glucose metabolism

Malnutrition is a major risk factor for death in children in developing countries (Faruque et al., 2008), and the mortality risk is higher in infants when they present with severe form of malnutrition (Pelletier et al., 1994, Naheed et al., 2009, Chisti et al., 2009c), especially in a set up with critical care medicine (Elusiyan et al., 2006). It has not received enough attention in developing countries. The primary therapy is very simple by immediate infusion of intravenous glucose. The occurrence of hypoglycemia is directly related to energy balance and determined by the availability of glucose, free fatty acids and ketone bodies in the tissue (Nuoffer and Mullis, 2005, Fluck et al., 2003, Mohnike and Aynsley-Green, 1993). An intact energy balance and maintenance of normal blood sugar concentration is dependent upon: an adequate caloric and qualitative dietary intake; a functionally intact hepatic glucogenolytic and gluconeogenic enzyme system; an adequate supply of endogenous gluconeogenic substrates (lactate, amino acids and glycerol); an adequate energy supply provided by the beta-oxidation of fatty acids to synthesize glucose and ketone bodies and a normal endocrine system (insulin, glucagon, catecholamines and growth hormone) for integrating and modulating these processes (Nuoffer and Mullis, 2005, Mohnike et al., 1993). Disturbances in each of these factors may lead to hypoglycemia. Glucose has an essential and fundamental importance for the brain metabolism. The major contribution of the brain to the basal metabolic rate is an important factor contributing to the frequency and severity of a hypoglycemic syndrome in the pediatric age (Nuoffer and Mullis, 2005, Mohnike et al., 1993). Cerebral glucose uptake occurs through a glucose transporter molecule and these molecules are carrier mediated and facilitate diffusion process that is dependent on blood glucose concentration but cerebral and cerebrospinal fluid (CSF) glucose uptake are not regulated by insulin (Sperling et al., 2008). Paucity of glucose transporter molecule can result in seizures due to reduced cerebral and CSF glucose concentrations although there might have normal blood glucose levels (Sperling et al., 2008, Mohnike et al., 1993). Thus, hypoglycemia should be considered as a medical emergency and treated very aggressively especially in children with other associated illnesses such as SAM, severe sepsis, septic shock, febrile neonates, prematurity and low birth weight in the critical care medicine ward.

9. Pathophysiology of hypoglycemia

Normal blood glucose is very narrowly regulated, usually from 4.4-5 mmol/L. Glucose levels increase transiently after meals to 6.6-7.7 mmol/L. Feedback systems return the glucose concentration rapidly back to the preprandial level, usually within 2 hours after the last absorption of carbohydrates (Fleisher, 2000, Halamek and Stevenson, 1998, Reid et al., 2003, Sperling et al., 2008).

Insulin and glucagon are the important hormones in the immediate feedback control system of glucose (Sperling et al., 2008). When blood glucose increases after a meal, the rate of insulin secretion increases and stimulates the liver to store glucose as glycogen (Halamek et al., 1997b). When cells (primarily liver and muscle) are saturated with glycogen, additional glucose is stored as fat (Reid et al., 2003).

When blood glucose levels fall, glucagon secretion functions to increase blood glucose levels by stimulating the liver to undergo glycogenolysis and release glucose back into the blood (Sperling et al., 2008, Halamek et al., 1997b).

In starvation, the liver maintains the glucose level via gluconeogenesis (Sperling et al., 2008). Gluconeogenesis is the formation of glucose from amino acids and the glycerol portion of fat. Muscle provides a store of glycogen and muscle protein breaks down to amino acids, which are substrates utilized in gluconeogenesis in the liver (Narayan et al., 2001). Circulating fatty acids are catabolized to ketones, acetoacetate, and B-hydroxybutyrate and can be used as auxiliary fuel by most tissues, including the brain (Fleisher, 2000, Sperling et al., 2008).

The hypothalamus stimulates the sympathetic nervous system, and epinephrine is secreted by the adrenals causing the further release of glucose from the liver (Haninger and Farley, 2001). Over a period of hours to days of prolonged hypoglycemia, growth hormone and cortisol are secreted and decrease the rate of glucose utilization by most cells of the body (Halamek and Stevenson, 1998).

In the newborn, serum glucose levels decline after birth until 1-3 hours due to an abrupt transition from the intrauterine life, then they spontaneously increase, ultimately characterized by the autonomous ability to maintain euglycemia. Liver glycogen stores become rapidly depleted within hours of birth, and gluconeogenesis, primarily from alanine, can account for 10% of glucose turnover in the newborn infant by several hours of age (Halamek and Stevenson, 1998).

Neonatal hypoglycemia (Halamek and Stevenson, 1998, Sperling et al., 2008)

- Inappropriate changes in hormone secretion
- Inadequate substrate reserve in the form of hepatic glycogen
- Inadequate muscle stores as a source of amino acids for gluconeogenesis
- Inadequate lipid stores for the release of fatty acids

Hypoglycemia in older infants and children (Sperling et al., 2008, Reid et al., 2003)

- The pathophysiology of hypoglycemia is analogous to that in adults.
- Glucose homeostasis is maintained by glycogenolysis in the immediate post feeding periods and by gluconeogenesis several hours after meals.

Hypoglycemia in severely malnourished children:

The pathophysiology of the hypoglycemia is poorly understood although there is popular belief that it is mainly due to severe infection in severely malnourished children. There is decreased endogenous glucose production (EGP) in severely malnourished children which is related to the degree of hypoalbuminemia and oxidative stress (Bandsma et al.). Severe malnutrition is associated with impaired glucose absorption and decreased glucose absorption correlates with oxidative stress in sick children who needs admission to the pediatric critical care medicine (Bandsma et al.). This potentially explains the etiology of hypoglycemia in severely malnourished children. Severe malnutrition in infants often causes depressed cell-mediated and humoral immune responses, associated with impairment of IgA production, chemotaxis, reduced mature T cells, and compromised phagocytic activity (Suskind and Suskind, 1990, Morgan, 1997). As a result, patients become highly susceptible to infectious disease, predominantly diarrhea, which is often associated with prolonged anorexia and vomiting (Feign. R and Garg, 1987). Failure of gluconeogenesis in such infants is a common phenomenon (Butler et al., 1989, Bennish et al., 1990) and potentially responsible for the development of fatal hypoglycemia.

10. Causes/etiology of hypoglycemia

Hypoglycemia events are usually accompanied by an increased heart rate with bounding pulse due to increased epinephrine secretion (Dubois et al., 1995). This leads the infant to be irritable, tremulous, and cranky (al-Rabeeah et al., 1995). In any case the brain energy supply is severely impaired; the mental status of the children is likely to be impaired with extreme inappropriate effect and mood, lethargy, seizure, or coma. Large body size for age in the neonate or older child suggests hyperinsulinism, although some children with hyperinsulinism are born prematurely and are small for gestational age (de Lonlay-Debeney et al., 1999, Stanley, 1997). Decreased subcutaneous fat as in severe malnutrition such as in severe wasting suggests inadequate glucose stores (de Lonlay-Debeney et al., 1999, Dubois et al., 1995). Poor linear growth may point to growth hormone deficiency, and midline facial and cranial abnormalities suggest pituitary hormone deficiencies (Dunne et al., 1997). Liver size should be assessed for evidence of glycogen-storage diseases. Etiology of hypoglycemia includes the following:

10.1 Hyperinsulinemia

Potential causes of hyperinsulinism in children include maternal diabetes in pregnancy, persistent hyperinsulinemic hypoglycemia of infancy, insulin-producing tumors, and child abuse (Stanley, 1997). Hyperinsulinism causes excess glucose use primarily by stimulating skeletal muscle to uptake glucose. This is aggravated by insulin-induced suppression of hepatic glycogenolysis and gluconeogenesis (al-Rabeeah et al., 1995, Stanley, 1997).

In neonates

Hyperinsulinism is the most common cause of hypoglycemia in neonates. However, in addition to hyperinsulinism, or persistent hyperinsulinemic hypoglycemia of infancy (PHHI), hypoglycemia occurs due to limited glycogen stores (eg, prematurity, intrauterine growth retardation), depleted glycogen stores (eg, stress in perinatal asphyxia, starvation), in ketotic hypoglycemia, easily depleted glycogen stores, in combination with inadequate production of glucose through gluconeogenesis, contribute to hypoglycemia (Cranmer, 2009, Guideline, 2004). Thus, fatty acid oxygenation is required to provide substrate for gluconeogenesis and ketogenesis. Ketones, the byproduct of fatty acid metabolism, are found in urine and represent the starved state. Increased glucose use (eg, hyperthermia, polycythemia, sepsis, growth hormone deficiency), decreased glycogenolysis, gluconeogenesis, or use of alternate fuels (eg, inborn errors of metabolism, adrenal insufficiency) (Cranmer, 2009, Guideline, 2004).

In infants

Hyperinsulinemia may be due to various genetic defects that cause a loss of glucose regulation of insulin secretion (Cosgrove et al., 2004, Tornovsky et al., 2004). This disorder is known as endogenous-persistent hyperinsulinemic hypoglycemia of infancy (previously termed nesidioblastosis) (Cosgrove et al., 2004, Stanley, 1997). No genetic defect is identified in 50% of patients with hyperinsulinism although unusual single nucleotide polymorphisms defects have been found that may be responsible in some infants (Di Candia et al., 2009).

Infants of mothers with diabetes also have high insulin levels after birth due to the high glucose exposure in utero; the poorer the glucose control during pregnancy, the greater the likelihood of hyperinsulinism in the infant (Stanley, 1997). In older children, hyperinsulinemia is rare, but an insulin-producing tumor is the most common cause (Stanley, 1997). Exogenous administration of insulin or oral hypoglycemic agents, either accidental or due to abuse, must be considered (Di Candia et al., 2009).

Overall criteria for the diagnosis of hyperinsulinism in the infant (Sperling et al., 2008)

- Hyperinsulinemia (plasma insulin > 2 μU/mL)
- Hypofattyacidemia (plasma free fatty acids < 1.5 mmol/L
- Hypoketonemia (plasma β-hydroxybuterate < 2.0 mmol/L)
- Inappropriate glycemic response to glucagon, 1 mg IV (delta glucose > 40 mg/dl))

10.2 Disorders of glucose underproduction

This includes inadequate glucose stores which are associated with prematurity, infants who are small for gestational age, SAM, and ketotic hypoglycemia (Di Candia et al., 2009).

Among them, children with SAM who need admission to the critical care medicine have paramount importance. We will focus our discussion at the later part of the chapter.

After insulin treatment in diabetes, the above mentioned disorders are the most common causes of hypoglycemia. These disorders are largely diagnoses of exclusion made after other causes of hypoglycemia are ruled out. Prematurity, infants who are small for gestational age, and SAM should be readily apparent based on the clinical situation. Ketotic hypoglycemia, which usually affects children with SAM and aged 18 months to 6 years, is usually due to disrupted food intake (Di Candia et al., 2009).

Glycogen-storage disease type 0 (due to glycogen synthase deficiency) is associated with fasting hypoglycemia because of the liver's inability to store glucose in the immediate postprandial state. Thus, the glucose load from the meal is anaerobically used rather than stored for later use. In this disorder, plasma glucose and lactate levels are high in the immediate postprandial state (Di Candia et al., 2009).

Glycogen-storage disease type I (Due to disorders of hepatic glucose production include glucose-6-phosphatase deficiency), glycogen-storage disease type III (due to debrancher deficiency), and glycogen-storage disease type VI (due to hepatic phosphorylase deficiency), galactosemia, hereditary fructose intolerance, and maple syrup urine disease interfere in glucose production through various defects, including blockage of glucose release or synthesis or blockage or inhibition of gluconeogenesis. Children with these diseases may adapt to their hypoglycemia because of its chronicity (Di Candia et al., 2009).

Hormonal abnormalities include panhypopituitarism, growth hormone deficiency, and cortisol deficiency (primary or secondary). As described above, growth hormone and cortisol play important roles in generating alternative fuels and stimulating glucose production. Because they are easily treatable abnormalities, early recognition is important (Di Candia et al., 2009).

Toxins and other illnesses (ethanol, salicylates, propranolol, malaria) also cause hypoglycemia. Ethanol inhibits gluconeogenesis in the liver and can thus cause hypoglycemia. This is particularly true in patients with insulin-treated diabetes who are unable to reduce insulin secretion in response to developing hypoglycemia. Salicylate intoxication causes both hyperglycemia and hypoglycemia. The latter is due to augmentation of insulin secretion and inhibition of gluconeogenesis (Di Candia et al., 2009).

11. Clinical features of hypoglycemia

Glucose usually provides the primary source for brain energy. Clinical manifestations are broad and can be from a combination of adrenergic stimulation or from decreased availability of glucose for the CNS. Unlike older children, infants are not able to verbalize their symptoms and are particularly vulnerable to hypoglycemia (Cranmer, 2009). Symptoms of hypoglycemia occur through two main clinical pathways. The first one is caused by activation of the autonomic nervous system, which causes symptoms such as anxiety, tremulousness, diaphoresis, tachycardia, pallor, hunger, nausea, and vomiting (Dunne et al., 2004). The symptoms of second one is due to neuroglycopenia (hypoglycorrhachia) and consists of headache, mental confusion, staring, behavioral changes, difficulty concentrating, visual disturbances (eg, decreased acuity, diplopia), dysarthria, seizures, ataxia, somnolence, coma, stroke (hemiplegia, aphasia), paresthesias,

dizziness, amnesia, decerebrate or decorticate posturing (Dunne et al., 2004). There are other nonspecific symptoms which include dry mouth, mouth tingling, headache, nausea, and blurred vision (Dunne et al., 2004).
During the first or second day of life, symptoms vary from asymptomatic to CNS and cardiopulmonary disturbances (Guideline, 2004).

Following high risk groups does need screening for hypoglycemia in the first hour of life (Guideline, 2004, Feign. R and Garg, 1987, Fleisher, 2000)

- Newborns who weigh more than 4 kg or less than 2 kg
- Large for gestational age infants who are above the 90th percentile, small for gestational age infants below the 10th percentile, and infants with intrauterine growth restriction
- Infants born to insulin-dependent mothers or mothers with gestational diabetes
- Gestational age less than 37 weeks
- Newborns suspected of sepsis or born to a mother suspected of having chorioamnionitis
- Newborns with symptoms suggestive of hypoglycemia, including jitteriness, tachypnea, hypotonia, poor feeding, apnea, temperature instability, seizures, lethargy

In addition, consider hypoglycemia screening in infants with following conditions: (Guideline, 2004).

- Significant hypoxemia
- Perinatal distress
- 5-minute APGAR scores less than 5
- Mother on terbutaline, beta-blockers, or oral hypoglycemic agents
- Isolated hepatomegaly
- Microcephaly
- Anterior midline defects
- Gigantism
- Macroglossia or hemihypertrophy; or any possibility of an inborn error of metabolism

The onset of hyperinsulinemia is from birth to 18 months (al-Rabeeah et al., 1995, de Lonlay-Debeney et al., 1999, Dubois et al., 1995, Dunne et al., 2004, Dunne et al., 1997).

- Insulin concentrations are inappropriately elevated at the time of documented hypoglycemia.
- Transient neonatal hyperinsulinism occurs in macrosomic infants of diabetic mothers who have diminished glucagon secretion and endogenous glucose production is significantly inhibited. Clinically, these infants are macrosomic and have increasing demands for feeding, intermittent lethargy, jitteriness, and frank seizures.
- Infants with prolonged neonatal hyperinsulinism can be described by small for gestational age, patients with perinatal asphyxia, neonates born to mothers with toxemia, have high rates of glucose use and often require dextrose infusion for a prolonged period of time

Ketotic hypoglycemia is an uncommon but dramatic illness. It is observed in children younger than 5 years who usually become symptomatic after an overnight or prolonged fast, especially with illness and poor oral intake. Children often present inexplicably lethargic or frankly comatose, having only marked hypoglycemia with ketonuria (Cranmer, 2009).

The symptoms often vary according to age of the children as follows (de Lonlay-Debeney et al., 1999, Daly et al., 2003, al-Rabeeah et al., 1995, Dubois et al., 1995, Schwartz, 1997b, Schwartz, 1997a, Luber et al., 1998):

In neonates-

- Restlessness
- Hypothermia
- Tremulousness
- Brisk Moro reflex
- Compromised activity
- Poor feeding
- Hypotonia
- Lethargy
- Apathy
- Jitteriness
- Seizures
- Congestive heart failure
- Respiratory difficulty
- Apnea
- Bradycardia
- Convulsion
- Coma and
- Sudden death

In older children-

- Dizziness
- Hunger
- Anxiousness
- Sweating
- Lethargy
- Poor feeding
- Confusion
- Irritability
- Convulsion
- Coma and
- Sudden death

Clinical signs of hypoglycemia in SAM

A large number of patients with hypoglycemia may not have any symptoms or may present with severe CNS and cardiopulmonary disturbances. However, in children with SAM who need the admission in the pediatric critical care medicine, the most common clinical manifestations can take account as

- Altered level of consciousness,
- Seizure,
- Vomiting,

- Unresponsiveness, and
- Lethargy.

Any child with SAM and acute illness should be evaluated for hypoglycemia, especially when history reveals lesser oral intake (Chisti et al., 2010). Persistent or repetitive hypoglycemia in infants and children has a major impact on normal brain development and function (al-Rabeeah et al., 1995, Bennish et al., 1990). Evidence suggests that hypoxemia potentiate hypoglycemia, causing brain damage that may permanently impair neurologic development (Bennish et al., 1990).

Hypoglycemia is often a sign of severe infection (Bennish et al., 1990). The child should be tested for hypoglycemia on admission or whenever lethargy, convulsions or hypothermia are found (Butler et al., 1989). If blood glucose cannot be measured, all children with SAM suspected to have hypoglycemia should be treated accordingly (Ahmed et al., 1999). Otherwise the children with severe malnutrition and hypoglycemia may die within few minutes (Chisti et al., 2010, Huq et al., 2007).

12. Differential diagnosis of hypoglycemia in children (de Lonlay-Debeney et al., 1999, Daly et al., 2003, al-Rabeeah et al., 1995, Dubois et al., 1995, Schwartz, 1997b, Schwartz, 1997a, Wyngaarden et al., Cosman et al., 1989, Stuckey et al., Wall, 2000, Olry, 2002, Belay et al., 1999, CDC, Dellinger et al., 2008)

- Adrenal Insufficiency and Adrenal Crisis
- Hypopituitarism
- Hypothyroidism and Myxedema Coma
- Munchausen Syndrome
- Reye Syndrome
- Plant Poisoning, Hypoglycemics
- Shock, Septic
- Toxicity, Alcohols
- Toxicity, salicylates

13. Laboratory studies

A bedside glucose level is a very cheap rapid diagnostic test, although it may lead to over treatment of hypoglycemia (Cranmer, 2009).

Serum or plasma glucose levels (Serum glucose level is higher than whole blood glucose level) (Cranmer, 2009)

- Arterial and capillary samples may overestimate the plasma glucose concentration by 10% in non-fasting patients.
- Whole blood estimation of glucose may underestimate the plasma glucose concentration by approximately 10-15% because RBCs contain relatively low concentrations of glucose.

Serum insulin: when blood glucose is less than 40 mg/dL, plasma insulin concentration should be less than 5 and no higher than 10 microunits/mL (Cranmer, 2009).

Urine (first voided urine dipstick for ketones) (Sperling et al., 2008, Reid et al., 2003)

- Absence of large ketones with hypoglycemia suggests that fat is not being metabolized from adipose tissue (hyperinsulinism) or that fat cannot be used for ketone body formation (enzymatic defects in fatty acid oxidation).
- Consider urine for organic acid analysis.

Newborn screening (Sperling et al., 2008, Schwartz, 1997b):

- Aminoacidemias
- Urea cycle disorders
- Organic acidurias and
- Fatty acid oxidation disorders by electrospray ionization-tandem mass spectrometry.

First and prompt recognition of these inborn errors of metabolism has the potential to reduce morbidity and mortality rates in these infants.

Imaging studies (Sperling et al., 2008):

- Celiac angiography to detect adenomas has limited success. There is potential risk of causing vascular trauma in infants younger than 2 years.

14. Consequencess associated with hypoglycemia (Schwartz, 1997b, Guideline, 2004, Cranmer, 2009)

Hypoglycemia is the most common metabolic problem in neonates. Still, the level or duration of hypoglycemia that is harmful to an infant's developing brain is not known. Major long-term sequelae include:

- Neurologic damage resulting in mental retardation
- Recurrent seizure
- Respiratory distress
- Developmental delay
- Heart failure and
- Personality disorders.

Some evidence suggests that severe hypoglycemia may impair cardiovascular function.

15. Management

In children without severe malnutrition (Cranmer, 2009, Cornblath and Ichord, 2000):

In the critical care ward, supportive therapy includes oxygen, establishing an intravenous (IV) line, and monitoring.

- If convulsion, unresponsive to correction of hypoglycemia should be managed with appropriate anticonvulsants.
- If there is marked acidosis (pH < 7.1) suggestive of shock or serious underlying disease and should be treated appropriately.
- The goal of treatment is to maintain a blood glucose level of at least 45 mg/dL (2.5 mmol/L).
- Children who drink but has intact airway protective reflexes, nasogastric administration of oral liquids containing sugar may be performed.

15.1 Medication

Hypoglycemia should be treated as soon as possible to prevent complications of neurologic damage. Early feeding of the newborn with breast milk or formula is encouraged. For those unable to drink, a nasogastric tube can be used. The mainstay of therapy for children that is alert with intact airway protection. For those who cannot protect their airway or are unable to drink, nasogastric, intramuscular, intraosseous, or intravenous (IV) routes can be used for the following drugs used to raise glucose levels (Sperling et al., 2008, Reid et al., 2003):

- Dextrose
- Glucagon
- Diazoxide and
- Octreotide

Case reports have shown that nifedipine may help maintain normoglycemia in children with persistent hyperinsulinemic hypoglycemia of infancy (PHHI) (Cranmer, 2009).
Cortisol should not be used because it has minimal acute benefit and may delay the diagnosis of the cause of hypoglycemia. Cortisol stimulates gluconeogenesis and causes decreased use of glucose, which leads to overall elevated blood glucose and may mask the true cause of hypoglycemia (Cranmer, 2009).

Anti-hypoglycemic agents (agents elevate blood glucose levels)

Dextrose

Choice of treatment as it is absorbed from the intestine resulting in rapid increase in blood glucose concentration when administered PO (Reid et al., 2003). Give IV dextrose to infants of diabetic mothers with transient neonatal hyperinsulinemia for several days until hyperinsulinemia abates (Sperling et al., 2008). Avoid hyperglycemia evoking prompt insulin release, which may produce rebound hypoglycemia. SGA infants and those with maternal toxemia or perinatal asphyxia require dextrose IV infusion rates >20 mg/kg/min to control levels (Halamek and Stevenson, 1998). Treatment may be necessary for 2-4 week .

Diazoxide

Aim to increase blood glucose by inhibiting pancreatic insulin release, and possibly through an extrapancreatic effect. Hyperglycemic effect starts within an hour and usually lasts a maximum of 8 h with normal renal function (Halamek and Stevenson, 1998, Sperling et al., 2008, Shirland, 2001).

Octreotide

Long-acting analog of somatostatin that suppresses insulin secretion for short-term management of hypoglycemia (Cranmer, 2009, Fontaine et al., 1972).

Glucagon (Glucagon Emergency Kit)

May be used to treat hypoglycemia secondary to hyperinsulinemia and administered to patients without initial IV access. Each mL contains 1 mg (ie, 1 unit). Maximal glucose concentration occurs between 5-20 min for IV administration and about 30 min for IM administration (Cranmer, 2009, Stanley, 1997).

Surgical opinion

If hypoglycemia is diagnosed in an infant younger than 3 months, surgical intervention may be necessary. Surgical exploration usually is undertaken in severely affected neonates who are unresponsive to glucose and somatostatin therapy (Halamek and Stevenson, 1998, Sperling et al., 2008).

In one most recently conducted study revealed that once the diagnosis is made and if medical therapy with diazoxide fails, one should assume that the infant has a K(ATP) channel defect and may require surgery (Palladino and Stanley). In this case, the infant should be referred to a center that specializes in 18-fluoro L-3,4-dihydroxyphenylalanine positron emission tomography scan. This report describes a center specializing in 18-fluoro L-3,4-dihydroxyphenylalanine positron emission tomography scan with a team of experts consisting of endocrinologists, nurse practitioners, geneticists, radiologists, pathologists, and a surgeon. It describes the center's paradigm for managing severe cases of congenital hypersplenism (H1) with surgery (Palladino and Stanley). On the other hand another indicated that in absence of response to the medical treatment with diazoxide a limited pancreatectomy permits to cure focal HI, while a diffuse HI requires a subtotal pancreatectomy with high risk of subsequent diabetes mellitus (Giurgea et al., 2005). However over all recommendation with risk benefit from the peer reviewed publications and text book are as follows (Halamek et al., 1997b, Sperling et al., 2008, Reid et al., 2003)

- Near total resection of 85-90% of the pancreas is recommended.
- Risks include the development of diabetes.

If hypoglycemia first manifests in infants aged 3-6 months, a therapeutic trial of octreotide, diazoxide, steroids, and frequent feedings can be attempted for as long as 2-4 weeks.

Management of hypoglycemia in children with SAM:

If the child is conscious and blood glucose is <3mmol/l or 54mg/dl:

50 ml bolus of 10% glucose or 10% sucrose solution (1 rounded teaspoon of sugar in 3.5 tablespoons water) is given orally or by nasogastric (NG) tube. The starter diet F-75 or "milk suzi" in children above 6 months of age / expressed breast milk (EBM) or "infant formula" for children under the age of 6 months of age is given every 30 min for two hours (giving one quarter of the two-hourly feed each time) (WHO, 1999, Ahmed et al., 1999). Thereafter, two-hourly feeds are continued for first 24-48 hours (Ahmed et al., 1999).

If the child is unconscious, lethargic or convulsing:

Sterile 10% glucose (5ml/kg) or 25% dextrose (2ml/kg) is given IV, followed by 50 ml of 10% glucose or sucrose by NG tube. Then the starter diet F-75 or "milk suzi"/EBM or "infant formula" is given as above (Ahmed et al., 1999, WHO, 1999). A number of studies revealed that continuous intravenous dextrose might require in case of uncontrolled hypoglycemia (Lilien et al., 1977, Lilien et al., 1980). One of the studies revealed that the treatment of neonatal hypoglycemia by constant infusion of glucose at the rate of 8 mg/kg/minute was studied in 22 hypoglycemic neonates. In that study, 18 neonates glucose levels rose above the hypoglycemic range within ten minutes of infusion and in three, within 30 to 50 minutes of infusion. The remaining neonate had hyperinsulinemia and responded only to diazoxide. Thus, constant glucose infusion was found to be useful therapeutically for neonatal hypoglycemia (Lilien et al., 1977). Results from the another study from India revealed that symptomatic hypoglycemia should always be treated with a continuous infusion of parenteral dextrose. Neonates needing dextrose infusion rates above 12 mg/kg/m should be investigated for refractory causes of hypoglycemia. Hypoglycemia has been linked to poor neuro-developmental outcome and therefore they recommended aggressive screening and treatment with continuous infusion of glucoes (Narayan et al., 2001).

Follow up (Cranmer, 2009, Cornblath and Ichord, 2000):
Any child with documented hypoglycemia not secondary to insulin therapy should be admitted in a critical care unit for careful monitoring and diagnostic testing.

16. Prognosis

The prognosis is good in asymptomatic neonates with hypoglycemia of short duration. Hypoglycemia recurs in 10-15% of infants after adequate treatment (Sperling et al., 2008). However, there are no published data on the prevalence of hypoglycemia in severe PEM after adequate treatment although it has been thought that it will be more than that of in infants. Rebound hypoglycemia is more common if intravenous fluid are extravasated or discontinued too early or do not offer oral glucose after IV infusion of glucose especially in case SAM (Sperling et al., 2008, Ahmed et al., 1999). Remission of congenital hyperinsulinism generally does not occur, but the severity of the disease may decrease with time. The prognosis of intellectual function could be worse if the symptoms stay for prolong duration and usually associated with neurological sequele (Sperling et al., 2008).

17. Patients care giver education

Provide genetic counseling for families with affected children, including information about a possible 25% risk of recurrence (DePuy et al., 2009).

18. Conclusion

Hypoglycemia in children especially in neonates and SAM is a medical emergency and should be tested for hypoglycemia on admission or whenever lethargy, convulsions, hypoxemia or hypothermia are found. IV infusion of glucose should be given very urgently in order to prevent life threatening consequences. If blood glucose cannot be measured, all neonates and children with SAM suspected to have hypoglycemia should be treated accordingly.

19. References

Newborn Nursery QI Committee. Neonatal hypoglycemia: initial and follow up management. Portland (ME): The Barbara
Bush Children's Hospital at Maine Medical Center; 2004 Jul. 4 p.

Adamson, S. J., Alessandri L. M., Badawi N., Burton P. R., Pemberton P. J. & Stanley F. (1995) Predictors of neonatal encephalopathy in full-term infants. *BMJ*, 311, 598-602.

Ahmed, T., Ali M., Ullah M. M., et al. (1999) Mortality in severely malnourished children with diarrhoea and use of a standardised management protocol. *Lancet*, 353, 1919-22.

Al-Rabeeah, A., Al-Ashwal A., Al-Herbish A., Al-Jurayyan N., Sakati N. & Abobakr A. (1995) Persistent hyperinsulinemic hypoglycemia of infancy: experience with 28 cases. *J Pediatr Surg*, 30, 1119-21.

Alkalay, A. L., Sarnat H. B., Flores-Sarnat L., Elashoff J. D., Farber S. J. & Simmons C. F. (2006) Population meta-analysis of low plasma glucose thresholds in full-term normal newborns. *Am J Perinatol,* 23, 115-9.

Bandsma, R. H., Mendel M., Spoelstra M. N., et al. Mechanisms behind decreased endogenous glucose production in malnourished children. *Pediatr Res,* 68, 423-8.

Bandsma, R. H., Spoelstra M. N., Mari A., et al. Impaired Glucose Absorption in Children with Severe Malnutrition. *J Pediatr.*

Belay, E. D., Bresee J. S., Holman R. C., Khan A. S., Shahriari A. & Schonberger L. B. (1999) Reye's syndrome in the United States from 1981 through 1997. *N Engl J Med,* 340, 1377-82.

Bennish, M. L., Azad A. K., Rahman O. & Phillips R. E. (1990) Hypoglycemia during diarrhea in childhood. Prevalence, pathophysiology, and outcome. *N Engl J Med,* 322, 1357-63.

Butler, T., Arnold M. & Islam M. (1989) Depletion of hepatic glycogen in the hypoglycaemia of fatal childhood diarrhoeal illnesses. *Trans R Soc Trop Med Hyg,* 83, 839-43.

Cdc Toxic hypoglycemic syndrome--Jamaica, 1989-1991. MMWR Morb Mortal Wkly Rep. Jan 31 1992;41(4):53-5.

Chertok, I. R., Raz I., Shoham I., Haddad H. & Wiznitzer A. (2009) Effects of early breastfeeding on neonatal glucose levels of term infants born to women with gestational diabetes. *J Hum Nutr Diet,* 22, 166-9.

Chisti, M. J., Ahmed T., Bardhan P. K. & Salam M. A. (2010) Evaluation of simple laboratory investigations to predict fatal outcome in infants with severe malnutrition presenting in an urban diarrhoea treatment centre in Bangladesh. *Trop Med Int Health,* 15, 1322-5.

Chisti, M. J., Ahmed T., Faruque A. S., Saha S., Salam M. A. & Islam S. (2009a) Factors associated with sclerema in infants with diarrhoeal disease: a matched case-control study. *Acta Paediatr,* 98, 873-8.

Chisti, M. J., Bardhan P. K., Huq S., et al. (2009b) High-dose intravenous dexamethasone in the management of diarrheal patients with enteric fever and encephalopathy. *Southeast Asian J Trop Med Public Health,* 40, 1065-73.

Chisti, M. J., Tebruegge M., La Vincente S., Graham S. M. & Duke T. (2009c) Pneumonia in severely malnourished children in developing countries - mortality risk, aetiology and validity of WHO clinical signs: a systematic review. *Trop Med Int Health,* 14, 1173-89.

Cornblath, M., Hawdon J. M., Williams A. F., et al. (2000) Controversies regarding definition of neonatal hypoglycemia: suggested operational thresholds. *Pediatrics,* 105, 1141-5.

Cornblath, M. & Ichord R. (2000) Hypoglycemia in the neonate. *Semin Perinatol,* 24, 136-49.

Cosgrove, K. E., Shepherd R. M., Fernandez E. M., et al. (2004) Genetics and pathophysiology of hyperinsulinism in infancy. *Horm Res,* 61, 270-88.

Cosman, F., Post K. D., Holub D. A. & Wardlaw S. L. (1989) Lymphocytic hypophysitis. Report of 3 new cases and review of the literature. *Medicine (Baltimore),* 68, 240-56.

Cowett, R. M. & Loughead J. L. (2002) Neonatal glucose metabolism: differential diagnoses, evaluation, and treatment of hypoglycemia. *Neonatal Netw,* 21, 9-19.

Cranmer, H. (2009) Pediatric Hypoglycemia. IN SHANNON, M., SLAPPER, D., WINDLE, M. L., WOLFRAM, W., HALAMKA, J. D. & BACHUR, R. D. (Eds.). eMedicine.

Daly, L. P., Osterhoudt K. C. & Weinzimer S. A. (2003) Presenting features of idiopathic ketotic hypoglycemia. *J Emerg Med,* 25, 39-43.

De Lonlay-Debeney, P., Poggi-Travert F., Fournet J. C., et al. (1999) Clinical features of 52 neonates with hyperinsulinism. *N Engl J Med,* 340, 1169-75.

Dellinger, R. P., Levy M. M., Carlet J. M., et al. (2008) Surviving Sepsis Campaign: international guidelines for management of severe sepsis and septic shock: 2008. *Crit Care Med,* 36, 296-327.

Depuy, A. M., Coassolo K. M., Som D. A. & Smulian J. C. (2009) Neonatal hypoglycemia in term, nondiabetic pregnancies. *Am J Obstet Gynecol,* 200, e45-51.

Deshpande, S. & Ward Platt M. (2005) The investigation and management of neonatal hypoglycaemia. *Semin Fetal Neonatal Med,* 10, 351-61.

Di Candia, S., Gessi A., Pepe G., et al. (2009) Identification of a diffuse form of hyperinsulinemic hypoglycemia by 18-fluoro-L-3,4 dihydroxyphenylalanine positron emission tomography/CT in a patient carrying a novel mutation of the HADH gene. *Eur J Endocrinol,* 160, 1019-23.

Dubois, J., Brunelle F., Touati G., et al. (1995) Hyperinsulinism in children: diagnostic value of pancreatic venous sampling correlated with clinical, pathological and surgical outcome in 25 cases. *Pediatr Radiol,* 25, 512-6.

Dunne, M. J., Cosgrove K. E., Shepherd R. M., Aynsley-Green A. & Lindley K. J. (2004) Hyperinsulinism in infancy: from basic science to clinical disease. *Physiol Rev,* 84, 239-75.

Dunne, M. J., Kane C., Shepherd R. M., et al. (1997) Familial persistent hyperinsulinemic hypoglycemia of infancy and mutations in the sulfonylurea receptor. *N Engl J Med,* 336, 703-6.

Elusiyan, J. B., Adejuyigbe E. A. & Adeodu O. O. (2006) Hypoglycaemia in a Nigerian paediatric emergency ward. *J Trop Pediatr,* 52, 96-102.

Faruque, A. S., Ahmed A. M., Ahmed T., et al. (2008) Nutrition: basis for healthy children and mothers in Bangladesh. *J Health Popul Nutr,* 26, 325-39.

Faustino, E. V. & Bogue C. W. Relationship between hypoglycemia and mortality in critically ill children. *Pediatr Crit Care Med,* 11, 690-8.

Feign. R, D. & Garg R. (1987) Interaction of infection and nutrition. IN 2ND (Ed.) *Text Book of Paediatric Infections.* Philadelphia

W.B/Saunders Company.

Fleisher, G. (2000) ed. Pediatric hypoglycemia. In:Textbook of Pediatric Emergency Medicine. Lippincott Williams & Wilkins; 2000

Fluck, C. E., Slotboom J., Nuoffer J. M., Kreis R., Boesch C. & Mullis P. E. (2003) Normal hepatic glycogen storage after fasting and feeding in children and adolescents with type 1 diabetes. *Pediatr Diabetes,* 4, 70-6.

Fontaine, G., Farriaux J. P. & Hongre J. F. (1972) [Value of diazoxide in the treatment of neonatal hypoglycemia]. *Nouv Presse Med,* 1, 50.

Giurgea, I., Ribeiro M. J., Boddaert N., et al. (2005) [Congenital hyperinsulinism in newborn and infant]. *Arch Pediatr,* 12, 1628-35.

Guideline (2004) Newborn Nursery QI Committee. Portland (ME): The Barbara Bush Children's Hospital at Maine Medical Center; 2004 Jul. Neonatal hypoglycemia: initial and follow up management *National Guideline Clearinghouse.*

Halamek, L. P., Benaron D. A. & Stevenson D. K. (1997a) Neonatal hypoglycemia, Part I: Background and definition. *Clin Pediatr (Phila),* 36, 675-80.

Halamek, L. P., Benaron D. A. & Stevenson D. K. (1997b) The value of neurophysiologic approaches in the anticipation and evaluation of neonatal hypoglycemia. *Acta Paediatr Jpn,* 39 Suppl 1, S33-43.

Halamek, L. P. & Stevenson D. K. (1998) Neonatal hypoglycemia, part II: pathophysiology and therapy. *Clin Pediatr (Phila),* 37, 11-6.

Haninger, N. C. & Farley C. L. (2001) Screening for hypoglycemia in healthy term neonates: effects on breastfeeding. *J Midwifery Womens Health,* 46, 292-301.

Huq, S., Hossain M. I., Malek M. A., Faruque A. S. & Salam M. A. (2007) Hypoglycaemia in under-five children with diarrhoea. *J Trop Pediatr,* 53, 197-201.

Ishiguro, A., Namai Y. & Ito Y. M. (2009) Managing "healthy" late preterm infants. *Pediatr Int,* 51, 720-5.

Jain, A., Aggarwal R., Jeevasanker M., Agarwal R., Deorari A. K. & Paul V. K. (2008) Hypoglycemia in the newborn. *Indian J Pediatr,* 75, 63-7.

Lilien, L. D., Grajwer L. A. & Pildes R. S. (1977) Treatment of neonatal hypoglycemia with continuous intravenous glucose infusion. *J Pediatr,* 91, 779-82.

Lilien, L. D., Pildes R. S., Srinivasan G., Voora S. & Yeh T. F. (1980) Treatment of neonatal hypoglycemia with minibolus and intraveous glucose infusion. *J Pediatr,* 97, 295-8.

Luber, S., Meldon S. & Brady W. (1998) Hypoglycemia presenting as acute respiratory failure in an infant. *Am J Emerg Med,* 16, 281-4.

Meier, P. P., Furman L. M. & Degenhardt M. (2007) Increased lactation risk for late preterm infants and mothers: evidence and management strategies to protect breastfeeding. *J Midwifery Womens Health,* 52, 579-87.

Mohnike, K. & Aynsley-Green A. (1993) [Hypoglycemia in childhood]. *Kinderarztl Prax,* 61, 316-22.

Mohnike, K., Starke I., Bannert N. & Heise H. R. (1993) [Differential diagnosis and therapy of hypoglycemia in childhood]. *Kinderarztl Prax,* 61, 192-201.

Morgan, G. (1997) What, if any, is the effect of malnutrition on immunological competence? *Lancet,* 349, 1693-5.

Naheed, A., Saha S. K., Breiman R. F., et al. (2009) Multihospital surveillance of pneumonia burden among children aged <5 years hospitalized for pneumonia in Bangladesh. *Clin Infect Dis,* 48 Suppl 2, S82-9.

Narayan, S., Aggarwal R., Deorari A. K. & Paul V. K. (2001) Hypoglycemia in the newborn. *Indian J Pediatr,* 68, 963-5.

Narchi, H. & Skinner A. (2009) Infants of diabetic mothers with abnormal fetal growth missed by standard growth charts. *J Obstet Gynaecol,* 29, 609-13.

Nuoffer, J. M. & Mullis P. E. (2005) [Hypoglycaemia--diagnosis and therapy in emergencies]. *Ther Umsch,* 62, 543-8.

Olry, R. (2002) Baron Munchhausen and the syndrome which bears his name: history of an endearing personage and of a strange mental disorder. *Vesalius,* 8, 53-7.

Palladino, A. A. & Stanley C. A. A specialized team approach to diagnosis and medical versus surgical treatment of infants with congenital hyperinsulinism. *Semin Pediatr Surg,* 20, 32-7.

Pelletier, D. L., Frongillo E. A., Jr., Schroeder D. G. & Habicht J. P. (1994) A methodology for estimating the contribution of malnutrition to child mortality in developing countries. *J Nutr,* 124, 2106S-2122S.

Reid, S. R. & Losek J. D. (2005) Hypoglycemia complicating dehydration in children with acute gastroenteritis. *J Emerg Med,* 29, 141-5.

Reid, S. R., Losek J. D. & Bosker G. (2003), ed. Hypoglycemia in infants and children. In: The Textbook of Primary and Acute Care Medicine. 2003.

Schaefer-Graf, U. M., Rossi R., Buhrer C., et al. (2002) Rate and risk factors of hypoglycemia in large-for-gestational-age newborn infants of nondiabetic mothers. *Am J Obstet Gynecol,* 187, 913-7.

Schwartz, R. P. (1997a) Hypoglycemia in infancy and childhood. *Indian J Pediatr,* 64, 43-55.

Schwartz, R. P. (1997b) Neonatal hypoglycemia: how low is too low? *J Pediatr,* 131, 171-3.

Shirland, L. (2001) When it is more than transient neonatal hypoglycemia: hyperinsulinemia--a case study challenge. *Neonatal Netw,* 20, 5-11.

Sperling, M. A., Behrman R. E. & Kliegman R. M. (2008) et al, eds. Hypoglycemia. In: Nelson Textbook of Pediatrics. 18th ed. 2008.

Stanley, C. A. (1997) Hyperinsulinism in infants and children. *Pediatr Clin North Am,* 44, 363-74.

Stuckey, B. G., Kent G. N., Ward L. C., Brown S. J. & Walsh J. P. Postpartum thyroid dysfunction and the long-term risk of hypothyroidism: results from a 12-year follow-up study of women with and without postpartum thyroid dysfunction. *Clin Endocrinol (Oxf),* 73, 389-95.

Suskind, D. M. K. & Suskind R. M. (1990) The malnourished child: an overview. IN SUSKIND. R, M. & SUSKIND. L (Eds.) *The Malnourished Child.* New York, Raven Press.

Tita, A. T., Landon M. B., Spong C. Y., et al. (2009) Timing of elective repeat cesarean delivery at term and neonatal outcomes. *N Engl J Med,* 360, 111-20.

Tornovsky, S., Crane A., Cosgrove K. E., et al. (2004) Hyperinsulinism of infancy: novel ABCC8 and KCNJ11 mutations and evidence for additional locus heterogeneity. *J Clin Endocrinol Metab,* 89, 6224-34.

Wall, C. R. (2000) Myxedema coma: diagnosis and treatment. *Am Fam Physician,* 62, 2485-90.

WHO (1999) Management of severe malnutrition: a Manual for physicians and other senior health workers. World Health Organization, Geneva

WHO (2005) Pocket book for hospital care of children: guidelines for the management of common illness with limited resources. WHO, Geneva

WHO.

Wight, N. E. (2006) Hypoglycemia in breastfed neonates. *Breastfeed Med,* 1, 253-62.
Wyngaarden, J. B., Smith L. H. & Bennett J. C. Adrenocortical hypofunction. Cecil Textbook of Medicine. 19th ed. WB Saunders; 1992:1271-1288.

Part 2

Section B

3

Brittle Diabetes: A Contemporary Review of the Myth and Its Realization

Christina Voulgari and Nicholas Tentolouris
First Department of Propaedeutic Medicine,
Athens University Medical School,
Laiko General Hospital, Athens,
Greece

1. Introduction

Type 1 Diabetes is an intrinsically unstable condition. A small group of patients with Type 1 Diabetes (3‰), mainly young women, suffer chronically by poor metabolic control, characterized by a severe instability of glycemic values with frequent and unpredictable hypoglycemic and/or diabetic ketoacidosis episodes which cannot be attributed to patients or clinicians errors. The quality of life of these patients is dramatically compromised in particular because of the frequency of acute events, hospital recoveries and precocious appearance of chronic complications. This clinical condition has been defined as "brittle diabetes" (Tattersall, 1977).

A precise quantification of these patients is difficult because diagnostic criteria are still not well defined and it is often difficult to verify errors of patients in terms of inappropriate conduct with the pathology. Metabolic instability is manifested most obviously by chaotic glycemic profiles, which show greater and more unpredictable variation than in "stable" patients with diabetes. Patients with brittle diabetes cannot be controlled adequately, even by closely supervised, intensive insulin regimens, including continuous subcutaneous and/or intravenous insulin infusion (Bertuzzi et al., 2007). Their care is often very expensive of time and resources, and their lives are constantly at risk from metabolic catastrophe. Management of these patients can also be frustrating and demoralizing for all concerned, including the patient's family and associates and the diabetes care team.

This review will focus on a contemporary "painting" of brittle diabetes beginning with a few historical notes leading to its definition, ongoing researched pathophysiologic substrate, common and life-threatening clinical manifestations, diagnosis and treatment.

2. Brittle diabetes: Historical notes

In 1942 the Chicago physician Woodyatt suggested that "The history of diabetes has been marked by recurrence of certain ideas which decline and disappear; only to go through a similar cycle again in an altered form in the new generation" (Woodyatt, 1942). This is particularly true of the concept of brittle diabetes which Woodyatt himself introduced in the 1940s. Although, he never wrote a paper on the subject, contemporaries understood it to refer to excessive fluctuations of blood sugar which could not be otherwise explained; the cardinal feature of brittle diabetes was unpredictability and unexpected hypoglycemic reactions. Also in the 1940s, practitioners of the newly formed psychosomatic movement took an interest in the effect of emotional factors on the course of diabetes and, in particular, patients who were "difficult" or "refractory". "Difficult" patients were marked by not following their doctor's instructions or having recurrent diabetic ketoacidosis.

By the 1950s the question was whether there were two distinct groups of patients; one whose lability could be cured by adjusting insulin, diet, and exercise, and another whose lability had an emotional origin. It remained a question whether in those patients in whom glycemic lability was attributed to an emotional cause, were in fact experiencing psychosocial problems as a consequence rather than a cause of the metabolic instability. Patients with factitious hypoglycemia, which remained undetected for weeks, suggested that neither close observation nor screening by a psychiatrist could rule out the factitious disease (Tattersall, 1997). Therefore in 1977 the definition of brittle diabetes was suggested by Tattersall for patients whose life was "constantly disrupted by episodes of hypo- or hyperglycemia, whatever their cause should be". This was widely accepted and there was a subtle shift towards regarding brittle diabetes as synonymous with recurrent ketoacidosis.

In the 1980s several groups investigated large series of such patients, using new methods to try to uncover a biochemical basis such as defective insulin absorption, accelerated degradation at insulin injection sites, and inappropriate secretion of various counterregulatory hormones (Schade et al., 1980; Fischer et al., 1980). Most of these patients were young overweight women and the eventual conclusion was that in most patients the instability was self-induced. In the 1980s recurrent, often warningless, hypoglycemia was recognized as a problem in its own right but in the current era it was reborn as also a problem of insulin pharmacokinetics, exact as Woodyatt originally conceived it.

3. Aetiology and pathophysiologic substrate: From the suspicion to ongoing research

Going back in literature, among the main causes of "brittleness" referenced are malabsorption, certain drugs (i.e. antipsychotics), defective insulin absorption or degradation, defect of hyperglycemic hormones especially glucocorticoid and glucagon, and above all delayed gastric emptying as a result of autonomic neuropathy (Vinik et al., 2003; Lehmann et al., 2003; Voulgari et al., 2010). Moreover, possible causes of hypoglycemic "brittleness" described are organic problems which comprise lost hypoglycemia warnings (Tattersall & Gill, 1991), such as alcohol abuse (Hepburn et al., 1990), renal failure, gastroparesis, hypopituitarism, and senile dementia (Potter et al., 1982).

Variable adherence to insulin treatment contributes to presentation of brittle type 1 diabetes in adolescents and young adults. The deterioration in glycemic control observed in patients aged 10-20 years is often associated with a significant reduction in the adherence index (the medically recommended insulin dose and cumulative volume of insulin prescriptions supplied for the calculation of the days of maximum possible insulin coverage per annum). The latter is inversely related to hospital admissions for diabetic ketoacidosis and all hospital admissions related to acute diabetes complications in young (<20 years) type 1 diabetes patients (Morris, 1990). Direct evidence of poor compliance with insulin therapy in young patients with type 1 diabetes and poor adherence to insulin treatment is a major factor that contributes to brittle diabetes with diabetic ketoacidosis in this age group.

Insulin requirements that apparently exceed 2.0 U/kg/day almost always indicate an underlying problem and frequently are suggestive of "brittleness". Causes of apparent or genuine insulin resistance in type 1 diabetes patients include: puberty (Amiel, 1996), overinsulinization (Rosenbloom & Giordano, 1977), the Mauriac Syndrome (Elder& Natarajan, 2010), chronic infections of the diabetic foot (Tentolouris et al., 1996; Tentolouris et al., 2010, Papanas & Maltezos, 2009), acromegaly (Elkeles et al., 1969), Cushing's Syndrome (Anagnostis et al., 2009), thyrotoxicosis (Jacobson et al., 1970) and phaeochromocytoma (Ishii et al., 2001). In few cases of recurrent diabetic ketoacidosis, there is some suggestion of a deliberate manipulation of diabetes control: patients with recurrent diabetic ketoacidosis are thought to be attention-seeking by omitting insulin due to marital problems and possible depression, and possibly personal gain from diabetic instability (Benbow et al., 2001); depression and manipulation are among the contributory factors to instability as well as chronic non-diabetic medical disease (Gill, 1992).

The aetiology of recurrent hypoglycemia includes impaired awareness of hypoglycemia, which can be associated with long-standing type 1 diabetes (Ryder et al., 1990), or induced by antecedent hypoglycemic episodes (Lager et al., 1986; Janssen et al., 2000), overinsulinization (Widom & Simonson, 1992), endocrinopathies (Hardy et al., 1994), and gastrointestinal diseases such as self-induced vomiting by patients with anorexia and/or bulimia (Lloyd et al., 1987; Stancin et al., 1989; Crow et al., 1999). Malabsorption, including celiac disease as it is analyzed later, which is associated with type 1 diabetes, can also cause decreased insulin requirements and unexpected and sometimes severe hypoglycemic episodes (Smith et al., 2000). Psychiatrically and psychological problems are more common than suspected. Psychosocial factors are very important and factitious "brittleness" may lead to a self-perpetuating condition. The factors reported are: as previously mentioned poor compliance (Pickup et al., 1983), family dysfunction (Diabetes Control and Complications Trial Research Group, 1993) and obsessional control of diabetes (Borch-Johnsen & Helweg-Larsen, 1993). Psychological problems (Tattersall & Gill, 1991), "life chaos" (Hepburn et al., 1990), factitious insulin overdose (Hepburn et al, 1990) and anorexia nervosa (Potter et al., 1982) also illustrate the aetiologic profile of hypoglycemic "brittleness". Suggested motives include escape from hostile situations to the security of hospital, attention seeking, and revenge on self or family and suicidal intent. Some patients induce hypoglycemia to"feel high" (Cassidy et al., 1999). Rarely cases of factitious overdose where insulin was given in excessive doses by a mother to her diabetic child (Munchausen's Disease by Proxy) are also referenced (Ludviksson et al., 1993; Gill & Lucas, 1999).

Acute psychological stress plays a role in the glycemic instability of some patients with brittle type 1 diabetes through an increased secretion of insulin-counteracting hormones. Psychological interviews showed that most patients with brittle diabetes perceive a link between life stress and their blood glucose control and they have much more difficulty in verbalizing their emotions (Dutour et al., 1996; Scantamburlo et al., 2001). Patients with brittle diabetes display distinct cardiovascular and neuroendocrine responses to psychological stress, as well as distinct psychological profiles (Jørgensen, 2007). Moreover, hormonal response to an acute psychological stress is more pronounced in brittle diabetes and might be one of its pathogenic factors (Dutour et al., 1996).

Psychosocial parameters interact with metabolic instability even in juvenile brittle type 1 diabetes. Feelings of dominance precede an increase of blood sugar variance, whereas depressive moods, anger and body symptoms are associated with metabolic instability

(Brosig et al., 2001). A family therapy session also results in an increase of the mean blood sugar variance. Multivariate time-series is a mean to demonstrate psychosomatic interrelations and may also contribute to an empirically rooted understanding of psychodynamic processes in psychosomatoses.

Schizophrenia, like other autoimmune disorders, is likely a heritable phenomenon, and a genetic liability in this disorder is hardly disputed. Research has indicated that physiologic connections between IFN-gamma and TNF-alpha are suggestive of a connection between the symptoms associated with schizophrenia and those of hypoglycemic events in type 1 diabetes patients (Kane et al., 2009). Autoimmune pathogeneses of schizophrenia have been hypothesized and the clinical delineation of a potentially corresponding subset of patients has been addressed in young female patients who carry the concomitant diagnoses of schizophrenia, brittle type 1 diabetes, and hypothyroidism. These patients when treated with corresponding antipsychotic medication on an acute basis, an apparent resolution of their brittle type 1 diabetes with the successful treatment of their psychotic disorder is observed (Balter et al., 2004; Ramaswamy et al., 2006). This well documented link between antipsychotic agents and changes in blood glucose may be of benefit in a subset of patients who suffer from both psychotic and diabetic disorders.

In autoimmune polyendocrinopathy with candidiasis and ectodermal dystrophy, autoimmune destruction of the pancreatic beta-cells with development of brittle type 1 diabetes is possible, but rarer than in the other polyglandular autoimmune syndromes (Lankisch et al., 2009). The pathogenesis of this unique autoimmune disease is unknown (Vogel et al., 1992). However, cases of young female patients with the diagnosis of autoimmune polyendocrinopathy, candidiasis and ectodermal dystrophy have been presented and characterized by psychosomatic abnormal development, teeth alterations, post-puberal gonadal failure with dystrophic hypoplasia of external genitalia, previous vaginal candidiasis, and slowly developing juvenile brittle diabetes with an early onset and severe complications (Iannello et al., 1997). Such patients (and their female maternal relatives) need a long-term follow-up in order to evaluate the function of endocrine glands and to initiate early treatment for hormonal deficits, as well as to detect the non-endocrine components of disease.

Most patients with brittle diabetes are in the second or third decade of life and they are typically admitted with diabetic ketoacidosis rather than hypoglycemia or mixed patterns of instability. A "second peak" of prevalence at the age of 60-70 years has been recorded though much smaller than the main peak at 15-30 years (Gill et al., 1996). Causes for this "second round" of "brittleness" include medical disease (14%), hypoglycemic unawareness (6%), and memory or behavioral problems (8%).

Brittle diabetes in older (≥70 years) patients with a history of insulin therapy using mainly human recombinant insulin is reported and is attributed to a high titer of insulin antibodies and a higher level of insulin resistance (Park et al., 2008). Steroid pulse therapy reduces the possible effect of the insulin antibodies on insulin resistance and glycemic instability, successfully decreases their titer and binding capacity, increased glucose infusion rate and improved glycemic control with reduced blood glucose excursion (Matsuyoshi et al., 2006). Alteration in insulin pharmacokinetics induced by insulin antibodies seems to be a cause of brittle diabetes. Steroid treatment might be useful for the improvement of glycemic control in such patients.

Brittle diabetes in the elderly patients with diabetes is most frequent characterized by recurrent hypoglycemia (Benbow et al., 2001). In elderly patients with brittle diabetes, contributing factors to instability are chronic, nondiabetic medical diseases. Unrecognized celiac disease is one such chronic disorder and recurrent hypoglycemia is ameliorated by adherence to a gluten-free diet, when coexisting colorectal disease has been ruled out by barium enema and colonoscopy. The fact that 19% of patients with adult celiac disease could be in the above 60 years of age group should alert us to the possibility of an association with brittle diabetes in older age as well (Mody et al., 2003). Furthermore, in the presence of otherwise unexplained brittle diabetes, the coexistence of iron-deficiency anemia should heighten suspicion, since this haematinic deficiency is the commonest extraintestinal manifestation of celiac disease with distinct episodes of microcytic and/or hypochromic anemia, responsive to iron supplements (Jolobe & Khin, 2002; Hershko & Skikne, 2009).

Brittle diabetes in the extremely elderly patients with diabetes (>80 years) is thought to be a depletion of endocrine insulin secretion due to marked beta-cell reduction and/or beta-cell exhaustion secondary to long term diabetes duration. It is usually characterized by frequent striking hypoglycemic episodes without clinical awareness. These patients often are presented with vascular dementia, visual disturbances, hearing difficulties and speech and motor disturbances. Daily detailed observation is required to care for such patients with brittle diabetes (Kawanishi & Miyashita 2003).

Sometimes, there is no obvious cause. Most patients with "idiopathic" brittle diabetes that oscillates between hypoglycemia and hyperglycemia have no obvious underlying cause, but many deliberately induce glycemic instability by interfering with their treatment. Nonetheless, organic causes of brittle diabetes are occasionally found and must always be sought, i.e. recurrent infections, especially if insulin dosage is not increased (Laffel et al., 2006; Voulgari & Tentolouris, 2010), endocrinopathies, i.e. hypoadrenalism (Gill & Williams, 2000), inappropriate treatment regimens or lifestyle, and pancreatic damage.

Diabetes after total pancreatectomy is commonly described as "brittle" with most series reporting outcomes after resection for pancreatitis alone (Jethwa et al, 2006). Brittle diabetes is also frequently developed in patients with chronic pancreatitis after partial pancreatectomy and its development is partially related to reduced pancreatic beta-cell area (Meier et al., 2009), as well as other clinical variables, i.e. pre-operative fasting glucose levels, HbA1c and body mass index (Schrader et al, 2010). This is further highlighted by the fact that different surgical procedures have an unequal impact on glucose control. Insulin secretion is diminished after pancreatic-head and pancreatic-tail resection, but post-challenge glucose concentrations can be ameliorated only after pancreatic-head resection (Menge et al., 2009).

Brittle diabetes in chronic pancreatitis due to the gradually loss of pancreatic parenchyma and the appearance of calcifications and of steatorrhea, is characterized by a high risk of hypoglycemia due to the decreasing output of insulin and glucagon. In most instances, measurement of fecal concentration of elastase may be sufficient to diagnose exocrine pancreatic insufficiency (Layer & Keller, 1999). Fecal fat analysis is useful to establish malabsorption and to monitor pancreatic enzyme replacement therapy (Dobrilla, 1989). Modern pancreatic preparations are also engineered and most patients reduce their steatorrhea, although in selected cases larger doses may be needed, depending on size of the meal and the severity of the disease. Efficacy of enzyme replacement therapy is influenced by the presence of diabetes and vise-versa (Hammer, 2010).

Acute tropical calculous pancreatitis was also reported as generative of brittle diabetes and oral pancreatic enzyme therapy was used for the glycemic control with favorable results regarding HbA1c, and fasting glucose levels (Mohan et al., 1998).

Recently, impaired metabolism of intestinally derived chylomicron remnants has been implicated in the development of atherosclerosis. A specific marker of chylomicron particle number (apoB48) has been associated with increased vascular disease such as obesity, metabolic syndrome, type 2 diabetes, and familial hypercholesterolemia (Otokozawa et al., 2009; Valdivielso et al, 2009). The role of these particles in the increased atherosclerotic risk associated with brittle type 1 diabetes is currently demonstrated. ApoB48 metabolism is shown to be altered in individuals with brittle diabetes even in the absence of classic dyslipidemia (Su et al., 2009). Disturbed plasma apoB48 remnants can potentially predict coronary artery disease in this population. Among the newest pathogenetic theories demonstrated is that plasma glucose levels in patients with brittle type 1 diabetes respond directly to the amount of transient electromagnetic fields ("dirty electricity") generated by everyday electronic equipment and wireless devices in their environment (Havas, 2008). In an electromagnetically clean environment, patients with type 1 diabetes require less insulin and have lower levels of plasma glucose (Li, 2005; Beale et al., 1997). Exposure to electromagnetic pollution in its various forms may explain the difficulty in glycemic control in patients with brittle diabetes who suffer from symptoms of electrical hypersensitivity (almost 35%). Reducing exposure to electromagnetic pollution by avoidance or with specially designed GS filters may enable some patients with diabetes to better regulate their blood sugar with less medication (National Toxicology Program, 2010). Figure 1 illustrates a summary of the cited causes of Brittle Diabetes.

4. Diagnosis and clinical manifestations

There are no universally agreed diagnostic criteria. Three forms of brittle diabetes have been described: recurrent diabetic ketoacidosis, predominant hypoglycemic forms and mixed instability (Figure 1). Previous studies have shown that over 90% of hospital admissions in patients with recurrent diabetic ketoacidosis or recurrent hypoglycemia are due to that particular type of glycemic instability (Gill, 1992). Hypoglycemic brittle diabetes makes up 17% of the total brittle spectrum, compared with 59% of ketoacidosis brittleness (Tattersall, 1991) and 24% (Gill, 1992) of mixed brittleness. Compared with patients with recurrent diabetic ketoacidosis, hypoglycemic brittle patients are significantly older; and are of approximately equal male: female ratio, compared with a female excess in recurrent diabetic ketoacidosis (Gill & Lucas, 1992). Also of interest is that patients with mixed brittleness are intermediate in both age and sex-ratio, between the groups with recurrent diabetic ketoacidosis and recurrent hypoglycemia. Idiopathic brittle diabetes is a label applied to those patients who remain poorly controlled despite modern intensified insulin regimens and have no obvious cause for their instability (Somogyi, 1959). Most display a pattern of general hyperglycemia with wide glycemic swings and recurrent episodes of ketoacidosis.

A scheme for investigating patients suspected for brittle diabetes is suggested in Figure 2. A thorough history and examination may elucidate drug-induced causes, infections or endocrine conditions (including puberty). Before moving on to more detailed investigations, the patients understanding of diabetes monitoring and treatment should be assessed. It should be reasonable to exclude chronic infections and specific endocrine diseases. If considered necessary insulin antibodies and insulin receptor antibodies should be measured. Should no cause for insulin resistance emerge, the possibility of factitious insulin

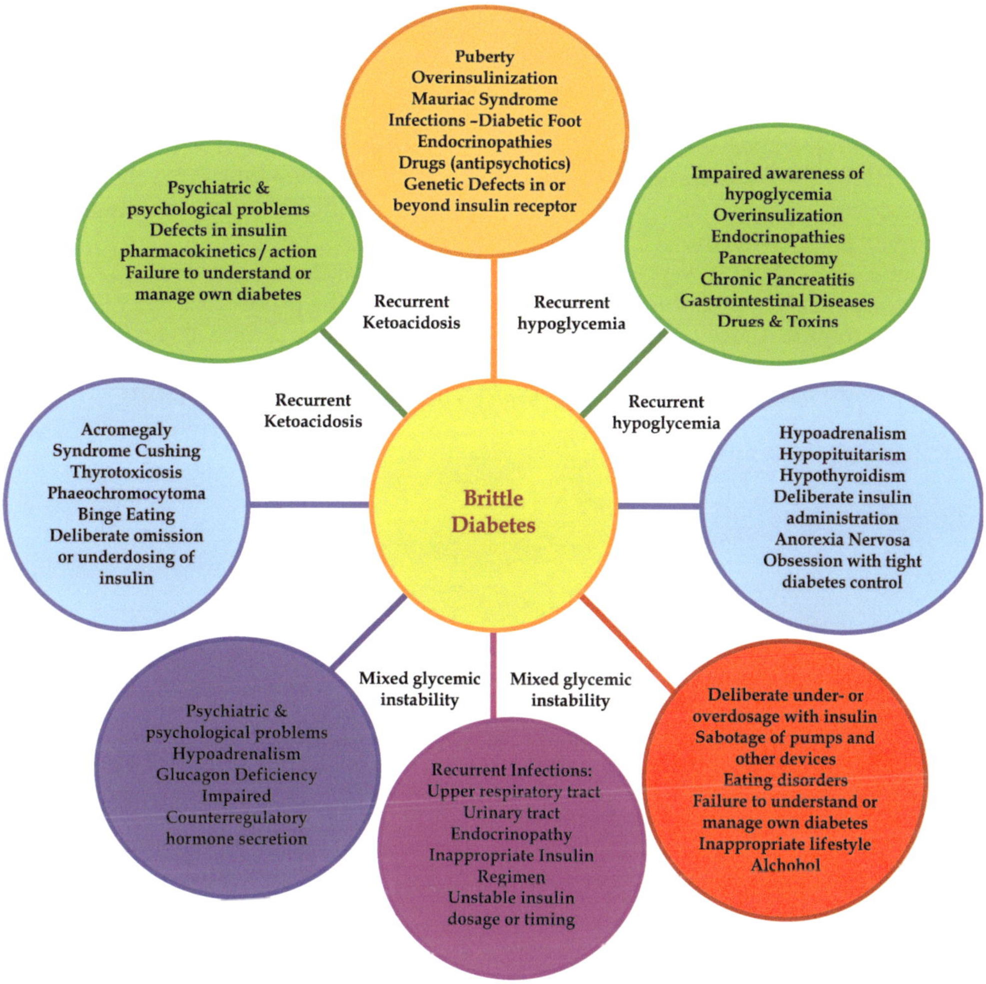
Puberty
Overinsulinization
Mauriac Syndrome
Infections -Diabetic Foot
Endocrinopathies
Drugs (antipsychotics)
Genetic Defects in or beyond insulin receptor
Psychiatric & psychological problems
Defects in insulin pharmacokinetics / action
Failure to understand or manage own diabetes
Impaired awareness of hypoglycemia
Overinsulization
Endocrinopathies
Pancreatectomy
Chronic Pancreatitis
Gastrointestinal Diseases
Drugs & Toxins
Recurrent Ketoacidosis
Recurrent hypoglycemia
Recurrent Ketoacidosis
Recurrent hypoglycemia
Acromegaly
Syndrome Cushing
Thyrotoxicosis
Phaeochromocytoma
Binge Eating
Deliberate omission or underdosing of insulin
Brittle Diabetes
Hypoadrenalism
Hypopituitarism
Hypothyroidism
Deliberate insulin administration
Anorexia Nervosa
Obsession with tight diabetes control
Mixed glycemic instability
Mixed glycemic instability
Psychiatric & psychological problems
Hypoadrenalism
Glucagon Deficiency
Impaired Counterregulatory hormone secretion
Recurrent Infections:
Upper respiratory tract
Urinary tract
Endocrinopathy
Inappropriate Insulin Regimen
Unstable insulin dosage or timing
Deliberate under- or overdosage with insulin
Sabotage of pumps and other devices
Eating disorders
Failure to understand or manage own diabetes
Inappropriate lifestyle
Alchohol

Fig. 1. Causes of Brittle Diabetes

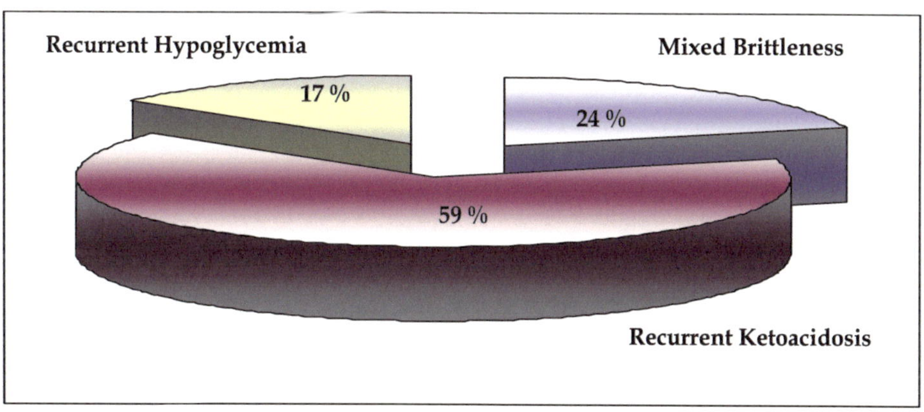

Fig. 2. The spectrum of Clinical Manifestations of Brittle Diabetes in Type 1 Diabetes Patients

resistance should be explored and an insulin challenge test should be performed (Serlin & Lash, 2009). Most patients who remain undiagnosed at this stage probably have factitious disease and may be skilled at manipulating their treatment, their families and physicians. Therefore, the test injections must be given by a member of the diabetes care team under conditions that guarantee the patients' cooperation. The need this must be explained to both patients and family. Hospital admission in such cases can provide formal psychological and psychiatric assessment of the patient and the family, without which investigation and management are incomplete.

It is essential to follow a logical protocol that initially excludes potentially remediable, organic causes. Cases remaining unexplained at the end of the process are most likely to be factitious in origin. Close observation during hospitalization is important: some brittle diabetes patients are skilled at stimulating hypoglycemia, possibly to gain attention or simply to obtain food that they desire (i.e. sweets) that are otherwise prohibited.

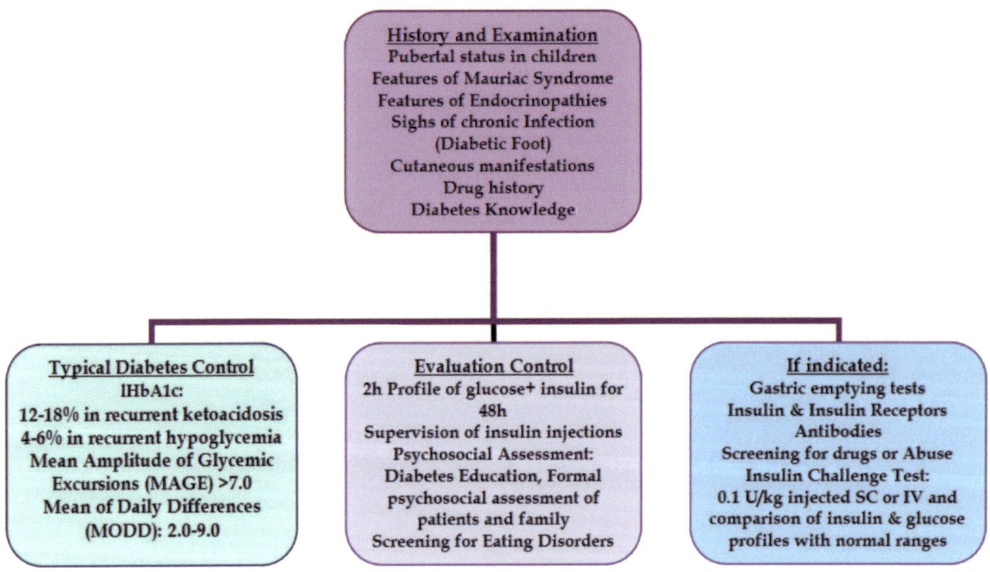

Fig. 3. Scheme for investigation of Brittle Diabetes

Among the life-threatening clinical manifestations, cases of spontaneous muscle infarction in young (mainly ≤30 years) women with a short duration (≤5 years) history of brittle type 1 diabetes that was not complicated by nephropathy, retinopathy or neuropathy have been described in the literature (Virally et al, 2007).

Spontaneous muscle infarction is a rare complication of diabetes, usually described in patients with multiple long-term diabetic complications (Woolley & Smith, 2006). Diabetic muscle infarction is more frequent in women (61.5%) and in type 1 diabetes (59%). The mean age of reported cases is 42.6 years, with a mean duration of diabetes of 14.3 years (Mathew et al., 2007). Multiple complications are usually present: 71% of patients have nephropathy (Madhan et al., 2000), 57% have retinopathy, and 54% suffer from autonomic neuropathy (Trujillo-Santos, 2003). Spontaneous diabetic muscle infarction is presented with necrosis of all muscle elements, with polymorphonuclear or mononuclear cellular infiltration and a varying but often limited degree of regeneration, depending on the age of the lesion. The presentation is usually acute, with pain and swelling localized to the thigh in most instances. Systemic signs such as pyrexia are infrequent. Laboratory tests (such as white cell count and creatinine kinase) and plain radiographs are not helpful, although the erythrocyte sedimentation rate is often elevated. The diagnosis, in the appropriate setting, is strongly suggested by magnetic resonance imaging, which shows increased signal intensity and asymmetry of the muscle on T2-weighted scanning as well as fluid in the tissue planes. Management consists of resting the muscle, analgesics, and gradual mobilization. Recurrence is common and may be seen in more than 50% of the patients. Long-term prognosis is poor, with most patients dying from cardiovascular complications of diabetes within 5 years of diagnosis. Therefore, a high index of suspicion, when a poorly controlled patient with diabetes presents with non-traumatic limb pain is needed (Mathew et al., 2007). All common causes of muscle infarction should be excluded, particularly microangiopathy and a hypercoagulable state. The differential diagnosis includes infection (pyomyositis, necrotic fasciitis), focal inflammatory myositis, vascular events, trauma, tumor and diabetic amyotrophy (Grigoriadis et al., 2000). When all of these are excluded, the possibility that the alternating states of transient acute hypoglycemia and hyperglycemia may be responsible for the myocardial infarction should be aroused and brought to the diagnostic table. "Brittleness" usually resumes after treatment with subcutaneous insulin infusion using a portable pump and no recurrence of muscle infarction is observed during the follow-up.

Although, integration of the patient's mental organization is an important part of all psychotherapeutic experiences and generally it is welcomed and thought well worth the effort needed to achieve it, however patients with brittle diabetes feel terrified by this process (Tallandini, 1999). They seem to think that integration involves a loss of the self: they feel it is dangerous and even resist it with psychotic-type defenses. For them, this reaction is always activated by separation, and it also appears prior to any developmental step they need to take- i.e. in recognizing self-boundaries, sexual identity, and facing the oedipal conflict. On all these occasions their reaction is to run away from treatment in a state of deep regression, feeling suicidal, and liable to seriously harm their self through the mistreatment of their diabetes (Hoffman, 2003).

Patients with long standing brittle diabetes with numerous episodes of diabetic ketoacidosis and frequent hypoglycemic episodes may present significant pathological changes in the gastric wall that affect all major components including muscle, neurons and interstitial cells of Cajal. Gastroparesis and severe malnutrition can occur in the presence of these changes, and may reflect vagal, central or hormonal influences (Pasricha et al., 2008). In juvenile brittle diabetes early diagnosed (in the first days of life) it is possible to develop severe secretory diarrhea. Extensive biochemical and serological investigation often fails to reveal the etiology of the diarrhea. Therapeutic trials with various agents (i.e. loperamide, cholestyramine, prednisone, indomethacin, and somatostatin analogue) often have no response. In some cases death from septicemia and malnutrition related to diarrhea and poor control of glycemia is reported before the completion of 1 year of age (Jonas et al., 1991; Roberts & Searle, 1995). Autopsy, may reveal absence of islets of Langerhans in the pancreas, and diffuse dysplastic changes in small and large intestinal mucosa. The entire alimentary tract may be lined by epithelia most typical of foregut mucosa: secretory-type glands, absent crypts of Lieberkuhn, and absent villi relating brittle type 1 diabetes with diffuse intestinal dysplasia independently or as part of a hyperimmunoglobulin syndrome (Peake et al., 1995).

Inhibition of the periodontal ligament cells which are the most important cells in the healing of wounds and the regeneration of periodontal tissues is the key explanation for the delayed periodontal regeneration and healing in patients with brittle diabetes with recurrent diabetic ketoacidosis (Kim et al., 2006). This is relevant to the increased number of infections that compromise more distant structures (via direct spread and distant spread), i.e. intracranial, retropharyngeal and pulmonary pleural infections and the dissemination by bloodstream that can lead to primary rheumatic problems and secondary deposits on the valves of the heart, i.e. endocarditis (Jiménez et al., 2004; Lazow, 2005).

Pulmonary edema, cerebral edema and multiple infarctions of the brain and cervical spinal cord develop more frequent in brittle type 1 diabetes than in "stable" type 1 diabetes patients during diabetic ketoacidosis, despite appropriate treatment. This may result in spastic quadraparesis and permanent disability (Dixon et al., 2006).

Some of the cutaneous manifestations of brittle diabetes include necrobiosis lipoidica diabeticorum, diabetic dermopathy, scleredema adultorum and acanthosis nigricans (Jabbour, 2003).

5. Quality of life: Struggling towards its achievement

The disruption of life, which is fundamental to the definition of brittle diabetes, obviously dependents on the patient's usual lifestyle and on numerous independent factors, including the admission policy of the diabetes care team. Emergency admissions due to poor diabetic control are much more common and prolonged than in "stable" patients, and it is not unusual for patients with brittle diabetes to spend several months each year in hospital. Pragmatic definitions of lifestyle disruption and "brittleness" include frequency and duration of hospitalization, more frequent psychosocial disruptions, pregnancy complications (Kent et al., 1994; Gill et al., 1996) and higher risk of death due to diabetic ketoacidosis, hypoglycemia, and renal failure (Tattersall et al., 1991).

Epidemiological studies in patients with brittle diabetes have established higher prevalence rates of psychiatric disorders, in particular mood and anxiety disorders. However, the prevalence rate and symptom profile of depression was found to be homogeneous between psychiatric patients with or without diabetes (Eiber et al., 1997).

Health-related quality of life is among the benefits of islet transplantation, because of a significant improvement in the dimensions of satisfaction and impact of diabetes (Benhamou et al., 2009). Therefore, its assessment may help in the selection of candidates with brittle diabetes for islet transplantation.

6. Management strategies in brittle diabetes

6.1 Qualification of glycemic variability

Several measures have been developed to quantify metabolic instability in brittle diabetes, which include assessment of the Mean Amplitude of the largest Glycemic Excursions (MAGE), the Mean of Daily Differences (MODD), Lability Index (LI), Low Blood Glucose Index (LBGI), Clarke's score, Hyposcore, and continuous blood glucose monitoring (Vantyghem & Press, 2006).

6.2 Continuous glucose monitoring systems: Indications, advantages, and limitations

Accurate and reliable devices sensing glucose on a near-continuous basis may facilitate specific therapeutic adjustments that need to be made to avoid hypo- and hyperglycemic excursions, thereby improving metabolic control. Patients with brittle diabetes, who are motivated to participate in their diabetes care and are technologically adept, may benefit from continuous glucose monitoring. Current continuous glucose monitoring systems indicate the glucose level, the direction and magnitude of change of glucose levels, and can be used to assess glycemic variability (De Block C et al., 2008). In addition, real-time continuous glucose monitoring sensors can serve as a tool to predict impending glucose excursions, thereby providing alarm signals of hypo- and hyperglycemic values warning the patient to take preventative actions (De Block C et al., 2008). Quality of life may also improve by using continuous glucose monitoring via reducing the fear of hypoglycemia (Weinzimer et al., 2004).

However, to successfully implement continuous glucose monitoring in daily practice, these devices must be accurate and reliable, and one must be aware of the limitations of current continuous glucose monitoring systems, that originate from physiological and technical aspects. Whether continuous glucose monitoring succeeds in ameliorating metabolic control and in reducing hypoglycemic episodes, as well as whether it improves quality of life in patients with brittle diabetes remains to be proven. Should this be the case, real-time continuous glucose monitoring may reduce chronic diabetic complications, and avoid hospitalizations, thereby reducing health care costs.

7. Treatment options

Therapy of brittle diabetes is based on education, glycemic control, intensive treatment and strict interaction between physicians and patients. Once psychogenic problems have been excluded, therapeutic strategies require firstly, the treatment of underlying organic causes of the "brittleness" whenever possible and secondly optimizing standard insulin therapy using analogues, multiple injections and consideration of continuous subcutaneous insulin infusion. However, patients with brittle diabetes characterized by recurrent diabetic ketoacidosis are often not improved by continuous subcutaneous insulin infusion, although there may be exceptions (Pickup & Keen, 2002). The introduction of insulin analogous, with either ultra-fast or ultra-slow action and the use of subcutaneous insulin pumps have significantly increased the possibility of treating most of these cases. However, there is a minority of patients resistant to therapy and alternative approaches are needed for these most severely affected patients. In similar cases, pancreas or islet transplantation represents an effective therapeutic option entailing good expected outcomes.

7.1 Lifestyle and education

Reduction of the rate of severe hypoglycemia has been noted with the Dose Adjustment for Normal Eating, a modern approach of advocating dietary freedom and appropriate flexibility of insulin doses, resulting in improved long-term metabolic control and better adherence to treatment goals (McIntyre, 2006).

The patient's ability to manage his or her own diabetes should be evaluated and reinforced if necessary, and guidelines drawn up with the patient's agreement for future treatment targets and follow-up. Any conclusions or diagnosis should be discussed in depth with the patient and family. Patients should be educated on self-management and insulin dose adjustments, since a main cause of brittle diabetes is failure of the patient to understand or manage his or her own diabetes (Rice, 2006). Effective education should provide knowledge within a context with which the patient can become familiar and should do justice to the unpredictability and complexity of actual life, as well as to the patient's own individuality

(Wroe, 2004). Efficacious education should transcend mechanical transmission of information to attain a deeper level of knowledge and inspire sustainable behavior changes and this is the only way to progress from incompliance to compliance and assimilation of fundamental principles, to active adherence, which is known to result in effective self-management (Lutfey et al., 1999). Thus, the patient is put in control to cope with the ever-changing situations of life (Papanas & Maltezos, 2008).

In recurrent hypoglycemia, all patients and their associates should be educated about the prevention and treatment of hypoglycemia (Dagogo-Jack, 2004). Moreover, appropriate information about hypoglycemia unawareness should take place upon diagnosis and regularly thereafter at follow-up consultations. Patients should be reminded to avoid usual behaviors that may contribute to hypoglycemia, such as taking excess insulin, delaying or missing meals, mistiming insulin/food intake around exercise, not monitoring before bed and appropriate increased food intake. Alcohol consumption can also lead to hypoglycemia and impair recovery from a hypoglycemic episode; the importance of not omitting food when drinking should be emphasized to patients. Additionally, patients should be advised to have a glucagon emergency kit on hand for severe hypoglycemic episodes (Aschner et al., 2010). Self monitoring of blood glucose can provide valuable information.

Although hypoglycemia avoidance restores awareness, it is difficult to be sustained. Hypoglycemia unawareness increases severe hypoglycemia risk. When adherence to treatment changes is compared by awareness status, reduced adherence to changes in insulin regimen in patients with hypoglycemia unawareness is compatible with habituation to hypoglycemic stress (Ly et al., 2009). Hypoglycemia unawareness in type 1 diabetes is largely secondary to recurrent therapeutic hypoglycemia, as assessed by neuroendocrine and symptom responses (Janssen et al., 2000) and cognitive function in patients with brittle type 1 diabetes and recurrent hypoglycemia (Bolli et al., 1998; Cryer et al., 2009). Reduced awareness of hypoglycemia in some patients with overzealous glycemic control may be partially restored by reducing insulin dosages and allowing mean blood glucose to rise (Fanelli et al., 1993). Respectively, after a short period (~2 weeks) of hypoglycemia prevention, the magnitude of symptom and neuroendocrine responses (with the exception of glucagon and norepinephrine) nearly normalizes, and cognitive function is deteriorated at the same glycemic threshold and to the same extent as in subjects without diabetes. At 3 months, the glycemic thresholds of symptom and neuroendocrine responses normalize, and some of the responses of glucagon are recovered (Fanelli et al., 1994). Hypoglycemia unawareness in type 1 diabetes is largely reversible and intensive insulin therapy together with a program of intensive education may substantially prevent hypoglycemia and at the same time maintain the glycemic targets of intensive insulin therapy in patients with brittle type 1 diabetes (Lager et al., 1986). Therapies aimed at reversing repetitive harmful behaviors may also be useful to restore hypoglycemia awareness, as well as protection from severe hypoglycemia.

7.2 Psychotherapy

Proven noncompliance to treatment requires careful handling. The "polarization" of brittle diabetic instability into hyperglycemic (recurrent diabetic ketoacidosis) or hypoglycemic behavior is well described, with relatively few displaying characteristics of "mixed brittleness" (Tattersall et al., 1991, Gill, 1992). Inpatient psychotherapy of patients with brittle diabetes and psychic reactions significantly stabilizes and improves blood glucose

after separation. Significant predictors for the average blood glucose are the therapist's vacation and the announcement of discharge from the hospital. A significant predictor for the daily blood glucose variation is mood (Milch et al., 2002). These results suggest the benefit of psychotherapy for young patients with brittle diabetes ((Mitchell et al., 2009).
Psychological therapy improves noncompliance as a primary cause of "brittleness" and in most cases patients are completed rehabilitated (Schade et al., 1985; Viner et al., 2003). However, in other groups the psychological management of "difficult" diabetes is less encouraging (Didjurgeit et al., 2002; Mitchell et al., 2009).

7.3 Alternative medicine

The Rauvolfia-Citrus tea is made by the boiling foliage of Rauvolfia vomitoria and the fruits of Citrus aurantium and is used to treat diabetes in Nigerian folk medicine. Chronic administration of the Rauvolfia-Citrus tea together with antidiabetic medication caused significant improvements in markers of glycemic control, such as blood glucose clearance, fasting and 2-h postprandial plasma glucose and HbA1c without adverse effects or hypoglycemia. Furthermore it ameliorated the fatty acid profile of skeletal muscle (Campbell-Tofte et al., 2010).
On healthy people vinegar delays gastric emptying and lowers postprandial blood glucose and insulin levels (Hlebowicz et al., 2008). The effect of 30 ml apple cider vinegar daily before breakfast on delayed gastric emptying rate on patients with brittle type 1 diabetes was assessed. Vinegar affected patients with diabetic gastroparesis by reducing the gastric emptying rate even further, with a concomitant disadvantage regarding to their glycemic control (Hlebowicz et al., 2007).

7.4 Insulin therapy

Intensive insulin treatment is defined by basal-prandial insulin therapy which tries to reproduce physiological insulin secretion. This requires 3 to 5 injections and self-monitoring of blood glucose 4 to 5 times a day. Patients who accept their disease and the demanding treatment regimen most often achieve glycemic treatment goals. Severe complications of diabetes can be avoided without increasing the risk of severe hypoglycemia. However, patients with brittle diabetes do not reach this objective (Jacqueminet et al., 2005). Besides the usual reasons affecting all patients with type 1 diabetes, i.e. diabetes itself, the idiosyncrasy of the patient, or the physician, in Brittle Diabetes the main obstacle which prevents patients from reaching the ideal glycemic target is more often related to psychological problems: difficulties in self-regulation, denial of diabetes presence, or phobia of hypoglycemia with avoidance behavior. Frequently, young women present eating disorders which can explain the poor diabetes control. The physician may be implicated in these poor glycemic results by not prescribing the right tools to obtain optimal glycemic control (staying with just two daily injections with premixed insulin) or by assigning glycemic targets inaccessible for the patient, or when an empathic relationship cannot be established between the patient and the physician. Patient empowerment is the key to the success of functional insulin treatment.
Cases of brittle type 1 diabetes in which recurrent hypoglycemia and peripheral edema were relieved after conversion from insulin lispro to insulin aspart have been reported (Tone et al., 2008) and stable glycemic control, as well as edema-free condition were maintained after conversion of insulin analogs. Several studies reported significantly fewer symptomatic

episodes of hypoglycemia with insulin aspart than with insulin lispro administrated by continuous subcutaneous insulin infusion in type 1 diabetes (Plank et al., 2002), which might be due to the differences in their pharmacokinetics and actions (O'Hare et al., 1983). On the other hand, plasma volume, intravascular albumin content and transcapillary escape rate of albumin change in response to hypoglycemia were also ameliorated by insulin conversion (Hilsted et al., 1991). Therefore, in cases of brittle type 1 diabetes, especially with peripheral edema, it may be worth using insulin analogs.

7.5 Insulin pump therapy

Though in use for more than 3 decades, insulin pumps are now being more commonly used because of their unique ability to continuously infuse insulin, closely mimicking that of physiological secretion from a normal pancreas. Unlike insulin shots with syringes, pump infusion sites need to be changed less frequently. Insulin pumps are reported to improve glycemic control, normalize blood glucose levels, reduce glycemic swings, and the dawn phenomenon. Fewer hypoglycemic episodes and a reduction in insulin dose per day are reported with insulin pump therapy as well as an improvement in sexual function, libido, and a significant relief of the intractable pain of peripheral neuropathy (Kesavadev et al., 2010). Quality of life is ameliorated by a reduction in the chronic fear of severe hypoglycemia, the more flexibility of lifestyle-no need to eat at fixed intervals, more freedom of lifestyle and easier participation in social and physical activity, and benefits for the patients' family (Cummins et al., 2010). The success of insulin pump therapy depends on selection of the right candidate, extensive education, motivation, and implementing the sophisticated programs with skill. Long-term follow-up of medical, psychological, and neurocognitive parameters in young patients with brittle diabetes have further summarized the same efficacy and safety of continuous subcutaneous insulin infusion in children ≤6 years of age (Eugster et al., 2006).

Insulin pump therapy can be initiated and used effectively in patients with brittle type 1 diabetes to improve metabolic control and quality of life. When diabetes and pump management are appropriately individualized, this kind of therapy can help patients with type 1 diabetes to achieve and to sustain metabolic control. Lifestyle flexibility, quality of life improvement, and independence can be maintained throughout young adulthood (Petrovski et al, 2007). Nocturnal glycemic control is improved with insulin pumps, and automatic basal rate changes help to minimize a pre-breakfast blood glucose increase (the "dawn phenomenon") often seen with injection therapy. Implantable pumps have advantages for patients who either weight more than 80kgs or have abnormalities of kidney or liver function or are highly sensitized. One study compared intraperitoneal insulin infusion through an implantable pump with intraportal islet transplantation (Vantyghem et al, 2009). Although the metabolic results (HbA1c, daily insulin need, glycemia) improved with both methods, they were significantly ameliorated with intraportal islet transplantation, though with more frequent side effects (hypoglycemia).

7.6 Islet transplantation

Islet cell transplantation is an attractive concept which holds great promise for the treatment of type 1 diabetes and for preventing brittle diabetes in patients undergoing pancreatic resection; given its potential high efficacy and that it is a relatively noninvasive procedure and a smart alternative to pancreas transplantation for restoring endogenous insulin secretion, islet cell transplantation may effectively control blood glucose for brittle type 1 diabetes, resulting in a marked reduction in hypoglycemic episodes and improvements in glycemic control. In addition, approximately 70% of transplanted patients with type 1 diabetes have achieved insulin independence (Matsumoto et al, 2005).

Isolated islet transplantation, which restores glucose sensing, should be considered in cases of hypoglycemic unawareness and/or lability especially if the body mass index is <25kg/m^2, but with current immunosuppressive protocols patients must have normal renal function and preferably no plans for pregnancy (Matsumoto et al., 2007). The main limiting factor of beta-cell function replacement by transplantation is so far represented by the potentially severe side effects of the immunosuppressant therapy necessary to avoid graft rejection and recurrence of autoimmunity.

Advances in islet isolation methods and immunosuppressive regimens are leading to expanded clinical trials to develop islet transplantation as a therapeutic option for patients with type 1 diabetes (Sumino et al., 2003). However, the isolation process is still potentially harmful to the islets (Bottino et al., 2004) because it may expose them to damaging factors that induce a general proinflammatory state. Moreover, after transplantation, islets are subject to hypoxia and early nonspecific inflammatory events, mostly mediated by the recipient's immune cells that can compromise beta-cell viability and function. Locally secreted chemoattractants and proinflammatory molecules might recruit and activate immune cells to the transplant site, mediating irreparable damage to the islet graft. Islet survival in the early post transplantation period is influenced by inflammatory events in and around islets.

CD40, a member of tumor necrosis factor receptor family expressed mainly in nonhematopoietic cells, is generally associated with inflammation. CD40 contributes not only to physiological cell-mediated responses, but also to immune pathological conditions such as autoimmune and vascular diseases, leading to a chronic inflammatory state. It has been previously reported that the CD40 molecule is expressed also in human pancreatic beta-cells and that expression can be upregulated by incubation with a cocktail of proinflammatory cytokines (Klein et al., 2005). CD40 signals in beta-cells upregulate secretion of interleukin (IL)-6, IL-8, macrophage inflammatory protein (MIP)-1, and MIP-1β (Barbé-Tuana et al., 2006). These results in vitro indicate that the CD40 receptor expressed by beta-cells could be activated in vivo inducing proinflammatory responses contributing to early islet graft loss after transplantation. In this regard, the use of specific blockers immediately after the isolation process could improve islet viability and perhaps clinical success rates.

Reducing the islet proinflammatory state has been demonstrated to reduce the early post-transplant complications and perhaps improve islet engraftment (Bertuzzi et al., 2004). Moreover, increased percentage of insulin-independence at 1-year post-transplant and decreased percentage of cardiovascular events has been achieved with corticosteroids-sparing protocols in pancreas islet allotransplantation in patients with brittle diabetes. Lympho-depleting induction antibodies, such as rabbit anti-thymocyte globulin or alemtuzumab, calcineurin inhibitors and mycophenolate or sirolimus have been widely used in successful trials. However, since most of the studies were uncontrolled trials of low-risk patients and therefore the grade of evidence is limited, large-scale prospective studies with long-term follow up are necessary to assess risks and benefits of corticosteroids-sparing regimens in pancreas transplantation before recommending such strategies as standard practice.

It is often reported that islets from more than one donor are required to achieved insulin independence, even when an acceptable islet mass was transplanted in the first infusion. The success of recent clinical trials for allogeneic islet transplantation as well as the increasing centers that perform auto-transplantation is showing that the beta-cell replacement therapy for the treatment of patients with diabetes or total pancreatectomy has been firmly established. It needs only to be improved and made more widely available to the millions of desperate patients with brittle diabetes who search for alternatives to a life of insulin injections, hypoglycemia and the risks of end-organ damage. Important issues to be addressed before this treatment is widely applicable, including difficulty in maintaining insulin independence, low islet isolation success rate, multiple donor requirements, and side effects associated with the use of immunosuppressants. Steady progress has been achieved in recent years in different areas in the pancreatic islet transplantation process including islet cell processing, preservation, and immune therapies that justify optimism.

Combined islet and donor CD34+ hematopoietic stem cell infusion using an 'Edmonton-like' immunosuppression (daclizumab, sirolimus, tacrolimus), with a single dose of anti-TNF alpha antibody (Infliximab) adds to the induction without ablative conditioning, and may lead to stable chimerism and graft tolerance in patients with Brittle Type 1 Diabetes receiving a single-donor allogeneic islet transplant (Mineo et al, 2008). A prospective phase 1/2 trial investigated the safety and reproducibility of allogeneic islet transplantation and tested a strategy to achieve insulin-independence with lower islet mass in C-peptide negative Brittle Type 1 Diabetes patients with hypoglycemic unawareness. All patients received an equal mean total number of islets. Both the Edmonton immunosuppression regimen (daclizumab, sirolimus, tacrolimus) and the University of Illinois protocol (etanercept, exenatide and the Edmonton regimen) induced insulin-independence. However, combined treatment of etanercept and exenatide improved islet graft function and facilitates achievement of insulin-independence with fewer islets (Gangemi et al, 2008).

Optimal primary graft function has been associated with prolonged graft survival and better metabolic control (HbA1c, mean glucose, glucose variability assessed with continuous glucose monitoring system, and glucose tolerance defined by an oral glucose tolerance test) after islet transplantation (Vantyghem et al., 2009). This result was not significantly influenced by HLA mismatches or by preexisting islet autoantibodies. A pancreas transplant alone in a nonuremic patient with Brittle Diabetes is a rare procedure because the tradeoff for insulin independence is lifelong immunosuppression. However, a technically successful pancreas transplant alone is currently the only treatment option that allows nonuremic patients with Brittle Diabetes to become insulin-independent in the long term. Risk factors for subsequent kidney failure (13% at 5 years posttransplant) are serum creatinine levels >1.5 mg/dL at the time of the pancreas transplant and recipient age<30 years (Gruessner et al., 2008).

Donor shortage is another dilemma. To address the issue of donor shortage, living donor islet transplantation and bioartificial islet transplantation using pig islets are being evaluated. Bioartificial islet transplantation could be the ultimate solution of the donor shortage. Currently, overcoming immunological hurdles, establishing reliable islet isolation methods, and controlling porcine endogenous retrovirus are the primary obstacles to the implementation of this treatment. If bioartificial islet transplant becomes a clinical reality, it may even be applicable in the treatment of select patients with Type 2 diabetes. Beta-Cell regeneration from naïve pancreas and beta-cell generation from embryonic stem cells or induced pluripotent stem cells are poised as the next-generation treatments for Type 1 diabetes (Matsumoto, 2010).

Preemptive simultaneous kidney-pancreas transplantation in patients with Type 1 Brittle Diabetes, severe diabetic autonomic neuropathy and nephrotic syndrome due to diabetic nephropathy, with near-normal exhibited function of the native kidneys leads to rapid and nearly complete diminution of proteinuria although the residual function of the patient's native kidneys was reduced from 60% at about 40% at 3 months after transplantation and slightly lower at 12 months after simultaneous kidney-pancreas transplantation (Sedlak et al, 2007). Besides kidney microcirculation, islet transplantation alone has also a beneficial effect on the retinal microcirculation, since recently an early, significant increase of arterial and venous retinal blood flow velocities was found 1-year after islet transplantation (Venturini et al., 2006).

However, whether islet transplantation should be aimed at restoring insulin independence or providing adequate metabolic control and restoration of diabetic microvascular complications is still debated (Badet et al., 2007). Updated summary of results from Edmonton procedure and experience with combined results from different institutions reported to the Collaborative Islet Transplant Registry have largely substantiated the reproducibility of the Edmonton procedure (Ryan et al., 2001). Complete insulin-independence is achieved in the majority of patients 1-year after transplant (more then 55%) but this state is not sustained permanently. Although only a minority (10%) of patients remained insulin-free after 5 years, more then 80% of them had still detectable levels of C-peptide and substantially improved glycemic control without episodes of hypoglycemia. Even though currently, the islet graft is still not a remedy for every patient with Brittle Diabetes, islet transplantation has already obtained "nonresearch" status and is close to having a biological license status approved by the FDA in the United States that would further stimulate progress in the field (Witkowski et al., 2006; Alejandro et al., 2008).

8. Conclusions

There are many complexities involved in treating patients with brittle diabetes and helping them to achieve and maintain their euglycemia. Therefore, adopting a team approach that involves a broad range of disciplines is essential. Depending on circumstances and available resources, the multidisciplinary team should include the patient, diabetes specialist, primary care physician, nurse, dietitian, podiatrist and psychologist/psychiatrist, as well as family and friends. All members of the team should work together to ensure continuity of care. Communication and coordination within the team are also imperative to ensure that all members share and are working towards the same treatment targets and recommendations.

9. References

Alejandro, R, Barton, FB, Hering, BJ, Wease, S; Collaborative Islet Transplant Registry Investigators. (2008). Update from the Collaborative Islet Transplant Registry. *Transplantation*, Vol.86, No.12, (December 2008); 1783-1788.

Amiel, SA. (1996). Studies in hypoglycaemia in children with insulin-dependent diabetes mellitus. *Hormone research*, Vol.45, No.6, pp.285-290

Anagnostis, P, Athyros, VG, Tziomalos, K, Karagiannis, A, Mikhailidis, DP. (2009). Clinical review: The pathogenetic role of cortisol in the metabolic syndrome: a hypothesis. *The Journal of clinical endocrinology and metabolism*, Vol.94, No.8, (August 2009), pp.2692-2701

Aschner, P, Horton, E, Leiter, LA, Munro, N, Skyler, JS; Global Partnership for Effective Diabetes Management. (2010). Practical steps to improving the management of type 1 diabetes: recommendations from the Global Partnership for Effective Diabetes Management. *International journal of clinical practice*, Vol.64, No.3, (February 2010), pp.305-315

Badet, L, Benhamou, PY, Wojtusciszyn, A, Baertschiger, R, Milliat-Guittard, L, Kessler, L, Penfornis, A, Thivolet, C, Renard, E, Bosco, D, Morel, P, Morelon, E, Bayle, F, Colin, C, Berney, T; GRAGIL Group. (2007). Expectations and strategies regarding islet transplantation: metabolic data from the GRAGIL 2 trial. *Transplantation*, Vol.84, No.1, July 2007, pp.89-96

Balter, J, Mofsen, R, Pinninti, N. (2004). Quetiapine in the successful treatment of psychosis and comorbid brittle diabetes mellitus: a case report. *International journal of psychiatry in medicine*, Vol.34,No.3, pp.259-266

Barbé-Tuana, FM, Klein, D, Ichii, H, Berman, DM, Coffey, L, Kenyon, NS, Ricordi, C, Pastori, RL. (2006). CD40-CD40 ligand interaction activates proinflammatory pathways in pancreatic islets. *Diabetes*, Vol.55, No.9, (September 2006), pp.2437-2445

Beale, IL, Pearce, NE, Conroy, DM, Henning, MA, Murrell, KA. (1997). Psychological effects of chronic exposure to 50 Hz magnetic fields in humans living near extra-high-voltage transmission lines. *Bioelectromagnetics*, Vol.18, No.8, (December 1997), pp.584-594

Benhamou, PY, Milliat-Guittard, L, Wojtusciszyn, A, Kessler, L, Toso, C, Baertschiger, R, Debaty, I, Badet, L, Penfornis, A, Thivolet, C, Renard, E, Bayle, F, Morel, P, Morelon, E, Colin, C, Berney, T; GRAGIL group. (2009). Quality of life after islet transplantation: data from the GRAGIL 1 and 2 trials. *Diabetic Medicine*, Vol.26, No.6, (June 2009), pp.617-621

Benbow, SJ, Walsh, A, Gill, GV. (2001). Brittle diabetes in the elderly. *Journal of the Royal Society of Medicine*, Vol.94, No.11, (November 2001), pp.578-580

Bertuzzi, F, Verzaro, R, Provenzano, V, Ricordi, C. (2007). Brittle type 1 diabetes mellitus. *Current medicinal chemistry*, Vol.14, No. 16, pp.1739-1744, ISSN: 0929-8673

Bertuzzi, F, Marzorati, S, Maffi, P, Piemonti, L, Melzi, R, de Taddeo, F, Valtolina, V, D'Angelo, A, di Carlo, V, Bonifacio, E, Secchi, A. (2004). Tissue factor and CCL2/monocyte chemoattractant protein-1 released by human islets affect islet engraftment in type 1 diabetic recipients. *The Journal of clinical endocrinology and metabolism*, Vol.89, No. 11, (November 2004), pp.5724-5728

Bolli, GB. (1998). Counterregulatory mechanisms to insulin-induced hypoglycemia in humans: relevance to the problem of intensive treatment of IDDM. *Journal of pediatric endocrinology & metabolism*, Vol.11, Suppl.1, (March 1998), pp.103-115

Bottino, R, Balamurugan, AN, Tse, H, Thirunavukkarasu, C, Ge, X, Profozich, J, Milton, M, Ziegenfuss, A, Trucco, M, Piganelli, JD. (2004). Response of human islets to isolation stress and the effect of antioxidant treatment. *Diabetes*, Vol.53, No.10, (October 2004), pp.2559-2568

Borch-Johnsen, K, Helweg-Larsen, K. Sudden death and human insulin: is there a link? (1993). *Diabetic medicine*, Vol.10, pp. 255-259

Brosig B, Leweke F, Milch W, Eckhard M, Reimer C. (2001). Psychosocial predictors of metabolic instability in brittle diabetes--a multivariate time series analysis.

Psychotherapie, Psychosomatik,medizinische Psychologie, Vol.51, No.6, (June 2001), pp.232-238

Campbell-Tofte, JI, Mølgaard, P, Josefsen, K, Abdallah, Z, Hansen, SH, Cornett, C, Mu, H, Richter, EA, Petersen, W, Nørregaard, JC, Winther, K. (2010). Randomized and double-blinded pilot clinical study of the safety and anti-diabetic efficacy of the Rauvolfia-Citrus tea, as used in Nigerian Traditional Medicine. *Journal of ethnopharmacology,* October 2010

Cassidy, EM, O'Halloran, DJ, Barry, S. (1999). Insulin as a substance of misuse in a patient with insulin dependent diabetes mellitus. *BMJ,* Vol.319, No.7222, November 1999, pp1417-1418

Crow, SJ, Keel, PK, Kendall, D. (1998). Eating disorders and insulin-dependent diabetes mellitus. *Psychosomatics,* Vol.39, No.3, (May-June 1998), pp.233-243

Cryer, PE. (2008). The barrier of hypoglycemia in diabetes. *Diabetes,* Vol.57, No.12, (December 2008), pp.3169-3176

Cummins, E, Royle, P, Snaith, A, Greene, A, Robertson, L, McIntyre, L, Waugh, N. (2010). Clinical effectiveness and cost-effectiveness of continuous subcutaneous insulin infusion for diabetes: systematic review and economic evaluation. *Health technology assessment (Winchester, England),* Vol.14, No.11, (February 2010), pp. iii-iv, xi-xvi, 1-181

Dagogo-Jack, S. (2004). Hypoglycemia in type 1 diabetes mellitus: pathophysiology and prevention. *Treatments in endocrinology,* Vol.3, No.2, pp.91-103

De Block, C, Vertommen, J, Manuel-y-Keenoy, B, Van Gaal, L. (2008). Minimally-invasive and non-invasive continuous glucose monitoring systems: indications, advantages, limitations and clinical aspects. *Current Diabetes Reviews,* Vol.4, No.3, (August 2008), pp.159-168

De Block, C, Manuel-y-Keenoy, B, Van Gaal, L. (2008) A review of current evidence with continuous glucose monitoring in patients with diabetes. *Journal of diabetes science and technology.* Vol.2, No.4, (July 2008), pp.718-727

Diabetes Control and Complications Trial Research Group. (1993). The effect of intensive treatment of diabetes on the development and progression of long-term complications in insulin-dependent diabetes mellitus. *The New England journal of medicine,* Vol 329, pp.977-986

Didjurgeit, U, Kruse, J, Schmitz, N, Stückenschneider, P, Sawicki, PT. (2002). A time-limited, problem - orientated psychotherapeutic intervention in Type 1 diabetic patients with complications: a randomized controlled trial. *Diabetic Medicine,* Vol.19, No.10, (October 2002), pp.814-821

Dixon, AN, Jude EB, Banerjee, AK, Bain, SC. (2006). Simultaneous pulmonary and cerebral oedema, and multiple CNS infarctions as complications of diabetic ketoacidosis: a case report. *Diabetic medicine* 2006, Vol.23, No.5, (May 2006), pp.571-573

Dobrilla, G. (1989). Management of chronic pancreatitis. Focus on enzyme replacement therapy. *International journal of pancreatology,* Vol.5, Supp.l, pp.17-29

Dutour, A, Boiteau, V, Dadoun, F, Feissel, A, Atlan, C, Oliver, C. (1996). Hormonal response to stress in brittle diabetes. *Psychoneuroendocrinology,* Vol. 21, No.6, (August 1996), pp.525-543

Eiber, R, Berlin, I, Grimaldi, A, Bisserbe, JC. (1997). Insulin-dependent diabetes and psychiatric pathology:general clinical and epidemiologic review. *Encéphale,* Vol.23, No.5, (September-October 1997), pp.351-357.

Elder, CJ, Natarajan, A. (2010). Mauriac syndrome--a modern reality. *Journal of pediatric endocrinology & metabolism,* Vol.23, No.3, (March 2010), pp.311-313

Elkeles, RS, Wright, AD, Lowy, C, Fraser, TR. (1969). Serum-insulin in acromegaly. *Lancet,* Vol.2, No.7621, (September 1969), pp.615-618

Eugster, EA, Francis, G; Lawson-Wilkins Drug and Therapeutics Committee. (2006). Position statement: Continuous subcutaneous insulin infusion in very young children with type 1 diabetes. *Pediatrics,* Vol.118 (No.4), (October 2006), pp. e1244-1249

Fanelli, CG, Epifano, L, Rambotti, AM, Pampanelli, S, Di Vincenzo, A, Modarelli, F, Lepore, M, Annibale, B, Ciofetta, M, Bottini, P, et al. (1993). Meticulous prevention of hypoglycemia normalizes the glycemic thresholds and magnitude of most of neuroendocrine responses to, symptoms of, and cognitive function during hypoglycemia in intensively treated patients with short-term IDDM. *Diabetes,* Vol.42, No.11, (November 1993), pp..1683-1689

Fanelli, C, Pampanelli, S, Epifano, L, Rambotti, AM, Di Vincenzo, A, Modarelli, F, Ciofetta, M, Lepore, M, Annibale, B, Torlone, E, et al. (1994). Long-term recovery from unawareness, deficient counterregulation and lack of cognitive dysfunction during hypoglycaemia, following institution of rational, intensive insulin therapy in IDDM. *Diabetologia,* Vol.37, No.12, (December 1994), pp.1265-1276

Fischer, U, Jutzi, E, Bombor, H, Freyse, EJ, Salzieder, E, Albrecht, G, Besch, W, Bruns, W. (1980). Assessment of an algorithm for the artificial B-cell using the normal insulin-glucose relationship in diabetic dogs and men. *Diabetologia;* Vol.18, No.2, pp.97-107

Gangemi, A, Salehi, P, Hatipoglu, B, Martellotto, J, Barbaro, B, Kuechle, JB, Qi, M, Wang, Y, Pallan, P, Owens, C, Bui, J, West, D, Kaplan, B, Benedetti, E, Oberholzer, J. (2008). Islet transplantation for brittle type 1 diabetes: the UIC protocol. *American journal of transplantation,* Vol. 8, No.6, (June 2008), pp. 1250-1261

Gill, GV. (1992). The spectrum of brittle diabetes. *Journal of the Royal Society of Medicine,* Vol.85, pp.259 -261

Gill, GV, Lucas, S, Kent, LA. (1996). Prevalence and characteristics of brittle diabetes in Britain. *QJM: monthly journal of the Association of Physicians,* Vol.89, No.11, (November 1996), pp.839-843

Gill, G & Lucas, S. (1999). Brittle diabetes characterized by recurrent hypoglycemia. *Diabetes & metabolism,* Vol.25, No.4, (September 1999), pp.308-311

Gill, GV, Williams, G. (2000). Brittle Addison's disease: a new variation on a familiar theme. *Postgraduate medical journal,* Vol.76, No.893, (March 2000), pp.166-167

Grigoriadis, E, Fam, AG, Starok, M, Ang, LC. (2000). Skeletal muscle infarction in diabetes mellitus. The *Journal of rheumatology,* Vol.27, No.4, (April 2000), pp.1063-1068

Gruessner, RW, Sutherland, DE, Kandaswamy, R, Gruessner, AC. (2008). Over 500 solitary pancreas transplants in nonuremic patients with brittle diabetes mellitus. *Transplantation,* Vol.15, No.85, (January 2008), pp.42-47

Hammer, HF. (2010). Pancreatic exocrine insufficiency: diagnostic evaluation and replacement therapy with pancreatic enzymes. *Digestive diseases (Basel, Switzerland)* , Vol.28, No.2, pp.339-343

Hardy, KJ, Burge, MR, Boyle, PJ, Scarpello, JH. (1994). A treatable cause of recurrent severe hypoglycemia. *Diabetes Care*, Vol.17, No.7, (July 1994), pp.722-724

Havas, M. (2008). Dirty electricity elevates blood sugar among electrically sensitive diabetics and may explain brittle diabetes. *Electromagnetic biology and medicine*, Vol.27, No.2, (June 2008), pp.135-146

Hedman, CA, Lindstrom, T, Arnqvist, HJ. (2001). Direct comparison of insulin lispro and aspart shows small differences in plasma insulin profiles after subcutaneous injection in type 1 diabetes. *Diabetes Care*, Vol.24, pp.1120-1121

Hepburn, DA, Patrick, AW, Eadington, DW, Ewing, DJ, Frier, BM. (1990). Unawareness of hypoglycaemia in insulin-treated diabetic patients: prevalence and relationship to autonomic neuropathy. *Diabetic medicine*, Vol. 7, pp.711-717

Hershko, C, Skikne, B. (2009). Pathogenesis and management of iron deficiency anemia: emerging role of celiac disease, helicobacter pylori, and autoimmune gastritis. *Seminars in hematology*, Vol.46, No.4, (October 2009), pp.339-350

Hilsted J, Frandsen H, Christensen NJ, Nielsen SL. (1991). Plasma volume changes during hypoglycaemia: the effect of autonomic blockade. *European Journal of Clinical Investigation*, Vol. 21, No.1, (February 1991), pp. 22–26

Hlebowicz, J, Darwiche, G, Björgell, O, Almér, LO. (2007). Effect of apple cider vinegar on delayed gastric emptying in patients with type 1 diabetes mellitus: a pilot study. BMC gastroenterology MC Gastroenteroy, Vol.20, No.7, (December 2007), p.46.

Hlebowicz J, Lindstedt S, Björgell O, Höglund P, Almér LO, Darwiche G. (2008). The botanical integrity of wheat products influences the gastric distention and satiety in healthy subjects. *Nutrition journal*, Vol.27, No.7, (April 2008), p.12

Hoffman, I. (2003). Identity maintenance in the affectively distant patient. *Journal of the American Psychoanalytic Association*. Spring, Vol.51, No.2, pp.491-515

Iannello, S, Campanile, E, Cipolli, D, Gallina, M, Merola, A, Puglisi, S, Tabita, V, Belfiore, F. (1997). A rare case of juvenile diabetes mellitus associated with APECED (autoimmune poly-endocrinopathy, candidiasis and ectodermal dystrophy) with strong X-linked familial inheritance. *Minerva endocrinologica*, Vol.22, No.2, (June 1997), pp.51-59

Ishii, C, Inoue, K, Negishi, K, Tane, N, Awata, T, Katayama, S. (2001). Diabetic ketoacidosis in a case of pheochromocytoma. *Diabetes research and clinical practice*, Vol.54, No.2, (November 2001), pp.137- 142

Jabbour, SA. (2003). Cutaneous manifestations of endocrine disorders: a guide for dermatologists. *American journal of clinical dermatology*, Vol.4, No.5, pp.315-331

Jacobson, R, Horenstein, M, Kassel, L. (1970). Hyperglycemia and hyperosmolarity in a brittle diabetic with thyrotoxicosis. *Diabetes, Vol. 19, No.1,* (January 1970), pp.70-71

Jacqueminet, S, Masseboeuf, N, Rolland, M, Grimaldi, A, Sachon, C. (2005). Limitations of the so-called "intensified" insulin therapy in type 1 diabetes mellitus. *Diabetes Metabolism*, Vol.31, No.4 (September 2005), pp.4S45-4S50

Janssen, MM, Snoek, FJ, Heine, RJ. (2000). Assessing impaired hypoglycemia awareness in type 1 diabetes: agreement of self- report but not of field study data with the autonomic symptom threshold during experimental hypoglycemia. *Diabetes Care*, April 2000, Vol.23, No.4, pp.529-532

Jethwa, P, Sodergren, M, Lala, A, Webber, J, Buckels, JA, Bramhall, SR, Mirza, DF. (2006). Diabetic control after total pancreatectomy. *Digestive and liver disease*, Vol.38, No.6, June 2006, pp.415-419

Jiménez, Y, Bagán, JV, Murillo, J, Poveda, R. (2004). Odontogenic infections. Complications. Systemic manifestations. *Medicina oral, patología oral y cirugía bucal*, Vol.9, Suppl:143-7, pp.139-143

Jolobe, OM & Khin, N. (2002). Brittle diabetes in the elderly. *Journal of the Royal Society of Medicine*, Vol.95, No.1, January 2002, p.58

Jonas MM, Bell MD, Eidson MS, Koutouby R, Hensley GT. (1991). Congenital diabetes mellitus and fatal secretory diarrhea in two infants *Journal of pediatric gastroenterology and nutrition*, Vol.13, No.4, (November 1991), pp.415-425

Jørgensen, HS. (2007). Studies on the neuroendocrine role of serotonin. *Danish medical bulletin*, Vol.54, No.4, (November 2007), pp.266-288

Kane, JM, Correll, CU, Goff, DC, Kirkpatrick, B, Marder, SR, Vester-Blokland, E, Sun, W, Carson, WH, Pikalov, A, Assunção-Talbott, S. (2009). A multicenter, randomized, double-blind, placebo-controlled, 16-week study of adjunctive aripiprazole for schizophrenia or schizoaffective disorder inadequately treated with quetiapine or risperidone monotherapy. *The Journal of clinical psychiatry*, Vol.70, No.10, (October 2009), pp.1348-1357

Kawanishi, K & Miyashita, H. (2003). A case of brittle diabetes in a 94-year-old man with vascular dementia, visual disturbance and hearing difficulty. *Nippon Ronen Igakkai zasshi. Japanese journal of geriatrics*, Vol.40, No.2, (March 2003), pp.156-159

Kent, L, Gill, GV, Williams, G. (1994). Mortality and outcome of patients with brittle diabetes and recurrent ketoacidosis. *Lancet*, Vol.344, No. 8925, (September 1994), pp.778-781

Kesavadev, J, Das, AK, Unnikrishnan, R 1st, Joshi, SR, Ramachandran, A, Shamsudeen, J, Krishnan, G, Jothydev, S, Mohan, V. (2010). Use of insulin pumps in India: suggested guidelines based on experience and cultural differences. *Diabetes technology & therapeutics*, Vol. 12, No.10, (October 2010), pp.823-831

Kim, HS, Park, JW, Yeo, SI, Choi, BJ, Suh, JY. (2006). Effects of high glucose on cellular activity of periodontal ligament cells in vitro. *Diabetes research and clinical practice*, Vol.74, No.1, (October 2006), pp.41-47

Klein, D, Barbé-Tuana, F, Pugliese, A, Ichii, H, Garza, D, Gonzalez, M, Molano, RD, Ricordi, C, Pastori, RL. (2005). A functional CD40 receptor is expressed in pancreatic beta cells. *Diabetologia*, Vol.48, No.2, (February 2005), pp.268-276

Laffel, LM, Wentzell, K, Loughlin, C, Tovar, A, Moltz, K, Brink, S. (2006). Sick day management using blood 3-hydroxybutyrate (3-OHB) compared with urine ketone monitoring reduces hospital visits in young people with T1DM: a randomized clinical trial. *Diabetic medicine*, Vol.23, No.3, (March 2006), pp.278-284

Lager, I, Attvall, S, Blohmé, G, Smith, U. (1986). Altered recognition of hypoglycaemic symptoms in type I diabetes during intensified control with continuous subcutaneous insulin infusion. *Diabetic Medicine*, Vol. 3, No.4, (July-August 1986), pp.322-325

Lankisch, TO, Jaeckel, E, Strassburg, CP. (2009). The autoimmune polyendocrinopathy-candidiasis-ectodermal dystrophy or autoimmune polyglandular syndrome type 1. Seminars in liver disease, Vol.29, No.3, (August 2009), pp.307-314

Layer, P, Keller, J. (1999). Pancreatic enzymes: secretion and luminal nutrient digestion in health and disease. *Journal of clinical gastroenterology*, Vol.28, No.1, January 1999, pp.3-10

Lazow, SK. (2005). Orofacial infections in the 21st century. *The New York state dental journal*, Vol.71, No.6, (November 2005), pp.36-41

Lehmann, R, Honegger, RA, Feinle, C, Fried, M, Spinas, GA, Schwizer, W. (2003). Glucose control is not improved by accelerating gastric emptying in patients with type 1 diabetes mellitus and gastroparesis. A pilot study with cisapride as a model drug. *Experimental and clinical endocrinology & diabetes*, Vol.111, No.5, (August 2003), pp.255-261

Li, L, Dai, Y, Xia, R, Chen, S, Qiao, D. (2005). Pulsed electric field exposure of insulin induces anti - proliferative effects on human hepatocytes. *Bioelectromagnetics*, Vol.26, No.8, (December 2005), pp.639-647

Lloyd, GG, Steel, JM, Young, RJ. (1987). Eating disorders and psychiatric morbidity in patients with diabetes mellitus. *Psychotherapy and psychosomatics*, Vol.48, No.1-4, pp.189-195

Ludviksson, BR, Griffin, J, Graziano, FM. (1993). Munchausen's syndrome: the importance of a comprehensive medical history. Wisconsin medical journal, Vol.92, Bo.3, (March 1993), pp.128-129

Lutfey, KE, Wishner, WJ. (1999). Beyond "compliance" is "adherence". Improving the prospect of diabetes care. *Diabetes Care*, Vol.22, No.4, (April 1999), pp. 4635-4639

Ly, TT, Gallego, PH, Davis, EA, Jones, TW. (2009). Impaired awareness of hypoglycemia in a population-based sample of children and adolescents with type 1 diabetes. *Diabetes Care*, Vol.32, No.10, (October 2009), pp.1802-1806

Madhan, KK, Symmans, P, Te Strake, L, van Der Merwe, W. (2000). Diabetic muscle infarction in patients on dialysis. *American journal of kidney diseases*, Vol.35, No.6, (June 2000), pp.1212-1216

Mathew, A, Reddy, IS, Archibald, C. (2007). Diabetic muscle infarction. *Emergency medicine journal*, Vol.24, No.7, July 2007, pp.513-514

Matsumoto, S, Okitsu, T, Iwanaga, Y, Noguchi, H, Nagata, H, Yonekawa, Y, Yamada, Y, Nakai, Y, Ueda, M, Ishii, A, Yabunaka, E, Shapiro, JA, Tanaka, K (2005). Insulin independence of unstable diabetic patient after single living donor islet transplantation. *Transplantation proceedings*, Vol.37, No.8, (October 2005), pp.3427-3429

Matsumoto, S, Noguchi, H, Naziruddin, B, Onaca, N, Jackson, A, Nobuyo, H, Teru, O, Naoya, K, Klintmalm, G, Levy, M. (2007). Improvement of pancreatic islet cell isolation for transplantation. *Proceedings (Baylor University. Medical Center)*, Vol.20, No.4, (October 2007), pp.357-362

Matsumoto S. (2010). Islet cell transplantation for Type 1 diabetes. *Journal of diabetes*, Vol.2, No.1, (March 2010), pp.16-22

Matsuyoshi, A, Shimoda, S, Tsuruzoe, K, Taketa, K, Chirioka, T, Sakamoto, F, Sakakida, M, Miyamura, N, Araki, E. (2006). A case of slowly progressive type 1 diabetes with unstable glycemic control caused by unusual insulin antibody and successfully treated with steroid therapy. *Diabetes research and clinical practice* , Vol. 72, No.3, June 2006, pp.238-243

McIntyre, HD. (2006). DAFNE (Dose Adjustment for Normal Eating): structured education in insulin replacement therapy for type 1 diabetes. *The Medical journal of Australia*, Vol.184, No.7, (April 2006), pp.317-318

Meier, JJ, Menge, BA, Breuer, TG, Müller, CA, Tannapfel, A, Uhl, W, Schmidt, WE, Schrader, H. Functional assessment of pancreatic beta-cell area in humans. *Diabetes*, Vol.58, No.7, (July 2009), pp.1595-1603

Menge, BA, Schrader, H, Breuer, TG, Dabrowski, Y, Uhl, W, Schmidt, WE, Meier, JJ. (2009). Metabolic consequences of a 50% partial pancreatectomy in humans. *Diabetologia*, Vol. 52, No.2, February 2009, pp.306-317

Milch, W, Leweke, F, Brosig, B, Reimer, C. (2002). Separation during inpatient psychotherapy and its impact on the regulation of blood glucose in a patient with Brittle Diabetes. *Zeitschrift für Psychosomatische Medizin und Psychotherapie*, Vol.48, No.3, pp.286-298

Mineo, D, Sageshima, J, Burke, GW, Ricordi, C. (2009). Minimization and withdrawal of steroids in pancreas and islet transplantation. *Transplant international*, Vol.22, No.1, (January 2009), pp.20-37

Mineo, D, Ricordi, C, Xu, X, Pileggi A, Garcia-Morales, R, Khan, A, Baidal, DA, Han, D, Monroy, K, Miller, J, Pugliese, A, Froud, T, Inverardi, L, Kenyon, NS, Alejandro, R. (2008). Combined islet and hematopoietic stem cell allotransplantation: a clinical pilot trial to induce chimerism and graft tolerance. *American journal of transplantation*, Vol. 8, No.6, (June 2008), pp.1262-1274

Mitchell, SJ, Hilliard, ME, Mednick, L, Henderson, C, Cogen, FR, Streisand, R. (2009). Stress among fathers of young children with type 1 diabetes. *Families, systems & health* , Vol.27, No.4, (December 2009), pp.314-324

Mody, RJ, Brown, PI, Wechsler, DS. (2003). Refractory iron deficiency anemia as the primary clinical manifestation of celiac disease. *The American journal of pediatric hematology/oncology*, Vol.25, No. 2, (February 2003), pp.169-172

Mohan V, Poongothai S, Pitchumoni CS. (1998). Oral pancreatic enzyme therapy in the control of diabetes mellitus in tropical calculous pancreatitis. *International journal of pancreatology*, Vol.24, No.1, (August 1998), pp.19-22

Morris, AD, Boyle, DI, McMahon, AD, Greene, SA, MacDonald, TM, Newton, RW. (1997). Adherence to insulin treatment, glycaemic control, and ketoacidosis in insulin-dependent diabetes mellitus. The DARTS/MEMO Collaboration. Diabetes Audit and Research in Tayside Scotland. Medicines Monitoring Unit. *Lancet*, Vol.350, No.9090, (November 1997), pp. 1505-1510

National Toxicology Program. (2010). Final Report on Carcinogens Background Document for Formaldehyde. *Report on carcinogens background document*, Vol.10, No.5981, (January 2010), p.i-512

Narendran, P, Creely, SJ, Syed, A, Tesfaye, S, Winer, J, Singh, BM. (2010). Aggressive and devastating neuropathy: the consequence of untreated slow-onset type 1 diabetes. *QJM*. July

O'Hare, JA, Ferriss, JB, Twomey, B, O'Sullivan, DJ. (1983). Poor metabolic control, hypertension and microangiopathy independently increase the transcapillary escape rate of albumin in diabetes, *Diabetologia*, Vol.25, No.3, (September 1983), pp. 260–263.

Otokozawa, S, Ai, M, Diffenderfer, MR, Asztalos, BF, Tanaka, A, Lamon-Fava, S, Schaefer, EJ. (2009). Fasting and postprandial apolipoprotein B-48 levels in healthy, obese, and hyperlipidemic subjects. *Metabolism*, Vol.58, No.11, (November 2009), pp. 1536-1542

Papanas, N, Maltezos, E. (2008). Education for dietary freedom in type 1 diabetes? Yes, it's possible. The *Diabetes educator*, Vol.34, No.1, (January-February 2008), pp.54-58

Papanas, N, Maltezos, E. (2009). The diabetic foot: a global threat and a huge challenge for Greece. *Hippokratia*, Vol.13, No.4, (October 2009), pp.199-204

Park, JY, Chong, AY, Cochran, EK, Kleiner, DE, Haller, MJ, Schatz, DA, Gorden, P. (2008). Type 1 diabetes associated with acquired generalized lipodystrophy and insulin resistance: the effect of long-term leptin therapy. *The Journal of clinical endocrinology and metabolism*, Vol.93, No.1, January 2008, pp. 26-31

Pasricha, PJ, Pehlivanov, ND, Gomez, G, Vittal, H, Lurken, MS, Farrugia, G. (2008). Changes in the gastric enteric nervous system and muscle: a case report on two patients with diabetic gastroparesis. *BMC gastroenterology*, Vol.30, No.8, (May 2008), p.21

Peake, JE, McCrossin, RB, Byrne, G, Shepherd, R. (1996). X-linked immune dysregulation, neonatal insulin dependent diabetes, and intractable diarrhoea. *Archives of disease in childhood. Fetal and neonatal edition*, Vol. 74, No.3, (May 1996), F195-199

Petrovski, G, Dimitrovski, C, Milenkovic, T. (2007) Insulin pump therapy with continuous glucose monitoring improves metabolic control in brittle type 1 diabetes. *Prilozi*, Vol.28, No.1, (July 2007), pp.129-135

Pickup, J, Williams, G, Johns, P, Keen, H. (1983). Clinical features of brittle diabetic patients unresponsive to optimised subcutaneous insulin therapy (continuous subcutaneous insulin infusion). *Diabetes Care*, 1983, Vol.6, pp. 279-284

Pickup, J, Keen, H. (2002). Continuous subcutaneous insulin infusion at 25 years: evidence base for the expanding use of insulin pump therapy in type 1 diabetes. *Diabetes Care*, Vol.25, No.3, pp.593-598

Plank, J, Wutte, A, Brunner, G, Siebenhofer, A, Semlitsch, B, Sommer, R, Hirschberger, S, Pieber, TR. (2002). A direct comparison of insulin aspart and insulin lispro in patients with type 1 diabetes. *Diabetes Care*, Vol.23, No.11, (November 2002), pp.2053-2057

Potter, J, Clarke, P, Gale, EAM, Dave, SH, Tattersall, RS. (1982). Insulin-induced hypoglycaemia in an accident and emergency department: the tip of an iceberg. *BMJ*, Vol. *285*, pp.1180-1182

Ramaswamy, K, Masand, PS, Nasrallah, HA. (2006). Do certain atypical antipsychotics increase the risk of diabetes? A critical review of 17 pharmacoepidemiologic studies. *Annals of clinical psychiatry*, Vol. 18, No.3, (July-September 2006), pp.183-194

Rice DM. Diabetes education... lost in translation? (2006). *Diabetes Educator*, Vol. 32, No.6, (November-December 2006), pp.823-824

Roberts, J, Searle, J. (1995). Neonatal diabetes mellitus associated with severe diarrhea, hyperimmunoglobulin E syndrome, and absence of islets of Langerhans. *Pediatric pathology & laboratory medicine*, Vol.15, No.3, (May-June 1995), pp.477-483

Rosenbloom AL, Giordano BP. (1977). Chronic overtreatment with insulin in children and adolescents. , *American journal of diseases of children* (1960), Vol.131, No.8 (August 1977), pp.881-885

Ryan, EA, Lakey, JR, Rajotte, RV, Korbutt, GS, Kin, T, Imes, S, Rabinovitch, A, Elliott, JF, Bigam, D, Kneteman, NM, Warnock, GL, Larsen, I, Shapiro, AM. (2001). Clinical outcomes and insulin secretion after islet transplantation with the Edmonton protocol. *Diabetes*, Vol.50, No.4, (April 2001), pp.710-9.

Ryder, RE, Owens, DR, Hayes, TM, Ghatei, MA, Bloom, SR. (1990). Unawareness of hypoglycaemia and inadequate hypoglycaemic counterregulation: no causal relation with diabetic autonomic neuropathy. *BMJ*, Vol.301, No.6755, October 1990, pp.783-787

Sabek, OM, Hamilton, DJ, Gaber, AO. (2009). Prospects for future advancements in islet cell transplantation. *Minerva chirurgica*; Vol.64, No.1, (February 2009), pp.59-73

Scantamburlo, G, Ansseau, M, Legros, JJ. (2001). Role of the neurohypophysis in psychological stress. *Encéphale*, Vol.27, No.3, (May-June 2001), pp.245-259

Schade, DS, Eaton, RP, Spencer, W. (1980). Normalization of plasma insulin profiles in diabetic subjects with programmed insulin delivery. *Diabetes Care*, (January-February 1980), Vol.3, No.1, pp.9-14

Schade DS, Eaton RP, Drumm DA, Duckworth WC. (1985). A clinical algorithm to determine the etiology of brittle diabetes. *Diabetes Care*, Vol.8, No.1, (January-February 1985), pp.5-11

Schrader, H, Menge, BA, Zeidler, C, Ritter, PR, Tannapfel, A, Uhl, W, Schmidt, WE, Meier, JJ. (2010). Determinants of glucose control in patients with chronic pancreatitis. *Diabetologia*, Vol.53, No.6, (June 2010), pp.1062-1069

Serlin, DC, Lash, RW. (2009). Diagnosis and management of gestational diabetes mellitus. *American family physician*, Vol. 80, No.1, (July 2009), pp.57-62

Smith, CB, Choudhary, P, Pernet, A, Hopkins, D, Amiel, SA. (2009). Hypoglycemia unawareness is associated with reduced adherence to therapeutic decisions in patients with type 1 diabetes: evidence from a clinical audit. *Diabetes Care*, Vol.32, No.7, (July 2009), pp. 1196-1198

Smith, CM, Clarke, CF, Porteous, LE, Elsori, H, Cameron, DJ. (2000). Prevalence of coeliac disease and longitudinal follow-up of antigliadin antibody status in children and adolescents with type 1 diabetes mellitus. *Pediatric diabetes*, Vol.1, No.4, December 2000, pp.199-203

Somogyi, M. (1959). Exacerbation of diabetes by excess insulin action. *The American journal of medicine*, Vol.26, No.2, (February 1959), pp.169-191

Stancin, T, Link, DL, Reuter, JM. (1989). Binge eating and purging in young women with IDDM. *Diabetes Care*, Vol12, No.9, (October 1989), pp.601-603

Su, JW, Lambert, JE, Clandinin, MT, Proctor, SD. (2009). Impaired postprandial metabolism of apolipoprotein B48-containing remnant particles in normolipidemic subjects with brittle type 1 diabetes. *Diabetes Care*, Vol.32, No.2, (February 2009), pp.e21

Sumino, H, Ichikawa, S, Kumakura, H, Takayama, Y, Kurabayashi, M. (2003). Genetic influence of hormone-replacement therapy on venous thromboembolism. *Lancet*, Vol.362, No.9391, (October 2003), p.1242.

Tallandini, MA. (1999). The dread of integration. Integrative processes in a chronically ill borderline patient. *The Psychoanalytic study of the child*, Vol.54, pp.289-315

Tattersall, RB, Gill, GV. (1991). Unexplained deaths of Type 1 diabetic patients. *Diabetic medicine*, Vol.*8*, pp.49-58

Tattersall, RB, Gregory, R, Selby, C, Kerr, D, Heller, S. (1991) Course of brittle diabetes: 12 year follow up. *BMJ*; Vol.302, No. 6787, (May 1991), pp.1240-1243

Tattersall, RB. (1997). Brittle Diabetes. *Clinics in endocrinology and metabolism*, Vol.6, No.2, (July 1997), pp.403-419

Tattersall, RB. (1997). Brittle diabetes revisited: the Third Arnold Bloom Memorial Lecture. *Diabetic Medicine*, Vol.14, No.2, (February 1997), pp.99-110

Tentolouris, N, Jude, EB, Smirnof, I, Knowles, EA, Boulton, AJ. (1999) Methicillin-resistant Staphylococcus aureus: an increasing problem in a diabetic foot clinic. *Diabetic Medicine*, Vol.16, No.9, September 1999, pp.767-771

Tentolouris, N, Voulgari, C, Liatis, S, Kokkinos, A, Eleftheriadou, I, Makrilakis, K, Marinou, K, Katsilambros N. (2010). Moisture status of the skin of the feet assessed by the visual test neuropad correlates with foot ulceration in diabetes. *Diabetes Care*, Vol.33, No.5, May 2010, pp.1112-1114

Tone, A, Shikata, K, Nakagawa, K, Hashimoto, M, Makino, H. (2008). A case of hypoglycemic brittle diabetes with peripheral edema successfully managed by conversion from insulin lispro to insulin aspart. *Diabetes research and clinical practice*, Vol.81, No.3, (September 2008), e15-e16

Trujillo-Santos, AJ. (2003). Diabetic muscle infarction: an underdiagnosed complication of long-standing diabetes. *Diabetes Care*, Vol.26, No.1, (January 2003), pp.211-215

Vaisrub, S. (1980). Pump and brittle circumstance. *JAMA*, Vol.13, No.243 (22), (June 1980), pp.2331-2332

Valdivielso, P, Puerta, S, Rioja, J, Alonso, I, Ariza, MJ, Sánchez-Chaparro, MA, Palacios, R, González-Santos, P. (2010). Postprandial apolipoprotein B48 is associated with asymptomatic peripheral arterial disease: a study in patients with type 2 diabetes and controls. *Clinica chimica Acta*, Vol.411, No.5-6, (March 2010), pp.433-437

Vantyghem, MC, Press, M. (2006). Management strategies for brittle diabetes. *Annales d'endocrinologie (Paris)*. Vol.67, No.4, (September 2006), pp.287-296

Vantyghem, MC, Kerr-Conte, J, Arnalsteen, L, Sergent, G, Defrance, F, Gmyr, V, Declerck, N, Raverdy, V, Vandewalle, B, Pigny, P, Noel, C, Pattou, F. (2009). Primary graft function, metabolic control, and graft survival after islet transplantation. *Diabetes Care*, Vol.32, No.8, (August 2009), pp.1473-1478

Vantyghem, MC, Marcelli-Tourvieille, S, Fermon, C, Duhamel, A, Raverdy, V, Arnalsteen, L, Kerr-Conte, J, Noel, C, Fontaine, P, Pattou, F. (2009). Intraperitoneal insulin infusion versus islet transplantation: comparative study in patients with type 1 diabetes. *Transplantation*, Vol.87, No.1 (January 2009), pp.66-71.

Venturini, M, Fiorina, P, Maffi, P, Losio, C, Vergani, A, Secchi, A, Del Maschio, A. (2006). Early increase of retinal arterial and venous blood flow velocities at color Doppler imaging in brittle type 1 diabetes after islet transplant alone. *Transplantation*, Vol.81, No.9, (May 2006), pp.1274-1277.

Viner, RM, Christie, D, Taylor, V, Hey, S. (2003). Motivational/solution-focused intervention improves HbA1c in adolescents with Type 1 diabetes: a pilot study. *Diabetic Medicine*, Vol.20, No.9, (September 2003), pp.739-742

Vinik, AI, Maser, RE, Mitchell, BD, Freeman, R. (2003). Diabetic autonomic neuropathy. *Diabetes Care*. Vol. 26, No.5, (May 2003), pp.1553-1579

Virally, M, Laloi-Michelin, M, Médeau, V, Meas, T, Kévorkian, JP, Mouly, S, Guillausseau, PJ. (2007). Muscle infarction in a young woman with brittle type 1 diabetes. *Diabetes & Metabolism*, Vol.33, No.6, (December 2007), pp.466-468

Vogel, A, Strassburg, CP, Obermayer-Straub, P, Brabant, G, Manns, MP. (2002). The genetic background of autoimmune polyendocrinopathy-candidiasis-ectodermal dystrophy and its autoimmune disease components. *Journal of molecular medicine*, Vol.80, No.4, (April 2002), pp.201-211

Voulgari, C, Tentolouris, N. (2010). The performance of a glucose-ketone meter in the diagnosis of diabetic ketoacidosis in patients with type 2 diabetes in the emergency room. *Diabetes technology & therapeutics*, Vol.12, No.7, July 2010, pp.529-535

Voulgari, C, Psallas, M, Kokkinos, A, Argiana, V, Katsilambros, N, Tentolouris, N. (2010). The association between cardiac autonomic neuropathy with metabolic and other factors in subjects with type 1 and type 2 diabetes. *Journal of diabetes and its complications* (August 2010)

Weinzimer, SA, Tamborlane, WV, Chase, HP, Garg, SK. (2004). Continuous glucose monitoring in type 1 diabetes. *Current diabetes reports*, Vol.4, No.2, (April 2004), pp.95-100

Widom B, Simonson DC. (1992). Intermittent hypoglycemia impairs glucose counterregulation. *Diabetes*, Vol.41, No.12, (December 1992), pp.1597-1602

Witkowski, P, Zakai, SB, Rana, A, Sledzinski, Z, Hardy, MA. (2006). Pancreatic islet transplantation, what has been achieved since Edmonton break-through. *Annals of transplantation*, Vol.11, No.2, pp.5-13, discussion 32-43

Woodyatt, RT (1942). The American Diabetes Association. *Science*, Vol.7, No.96 (2484), (August 1942), pp.138

Woolley, SL, Smith, DR. (2006). Acute compartment syndrome secondary to diabetic muscle infarction: case report and literature review. *European journal of emergency medicine*, Vol. 13, No.2, (April 2006), pp.113-116

Wroe, J. (2004). The second international DAWN summit: a call to action to improve psychosocial care for people with diabetes. *Practical Diabetes International*, Vol.21, pp.201 -208

4

Hypoglycemia in Critically Ill Patients

Cornelia Hoedemaekers and Johannes van der Hoeven
Radboud University Nijmegen Medical Centre,
Department of ICU Nijmegen,
The Netherlands

1. Introduction

Dysglycemia is common in critically ill patients. Both hyperglycemia and hypoglycemia are independent risk factors for increased morbidity and mortality. Hypoglycemia severity may even have a 'dose-response' relationship with increased mortality(Bagshaw et al., 2009). Acute hypoglycemia induces a systemic, counter-regulatory stress response that leads to an increase in blood norepinephrine, epinephrine, glucagon, growth hormone, and cortisol concentrations. Risk factors that are associated with the occurrence of hypoglycemia in ICU patients include severity of illness, strict glucose control, continuous veno-venous hemodialysis, decrease of nutrition without adjustment for insulin infusion, a prior diagnosis of diabetes mellitus, sepsis, and need for inotropic support (Arabi et al, 2009;Krinsley & Grover, 2007;Vriesendorp et al. ,2006).

The association between hyperglycemia and mortality seems population dependent, with the strongest association in patients in the cardiac, cardiothoracic and neurological ICU(Whitcomb et al., 2005). During acute illness, hyperglycemia might exert an even more deleterious effect on ICU patients without diabetes than among patients with diabetes(Capes et al., 2000;Krinsley 2006;Rady et al., 2005). Unlike nondiabetic patients, diabetic patients show no clear association between hyperglycemia during intensive care unit stay and mortality and markedly lower odds ratios of death at all levels of hyperglycemia. These findings suggest that, in critically patients with diabetes mellitus, hyperglycemia may have different biological and/or clinical implications(Egi et al., 2008).

Recently, variability of glucose concentrations has been identified as an additional factor that may contribute to the mortality and morbidity of dysglycemia. A retrospective evaluation of over 7000 patients identified glycemic variability, defined as the standard deviation of each patient's mean glucose level during ICU stay, as a stronger predictor of mortality than hyperglycemia(Egi et al., 2006). High glucose variability during ICU stay was associated with increased mortality in patients without diabetes, even after adjustment for severity of illness and mean glucose concentration(Krinsley 2009). In contrast, there was no independent association of glucose variability with mortality among patients with diabetes. Glucose variability contributes to ICU mortality and in-hospital death by increasing oxidative stress, neuronal damage, mitochondrial damage, and coagulation activation.

The relation between glucose concentration and outcome is complex and not linear. The interaction between glucose concentrations and outcome may arise from independent and synergistic domains of glycemic control including central tendency (such as mean and median glucose values), variability and the minimum glucose value (Mackenzie et al., 2011). Using these different metrics of glycemic control, a population-specific relationship between metrics of outcome was demonstrated in patients in a surgical, trauma, cardiac and neurological ICU. This relationship had a dose response component with an n-shape curve in neurological ICU patients, suggesting a survival advantage during hyperglycemia in these patients.

Strict glycemic control may improve morbidity and mortality in critically ill patients. Intensive glucose control is however associated with a higher incidence of hypoglycemia compared to conventionally treated patients. This increased risk of hypoglycemia may limit the use of strict glucose control in critically ill neurological patients, since hypoglycemia is a well known cause of secondary brain injury. In this review we will describe the different aspects of dysglycemia and glycemic control in critically ill patients, with a special emphasis on the critically ill neurological patients.

2. Glucose homeostasis in critically ill patients

Glucose homeostasis is a physiologically well-balanced mechanism depending on coordinated and simultaneously ongoing processes involving insulin secretion by the pancreas, hepatic and renal glucose output and glucose uptake by splanchnic (liver and gut) and peripheral tissues. Cellular uptake of glucose occurs via insulin- or noninsulin-dependent mechanisms. The noninsulin-dependent pathway is the major mechanism of glucose uptake in the basal state, accounting for 75-85% of the total post-prandial glucose uptake and is mainly directed at the brain(Gottesman et al., 1983).

The brain plays a central role in the orchestration of the changes in blood glucose and the appropriate counterregulatory responses (reviewed in (Watts & Donovan, 2010)). Some neurons possess specialized mechanisms that allow them to act as glucosensors and alter their firing rates with fluctuating ambient glucose concentrations. These neurons are predominantly located in the hypothalamus and hindbrain. Important glucosensing elements are also present in the hepatic portal/mesenteric vein, gut, carotid body and oral cavity. Information from the glucosensing elements is processed by neurons in the hypothalamus and hindbrain. These neurons regulate the counterregulatory responses and provide direct input to the appropriate neuroendocrine motor and preganglionic neurons in the hypothalamus, hindbrain, and autonomic ganglia. Their output in turn controls and/or modulates effector cells in the adrenal medulla (chromaffin cells), anterior pituitary (corticotopes and somatotropes), and pancreatic islets (α- and β-cells).

Severe illness induces a stress response with alterations in the glucose metabolism including enhanced peripheral glucose uptake and utilization, hyperlactatemia, increased glucose production, depressed glycogenesis, glucose intolerance, and insulin resistance(Mizock, 1995). Stress hyperglycemia is caused by a highly complex interplay between counterregulatory hormones such as cortisol, epinephrine, norepinephrine and glucagon, leading to an increase in hepatic and renal glucose production and insulin resistance (reviewed in (Dungan et al., 2009)). The hepatic gluconeogenesis that is induced by glucagon, cortisol and epinephrine is the key source of glucose production. The kidney is responsible for approximately 20% of the glucose production under resting conditions(Meyer et al., 2002). During stress, however, cathecholamines can increase the renal contribution to glucose production up to 40% by increasing substrate availability and the gluconeogenic efficiency of the kidney(Meyer et al., 2003). Glucagon increases both gluconeogenesis and glycogenolysis in the liver, but has no effect on the kidney. Cytokines such as IL-6 and TNF-α also contribute to the synthesis of glucose by regulation of key enzymes such as glucose 6-phosphatase (G6Pase) involved in the gluconeogenesis(Blumberg et al., 1995a;Blumberg et al., 1995b). Insulin suppresses glucose release in both the liver and kidney by direct enzyme activation/deactivation, as well as by reducing the availability of gluconeogenic substrates and actions on gluconeogenic activators. Glycogenolysis and reduced glycogen synthesis in the liver probably contribute only to a small extent to the stress induced hyperglycemia.

Insulin resistance is characterized by raised plasma levels of insulin, organ-specific alterations in glucose utilization, and impaired insulin-mediated uptake(Brealey & Singer 2009). The insulin resistance occurs at several levels and is mainly driven by the inflammatory response. TNF-α can activate protein kinase B, resulting in phosphorylation of the insulin receptor thereby reducing the glucose uptake(Fan et al., 1996;Ueki et al., 2004). In addition, a number of animal models measured a significant reduction in the number of insulin receptors(McCowen et al., 2001).

3. Glucose in critically ill neurological patients: Friend or foe?

3.1 Glucose is fuel for the brain

Under normal conditions, the human brain is an obligate glucose consumer and depends almost entirely on the availability of systemic glucose to maintain its normal metabolism. Glucose concentration in brain normally shows a linear relationship to blood concentrations with normal human blood glucose levels ranging between 70-128 mg/dL and the corresponding normal brain concentrations ranging from roughly 14.4-41.4 mg/dL (Gruetter et al., 1998).

Autoradiography and PET have shown that the rate of glucose consumption differs between brain regions, with higher values in grey matter, and also varies with time, with active areas capturing more glucose compared to inactive areas(Raichle & Mintun, 2006). In critically ill neurological patients the metabolic demand of the brain is increased, resulting in a relative deficiency in cerebral extracellular glucose(Bergsneider et al., 1997;Hutchinson et al., 2009).

Glucose is transported from the blood across the endothelial cells in the blood-brain barrier and across the plasma membranes of neurons and glia cells. Rapid breakdown of glucose by the brain creates a concentration gradient between the cerebrospinal fluid and the blood, resulting in a driving force of glucose towards the brain. Glucose is transported to the brain by facilitated glucose transport that is mediated by members of the glucose transporter (GLUT) protein family. Several GLUT isoforms have been identified in the brain: GLUT1 is highly expressed on endothelial cells at the blood-brain-barrier and in astrocytes, whereas GLUT3 is detected in neurons and GLUT5 in microglia (Vannucci et al., 1997).

During normal activity, glucose is the predominant energy substrate for neurons. The metabolic coupling between neurons and astrocytes preserves energy homeostasis in the brain during increased neuronal activity. Activation of neurons is accompanied by an increase in local cerebral blood flow, thus increasing the delivery of energy substrates. Glucose metabolism itself is also tightly coupled to neuronal activity: activation of astrocytes by glutamate, that is released by neurons, results in increased production of lactate by astrocytes that can be used as fuel by neurons to meet their energy demand (the astrocyte-neuron lactate shuffle)(Pellerin et al., 2007;Pellerin & Magistretti, 2004;Rothman et al., 1999). This astrocyte-neuron lactate shuffle also contributes to neurotransmitter recycling and restoration of neuronal membrane potentials. Recent studies indicate that the human brain has the capacity to support up to 10% of its energy metabolism with lactate. Lactate in plasma can cross the blood-brain barrier through monocarboxylate transporters(Simpson et al., 2007). Plasma lactate may become a significant source of fuel in conditions of increased plasma lactate levels or when blood glucose levels are reduced, accounting for up to 60% of the energy metabolism(Boumezbeur et al., 2010).

Glycogen metabolism is also under the control of metabolic coupling. Glycogen is predominantly localized in the peripheral astrocytic processes surrounding the neuronal elements and serves as an endogenous source of energy for these cells and for neurons during extreme energy failure. Neurochemical signals from neurons and astrocytes trigger glycogenolysis. In astrocytes, glucose derived from glycogenolysis is used for both oxidative metabolism and for production of lactate(Benarroch, 2010). This lactate serves as an energy substrate for oxidative metabolism in neurons.

Since the brain relies upon plasma glucose as its primary energy source, a reduced blood glucose concentration promptly induces a complex counter regulatory response aiming at recovery of plasma glucose concentrations. Glucagon and epinephrine are released after a small decrease in glucose concentration, followed by activation of the autonomic nervous system. This hypoglycemia induced systemic stress response is accompanied by an increasing cerebral blood flow and altered cerebral metabolism with increased glycogenolysis. Depending on the duration and severity, the effects of hypoglycemia span from mild changes in EEG signals to irreversible brain injury and coma. Not all neurons are equally sensitive to hypoglycemic injury. Neurons in the cerebral cortex and the hippocampus are affected preferentially, followed by neurons in the basal ganglia and the thalamus. Neurons in the brain stem, the cerebellum, and the spinal cord are generally spared, as are glial cells and white matter tracts (Auer et al., 1989). The hypoglycemic neuronal damage is not a direct result of energy failure but mainly caused by an excitotoxic amino acid mediated increase in intracellular calcium, production of reactive oxygen species and apoptosis (Suh et al., 2007).

In acute brain injury, the hypoglycemic threshold is lower compared to normal brain and even mild hypoglycemia can induce neuroglycopenia. In patients after traumatic brain injury, arterial glucose levels < 108 mg/dL resulted in decreased brain glucose concentrations with an increased cerebral uptake of glucose(Meierhans et al., 2010). Microdialysis markers of brain metabolic distress were significantly reduced at brain glucose concentrations > 18 mg/dL, reaching the lowest levels at arterial blood glucose levels between 108-162 mg/dL. From this study it was concluded that arterial blood glucose concentrations between 108-162 mg/dL were optimal in traumatic brain injury. In addition, low brain glucose concentrations are associated with recurrent, spontaneous, spreading depolarizations in pericontusional tissue, resulting in a further reduction in brain glucose concentration and an ongoing brain damage (Feuerstein et al., 2010;Parkin et al., 2005).

3.2 Glucose is toxic to the brain

Stress-related hyperglycaemia, previously considered to be a protective physiological response to meet the increased demands of an injury, is associated with a poor outcome in critically ill patients. This association of poor outcome and hyperglycemia has been consistently confirmed across multiple studies and different disease entities such as traumatic brain injury (Jeremitsky et al., 2005;Lam et al., 1991;Rovlias & Kotsou, 2000;Salim et al., 2009), intracranial hemorrhage (Fogelholm et al., 2005;Godoy et al., 2008;Godoy et al., 2009;Godoy & Di, 2007;Kimura et al., 2007;Passero et al., 2003) and subarachnoid hemorrhage (Badjatia et al., 2005;Frontera et al., 2006;Kruyt et al., 2008;Kruyt et al., 2009;Lanzino et al., 1993).

Hyperglycemia is associated with many detrimental effects, including reduced immune function, increased inflammation and coagulation, and modulation of the endothelium. Plasma concentrations of pro-inflammatory cytokines are increased during hyperglycemia, while insulin reduces the pro-inflammatory cytokine response and restores the pro- and anti-inflammatory balance (Turina et al., 2005). Glucose increases basal TNFα and IL-6 production in human monocytes *in-vitro* (Morohoshi et al., 1996). Similarly, a glucose-dependent increased production of TNFα by peripheral blood cells *in-vitro* after stimulation with lipopolysaccharide was measured, whereas glucose does not influence the production of the anti-inflammatory cytokine IL-10 (Hancu et al., 1998). *In-vivo* induced hypoglycaemia in hypoglycaemic human clamp models resulted in a down-modulation of lipopolysaccharide -induced TNFα synthesis(de Galan et al., 2003). Hyperglycemia increases the expression of tissue factor, which has both proinflammatory and procoagulant functions(Brealey & Singer, 2009). Hyperglycemia induces endothelial dysfunction through several damaging pathways, including the polyol/sorbitol/aldose reductase pathway, the protein kinase C pathway, the accumulation of non-enzymatic glycation end products and by increased oxidative stress, ultimately leading to increased expression of endothial cytokines and adhesion molecules (van den Oever et al., 2010). Insulin infusion restores normoglycemia in critically ill patients and improves and restores host defence, haemodynamics and coagulation abnormalities.

The deleterious effects of acute hyperglycemia on brain injury has been demonstrated in a large number of animal studies (reviewed in (Ergul et al., 2009)). Hyperglycemia increases infarct volume in focal models of ischemia and aggravates necrosis in global ischemia/reperfusion models. In addition, hyperglycemia contributes to the vascular damage during ischemia/reperfusion injury, resulting in increased hemorrhagic transformation during reperfusion(de Court et al., 1989;de Court et al., 1988). Marked blood-brain barrier disruption with formation of brain edema has been found in hyperglycemic rats after temporary and permanent middle cerebral artery occlusion(Kamada et al., 2007). In diabetes adaptive protective mechanisms gradually develop, protecting the subject against acute hyperglycemia. Diabetes promotes neovascularization, remodeling and increases in vascular tone limiting cerebral perfusion(Ergul et al., 2009). Resulting hypoxia and/or metabolic changes mediate ischemic tolerance via neuronal preconditioning but decreases vascular ischemic tolerance leading to increased and accelerated hemorrhagic transformation and development of edema in the event of an ischemic event. Acute hyperglycemia also increases vascular tone and disrupts vascular integrity but in the absence of sufficient time to stimulate adaptive protective mechanisms, the magnitude of neuronal damage is greater.

Cerebral ischemia results in widespread activation of the systemic inflammatory system (Offner et al., 2006). Systemic inflammatory mediators such as cytokines and adhesion molecules can activate microglial cells and perivascular macrophages and contribute to irreversible brain ischemia(Bemeur et al., 2007). After the initial activation of the innate immune response, inflammatory cells from the periphery are mobilized and contribute to microvessel obstruction, edema formation, cellular necrosis and tissue infarction.

Hyperglycemia enhances neutrophil infiltration and increases cytokine expression in several animal models of cerebral ischemia and likely exacerbates the ischemic injury(Bemeur et al., 2005).

4. Glucose control in critically ill patients

4.1 Intensive insulin therapy

A number of randomized controlled trials have been performed on the effects of strict glucose control in critically ill patients. Two single centre trials were performed in Leuven by van den Berghe et al(Van den Berghe et al., 2001;Van den Berghe et al., 2006a), followed by a number of multicentre trials. The first Leuven trial compared maintenance of blood glucose levels between 80 and 110 mg/dl versus 180 and 200 mg/dl in critically ill patients in a surgical ICU(Van den Berghe et al., 2001). In this trial strict glucose control resulted in a 42% reduction in mortality compared with conventional treatment. Septic patients and patients with an ICU stay > 5 days showed the largest reduction in mortality. In the second trial from Leuven performed in medical ICU patients no mortality benefit was demonstrated in the overall intention to treat analysis(Van den Berghe et al., 2006a). A reduction in hospital mortality from 52.5 to 43.0 percent was found in patients treated with intensive insulin therapy who stayed in the ICU for 3 days or more. Among patients treated < 3 days in the ICU, mortality was higher in the insulin group compared to the conventional group. The incidence of hypoglycemia was higher in the intervention group compared to the conventional treatment in both trials. Pooling the two datasets of both Leuven trials revealed that intensive insulin therapy reduced morbidity and mortality in a mixed surgical/medical ICU population, especially when continued for at least 3 days, without causing harm to patients treated for < 3 days(Van den Berghe et al., 2006b). The subgroup of patients with a prior history of diabetes did not appear to benefit. Blood glucose maintained at < 110 mg/dl was more effective that at 110-150 mg/dl, but also carried the highest risk of hypoglycemia.

How strict control of blood glucose reduces morbidity and mortality is unknown, but the mechanism may be related either to a direct effect of normalization of hyperglycemia or to the concomitantly higher insulin levels. *Post hoc* multivariate logistic regression analysis of the study by van den Berghe *et al.* suggests that the lowered blood glucose level rather than the insulin dose is related to the reduction in mortality (Van den Berghe et al., 2003). Apart from glucose lowering, insulin has a number of nonglycemic metabolic effects that may be important in critical illness (reviewed in (Honiden & Inzucchi, 2010)). Insulin can modulate inflammation via the mannose binding lectin pathway, via NF-kB and via modulation of pro- and anti-inflammatory cytokines. It can reduce free fatty acids and reverse the state of dyslipidemia in critical illness, regulate apotosis, prevent endothelial dysfunction and hypercoagulation, decrease neutrophil chemotaxis and leukocyte adhesion and prevent excessive nitric oxide which may help regulate oxidative stress.

A retrospective analysis of the databases of the two Leuven trials assessed the effect of intensive insulin therapy on blood glucose amplitude variation and pattern irregularity in critically ill patients(Meyfroidt et al., 2010). The Leuven intensive insulin therapy strategy increased mean daily delta blood glucose while not affecting standard deviation blood glucose. Increased blood glucose amplitude variation and pattern irregularity were associated with mortality, irrespective of blood glucose level. In contrast, the reduced mortality observed with intensive insulin therapy in the Leuven trials could not be attributed to an effect on blood glucose amplitude variation.

After these landmark studies by Van den Berghe in 2001 and 2006, tight glycemic control was adopted as standard care in a large number of ICUs. However, subsequent randomized controlled multicentre trials were unable to replicate the results of these landmark trials. The Glucontrol study compared strict glucose control (blood glucose concentrations 80-110 mg/dL) to a target glucose between 140-180mg/dL, in an attempt to prevent the adverse effects of severe hyperglycemia, while reducing the risks of hypoglycemia(Preiser et al., 2009). This multicentre study was stopped early due to the high rate of protocol violations. Strict glucose control failed to induce any clinical benefit, but was associated with a higher incidence of hypoglycemia. The VISEP trial was a multicenter, two-by-two factorial trial, that randomly assigned patients with severe sepsis to receive either intensive insulin therapy to maintain euglycemia or conventional insulin therapy and either a low-molecular-weight hydroxyethyl starch or modified Ringer's lactate for fluid resuscitation(Brunkhorst et al., 2008). After the first safety analysis, involving 488 patients intensive insulin therapy was terminated early by the data and safety monitoring board, owing to an increased number of hypoglycemic events (12.1%), as compared with conventional insulin therapy (2.1%). No differences in mortality and morbidity between the intensive and conventional treatments groups were found, but patients in the intensive-therapy group tended to have longer stays in the ICU than did patients in the conventional therapy group. The NICE-SUGAR trial was a large, international, randomized trial comparing intensive glucose control, with a target blood glucose range of 81 to 108 mg/dl to conventional glucose control, with a target < 180 mg/dl(Finfer et al. 2009). Intensive glucose control increased the absolute risk of death at 90 days by 2.6 percentage points; this represents a number needed to harm of 38. The difference in mortality remained significant after adjustment for potential confounders. Severe hypoglycemia was significantly more common with intensive glucose control. Given this lack of reproducible results in a heterogeneous group of ICU patients, and concerns over excessive hypoglycemia, extremely tight glucose control cannot be considered standard of care in ICU patients.

The multicentre trials were unable to replicate the findings of the 2 Leuven trials and raised the possibility that intensive insulin therapy may even increase the risk of mortality and morbidity in ICU patients. The explanation for the disparate findings seems multifactorial. In the Leuven studies the rate of use of total parenteral nutrition was higher compared to the other studies. Intensive insulin therapy may increase mortality in patients receiving enteral nutrition, possibly related to the adverse effects associated with hypoglycemia(Marik & Preiser, 2010). In turn, high dose parenteral glucose administration in the absence of intensive insulin therapy results in hyperglycemia with associated organ failure and death. In the Leuven studies, adjustments of insulin dosage were exclusively based on blood glucose measured on arterial blood via a point-of-care blood gas/glucose analyzer, whereas other studies used samples obtained from different sites and measured with different devices. The conventional treatment differed among the studies(Gunst & Van den Berghe, 2010). In the Leuven studies higher glucose values were tolerated compared to the other trials and the beneficial effects of intensive insulin therapy in these studies may be obtained by preventing excessive hyperglycemia.

4.2 Intensive insulin therapy in brain injury

Hyperglycemia at the time of brain injury is associated with increased morbidity and mortality. A planned subgroup analysis in patients with isolated brain injury of the first

Leuven study revealed that intensive insulin therapy resulted in lower intracranial pressures, less seizures and a better long-term rehabilitation. Strict glucose control also protected general ICU patients against critical illness polyneuropathy.
A number of small studies on glucose control in critically ill neurological patients have been published, but most of these trials were too small to achieve sufficient statistical power to demonstrate possible effects on neurological outcome or mortality. Intensive insulin therapy did not change the incidence of vasospasm, neurological outcome or mortality rates in patients with acute subarachnoid hemorrhage(Bilotta et al., 2007). A decrease in infection rate from 42 to 27% was observed in the patients with strict glucose control compared to conventional glucose control. No differences in neurological outcome or mortality rates were found in patients after severe traumatic brain injury(Bilotta et al., 2008;Coester et al., 2010). A trial in 483 patients undergoing elective or emergency brain surgery revealed that intensive insulin therapy significantly reduced the length of stay in the ICU (6 vs. 8 days), and the infection rate (25.7% vs. 39.3%) without a significant effect on neurological outcome or survival at 6 months(Bilotta et al., 2009). In the UK Glucose Insulin in Stroke Trial (GIST-UK) patients presenting within 24 hours of stroke onset were randomly assigned to receive glucose-potassium-insulin infusion aiming at a capillary glucose between 72-126 mg/dL or no glucose intervention(Gray et al., 2007). The trial was stopped due to slow enrolment after 933 patients were recruited. There was no significant reduction in mortality or neurological disability at 90 days, although the study was underpowered and alternative results could not be excluded. The Treatment of Hyperglycemia in Ischemic Stroke (THIS) trial revealed similar results(Bruno et al., 2008). Strict versus moderate glucose control did not improve outcome in patients after resuscitation from ventricular fibrillation(Oksanen et al., 2007). Intensive or conventional control of blood glucose levels in mechanically ventilated adult neurologic ICU patients resulted in a non-significant increase in mortality in the patients in the intensive insulin group (36 vs 25%), with no differences in functional outcome(Green et al., 2010).
The results from the studies on strict glucose control in unselected critically ill patients may not be directly applicable to patients with critical neurological disease because of the high sensitivity of the brain to the effects of hypoglycemia. Tight glucose control was complicated by an increased number of hypoglycemic events in all trials in critically ill neurological patients. Since studies in patients with acute brain injury did not show a beneficial effect of strict glucose control on mortality or neurological outcome, the markedly increased risk of hypoglycemia limits the safe use of intensive insulin therapy these patients.

5. Glucose monitoring in the ICU setting

Detection of hypoglycemia is difficult in ICU patients since these patients are often sedated and incapable of communicating, thereby masking clinical symptoms and signs. Frequent glucose measurement is therefore required to titrate the amount of insulin and detect episodes of hypoglycemia. For practical reasons bedside point of care (POCT) devices are frequently used. The accuracy of the POCT monitoring is influenced in several ways, including both preanalytic and analytic parameters. Glucose concentrations may differ according to the blood sampling site (venous, arterial or capillary blood). In critically ill patients, capillary blood glucose measured by fingerstick is inaccurate(Critchell et al., 2007;Kanji et al., 2005). Capillary sampling led to both overestimation(Kanji et al., 2005) and underestimation(Atkin et al., 1991) of blood glucose values. The presence of shock, use of vasopressors and upper extremity edema were associated with the occurrence of inaccurate readings.

The reliability of the POCT devices itself in critically ill patients is also poor. In a prospective observational study the performance of 3 different POCT devices was tested and compared with the glucose oxidase method in arterial blood samples(Hoedemaekers et al., 2008). To minimize preanalytical bias the measurements were performed simultaneously by an experienced laboratory technician under controlled circumstances using a single arterial blood sample. Paired samples from all 3 tested devices were inaccurate in 4.9-13.4% of measurements. Inaccurate glucose readings were most frequently falsely elevated, and occurred over the entire range of blood glucose values. Patients with inaccurate POCT glucose results were significantly older, had a higher disease severity score, and a higher ICU mortality compared with patients with accurate glucose values. The mechanism underlying the differences in glucose values between the different POCT systems and the glucose oxidase method in critically ill patients is unknown. Accu-Chek uses the glucosedehydrogenase-pyrroloquinolinequinone method for glucose determination, which is not specific for glucose. This method misinterprets maltose, icodextrine (which is converted to maltose), galactose, and xylose as glucose, leading to erroneously elevated glucose levels (Schleis, 2007). In addition, a large number of drugs commonly used in the treatment of critically ill patients, such as acetaminophen, dopamine, and mannitol, interfere with a number of POCT test systems. Changes in hematocrit concentration can influence the results of POCT measurements. Depending on the point-of-care testing device that is used both overestimation and underestimation of the glucose values can occur in patients with low hematocrit levels(Karon et al., 2008). Glucose measurement in the ICU setting using these bedside devices can be inaccurate and potentially dangerous: inaccurate glucose readings are most frequently falsely elevated, resulting in misinterpretation of high glucose values with subsequent inappropriate insulin administration or masking of true hypoglycemia.
In the past decade continuous glucose measurement devices have been developed in order to make glycemic management safer and more efficient. Due to concerns regarding altered perfusion in critical illness, many have questioned the accuracy of such devices in ICUs. So far, both excellent and poor performance has been reported in ICU patients (Bridges et al,. 2010;Corstjens et al., 2006;Holzinger et al., 2009;Price et al., 2008). Until these matters are solved, continuous monitoring of interstitial glucose values should be used with caution in the ICU.

6. Conclusion

Glucose control in the ICU is markedly different from that in an out-patient clinic. Severe illness induces dysglycemia, with potential detrimental effects of low, high and variable glucose values. The injured brain is particularly susceptible for changes in glucose concentrations. strict glucose control is not proven beneficial in neurological ICU patients and has a unacceptable risk of hypoglycemia. Glucose control in the neurological ICU should be focused on maintenance of a steady level of glucose between 8-10 mmol/l, avoiding large fluctuations. Glucose monitoring in neurological ICU patients is difficult and requires special attention.

7. References

Arabi, Y. M., H. M. Tamim, and A. H. Rishu. (2009). Hypoglycemia with intensive insulin therapy in critically ill patients: predisposing factors and association with mortality. *Crit Care Med.* 37:2536-2544.

Atkin, S. H., A. Dasmahapatra, M. A. Jaker, M. I. Chorost, and S. Reddy. (1991). Fingerstick glucose determination in shock *Ann.Intern.Med.* 114:1020-1024.

Auer, R. N., J. Hugh, E. Cosgrove, and B. Curry. (1989). Neuropathologic findings in three cases of profound hypoglycemia. *Clin.Neuropathol.* 8:63-68.

Badjatia, N., M. A. Topcuoglu, F. S. Buonanno, E. E. Smith, R. G. Nogueira, G. A. Rordorf, B. S. Carter, C. S. Ogilvy, and A. B. Singhal. (2005). Relationship between hyperglycemia and symptomatic vasospasm after subarachnoid hemorrhage. *Crit Care Med.* 33:1603-1609.

Bagshaw, S. M., R. Bellomo, M. J. Jacka, M. Egi, G. K. Hart, and C. George. (2009). The impact of early hypoglycemia and blood glucose variability on outcome in critical illness. *Crit Care* 13:R91.

Bemeur, C., L. Ste-Marie, P. Desjardins, L. Vachon, R. F. Butterworth, A. S. Hazell, and J. Montgomery. (2005). Dehydroascorbic acid normalizes several markers of oxidative stress and inflammation in acute hyperglycemic focal cerebral ischemia in the rat. *Neurochem.Int.* 46:399-407.

Bemeur, C., L. Ste-Marie, and J. Montgomery. (2007). Increased oxidative stress during hyperglycemic cerebral ischemia *Neurochem.Int.* 50:890-904.

Benarroch, E. E. (2010). Glycogen metabolism: metabolic coupling between astrocytes and neurons. *Neurology* 74:919-923.

Bergsneider, M., D. A. Hovda, E. Shalmon, D. F. Kelly, P. M. Vespa, N. A. Martin, M. E. Phelps, D. L. McArthur, M. J. Caron, J. F. Kraus, and D. P. Becker. (1997). Cerebral hyperglycolysis following severe traumatic brain injury in humans: a positron emission tomography study. *J.Neurosurg.* 86:241-251.

Bilotta, F., R. Caramia, I. Cernak, F. P. Paoloni, A. Doronzio, V. Cuzzone, A. Santoro, and G. Rosa. (2008). Intensive insulin therapy after severe traumatic brain injury: a randomized clinical trial. *Neurocrit.Care* 9:159-166.

Bilotta, F., R. Caramia, F. P. Paoloni, R. Delfini, and G. Rosa. (2009). Safety and efficacy of intensive insulin therapy in critical neurosurgical patients. *Anesthesiology* 110:611-619.

Bilotta, F., A. Spinelli, F. Giovannini, A. Doronzio, R. Delfini, and G. Rosa. (2007). The effect of intensive insulin therapy on infection rate, vasospasm, neurologic outcome, and mortality in neurointensive care unit after intracranial aneurysm clipping in patients with acute subarachnoid hemorrhage: a randomized prospective pilot trial. *J.Neurosurg.Anesthesiol.* 19:156-160.

Blumberg, D., S. Hochwald, M. F. Brennan, and M. Burt. (1995a). Interleukin-6 stimulates gluconeogenesis in primary cultures of rat hepatocytes. *Metabolism* 44:145-146.

Blumberg, D., S. Hochwald, M. Burt, D. Donner, and M. F. Brennan. (1995b). Tumor necrosis factor alpha stimulates gluconeogenesis from alanine in vivo. *J.Surg.Oncol.* 59:220-224.

Boumezbeur, F., K. F. Petersen, G. W. Cline, G. F. Mason, K. L. Behar, G. I. Shulman, and D. L. Rothman. (2010). The contribution of blood lactate to brain energy metabolism in humans measured by dynamic 13C nuclear magnetic resonance spectroscopy. *J.Neurosci.* 30:13983-13991.

Brealey, D. and M. Singer. (2009). Hyperglycemia in critical illness: a review. *J.Diabetes Sci.Technol.* 3:1250-1260.

Bridges, B. C., C. M. Preissig, K. O. Maher, and M. R. Rigby. (2010). Continuous glucose monitors prove highly accurate in critically ill children. *Crit Care* 14:R176.

Brunkhorst, F. M., C. Engel, F. Bloos, A. Meier-Hellmann, M. Ragaller, N. Weiler, O. Moerer, M. Gruendling, M. Oppert, S. Grond, D. Olthoff, U. Jaschinski, S. John, R. Rossaint, T. Welte, M. Schaefer, P. Kern, E. Kuhnt, M. Kiehntopf, C. Hartog, C. Natanson, M. Loeffler, and K. Reinhart. (2008). Intensive insulin therapy and pentastarch resuscitation in severe sepsis. *N.Engl.J.Med.* 358:125-139.

Bruno, A., T. A. Kent, B. M. Coull, R. R. Shankar, C. Saha, K. J. Becker, B. M. Kissela, and L. S. Williams. (2008). Treatment of hyperglycemia in ischemic stroke (THIS): a randomized pilot trial. *Stroke* 39:384-389.

Capes, S. E., D. Hunt, K. Malmberg, and H. C. Gerstein. (2000). Stress hyperglycaemia and increased risk of death after myocardial infarction in patients with and without diabetes: a systematic overview. *Lancet* 355:773-778.

Coester, A., C. R. Neumann, and M. I. Schmidt. (2010). Intensive insulin therapy in severe traumatic brain injury: a randomized trial. *J.Trauma* 68:904-911.

Corstjens, A. M., J. J. Ligtenberg, der Horst van, I, R. Spanjersberg, J. S. Lind, J. E. Tulleken, J. H. Meertens, and J. G. Zijlstra. (2006). Accuracy and feasibility of point-of-care and continuous blood glucose analysis in critically ill ICU patients. *Crit Care* 10:R135.

Critchell, C. D., V. Savarese, A. Callahan, C. Aboud, S. Jabbour, and P. Marik. (2007). Accuracy of bedside capillary blood glucose measurements in critically ill patients. *Intensive Care Med.* 33:2079-2084.

de Court, M. Kleinholz, K. R. Wagner, and R. E. Myers. (1989). Fatal strokes in hyperglycemic cats. *Stroke* 20:1707-1715.

de Court, R. E. Myers, and L. Schoolfield. (1988). Hyperglycemia enlarges infarct size in cerebrovascular occlusion in cats. *Stroke* 19:623-630.

de Galan, B. E., M. G. Netea, P. Smits, and J. W. van der Meer. (2003). Hypoglycaemia downregulates endotoxin-induced production of tumour necrosis factor-alpha, but does not affect IL-1beta, IL-6, or IL-10. *Cytokine* 22:71-76.

Dungan, K. M., S. S. Braithwaite, and J. C. Preiser. (2009). Stress hyperglycaemia. *Lancet* 373:1798-1807.

Egi, M., R. Bellomo, E. Stachowski, C. J. French, and G. Hart. (2006). Variability of blood glucose concentration and short-term mortality in critically ill patients. *Anesthesiology* 105:244-252.

Egi, M., R. Bellomo, E. Stachowski, C. J. French, G. K. Hart, C. Hegarty, and M. Bailey. (2008). Blood glucose concentration and outcome of critical illness: the impact of diabetes. *Crit Care Med.* 36:2249-2255.

Ergul, A., W. Li, M. M. Elgebaly, A. Bruno, and S. C. Fagan. (2009). Hyperglycemia, diabetes and stroke: focus on the cerebrovasculature. *Vascul.Pharmacol.* 51:44-49.

Fan, J., Y. H. Li, M. M. Wojnar, and C. H. Lang. (1996). Endotoxin-induced alterations in insulin-stimulated phosphorylation of insulin receptor, IRS-1, and MAP kinase in skeletal muscle. *Shock* 6:164-170.

Feuerstein, D., A. Manning, P. Hashemi, R. Bhatia, M. Fabricius, C. Tolias, C. Pahl, M. Ervine, A. J. Strong, and M. G. Boutelle. (2010). Dynamic metabolic response to multiple spreading depolarizations in patients with acute brain injury: an online microdialysis study. *J.Cereb.Blood Flow Metab* 30:1343-1355.

Finfer, S., D. R. Chittock, S. Y. Su, D. Blair, D. Foster, V. Dhingra, R. Bellomo, D. Cook, P. Dodek, W. R. Henderson, P. C. Hebert, S. Heritier, D. K. Heyland, C. McArthur, E. McDonald, I. Mitchell, J. A. Myburgh, R. Norton, J. Potter, B. G. Robinson, and J. J. Ronco. (2009). Intensive versus conventional glucose control in critically ill patients. *N.Engl.J.Med.* 360:1283-1297.

Fogelholm, R., K. Murros, A. Rissanen, and S. Avikainen. (2005). Admission blood glucose and short term survival in primary intracerebral haemorrhage: a population based study. *J.Neurol.Neurosurg.Psychiatry* 76:349-353.

Frontera, J. A., A. Fernandez, J. Claassen, M. Schmidt, H. C. Schumacher, K. Wartenberg, R. Temes, A. Parra, N. D. Ostapkovich, and S. A. Mayer. (2006). Hyperglycemia after SAH: predictors, associated complications, and impact on outcome. *Stroke* 37:199-203.

Godoy, D. A. and Napoli M. Di. (2007). Hyperglycemia in acute phase of spontaneous intracerebral hemorrhage (sICH). *J.Neurol.Sci.* 263:228-229.

Godoy, D. A., G. R. Pinero, S. Svampa, F. Papa, and Napoli M. Di. (2008). Hyperglycemia and short-term outcome in patients with spontaneous intracerebral hemorrhage. *Neurocrit.Care* 9:217-229.

Godoy, D. A., G. R. Pinero, S. Svampa, F. Papa, and Napoli M. Di. (2009). Early hyperglycemia and intravenous insulin-the rationale and management of hyperglycemia for spontaneous intracerebral hemorrhage patients: is time for change? *Neurocrit.Care* 10:150-153.

Gottesman, I., L. Mandarino, and J. Gerich. (1983). Estimation and kinetic analysis of insulin-independent glucose uptake in human subjects. *Am.J.Physiol* 244:E632-E635.

Gray, C. S., A. J. Hildreth, P. A. Sandercock, J. E. O'Connell, D. E. Johnston, N. E. Cartlidge, J. M. Bamford, O. F. James, and K. G. Alberti. (2007). Glucose-potassium-insulin infusions in the management of post-stroke hyperglycaemia: the UK Glucose Insulin in Stroke Trial (GIST-UK). *Lancet Neurol.* 6:397-406.

Green, D. M., K. H. O'Phelan, S. L. Bassin, C. W. Chang, T. S. Stern, and S. M. Asai. (2010). Intensive versus conventional insulin therapy in critically ill neurologic patients. *Neurocrit.Care* 13:299-306.

Gruetter, R., K. Ugurbil, and E. R. Seaquist. (1998). Steady-state cerebral glucose concentrations and transport in the human brain. *J.Neurochem.* 70:397-408.

Gunst, J. and Berghe G. Van den. (2010). Blood glucose control in the intensive care unit: benefits and risks. *Semin.Dial.* 23:157-162.

Hancu, N., M. G. Netea, and I. Baciu. (1998). High glucose concentrations increase the tumor necrosis factor-alpha production capacity by human peripheral blood mononuclear cells. *Rom.J.Physiol* 35:325-330.

Hoedemaekers, C. W., J. M. Klein Gunnewiek, M. A. Prinsen, J. L. Willems, and J. G. Van der Hoeven. (2008). Accuracy of bedside glucose measurement from three glucometers in critically ill patients. *Crit Care Med.* 36:3062-3066.

Holzinger, U., J. Warszawska, R. Kitzberger, H. Herkner, P. G. Metnitz, and C. Madl. (2009). Impact of shock requiring norepinephrine on the accuracy and reliability of subcutaneous continuous glucose monitoring. *Intensive Care Med.* 35:1383-1389.

Honiden, S. and S. E. Inzucchi. (2010). Glucose Controversies in the ICU. *J.Intensive Care Med.*

Hutchinson, P. J., M. T. O'Connell, A. Seal, J. Nortje, I. Timofeev, P. G. Al-Rawi, J. P. Coles, T. D. Fryer, D. K. Menon, J. D. Pickard, and K. L. Carpenter. (2009). A combined microdialysis and FDG-PET study of glucose metabolism in head injury. *Acta Neurochir.(Wien.)* 151:51-61.

Jeremitsky, E., L. A. Omert, C. M. Dunham, J. Wilberger, and A. Rodriguez. (2005). The impact of hyperglycemia on patients with severe brain injury. *J.Trauma* 58:47-50.

Kamada, H., F. Yu, C. Nito, and P. H. Chan. (2007). Influence of hyperglycemia on oxidative stress and matrix metalloproteinase-9 activation after focal cerebral ischemia/reperfusion in rats: relation to blood-brain barrier dysfunction. *Stroke* 38:1044-1049.

Kanji, S., J. Buffie, B. Hutton, P. S. Bunting, A. Singh, K. McDonald, D. Fergusson, L. A. McIntyre, and P. C. Hebert. (2005). Reliability of point-of-care testing for glucose measurement in critically ill adults. *Crit Care Med.* 33:2778-2785.

Karon, B. S., L. Griesmann, R. Scott, S. C. Bryant, J. A. Dubois, T. L. Shirey, S. Presti, and P. J. Santrach. (2008). Evaluation of the impact of hematocrit and other interference on the accuracy of hospital-based glucose meters. *Diabetes Technol.Ther.* 10:111-120.

Kimura, K., Y. Iguchi, T. Inoue, K. Shibazaki, N. Matsumoto, K. Kobayashi, and S. Yamashita. (2007). Hyperglycemia independently increases the risk of early death in acute spontaneous intracerebral hemorrhage. *J.Neurol.Sci.* 255:90-94.

Krinsley, J. S. (2006). Glycemic control, diabetic status, and mortality in a heterogeneous population of critically ill patients before and during the era of intensive glycemic management: six and one-half years experience at a university-affiliated community hospital. *Semin.Thorac.Cardiovasc.Surg.* 18:317-325.

Krinsley, J. S. (2009). Glycemic variability and mortality in critically ill patients: the impact of diabetes. *J.Diabetes Sci.Technol.* 3:1292-1301.

Krinsley, J. S. and A. Grover. (2007). Severe hypoglycemia in critically ill patients: risk factors and outcomes. *Crit Care Med.* 35:2262-2267.

Kruyt, N. D., G. J. Biessels, R. J. de Haan, M. Vermeulen, G. J. Rinkel, B. Coert, and Y. B. Roos. (2009). Hyperglycemia and clinical outcome in aneurysmal subarachnoid hemorrhage: a meta-analysis. *Stroke* 40:e424-e430.

Kruyt, N. D., Y. W. Roos, S. M. Dorhout Mees, W. M. van den Bergh, A. Algra, G. J. Rinkel, and G. J. Biessels. (2008). High mean fasting glucose levels independently predict poor outcome and delayed cerebral ischaemia after aneurysmal subarachnoid haemorrhage. *J.Neurol.Neurosurg.Psychiatry* 79:1382-1385.

Lam, A. M., H. R. Winn, B. F. Cullen, and N. Sundling. (1991). Hyperglycemia and neurological outcome in patients with head injury. *J.Neurosurg.* 75:545-551.

Lanzino, G., N. F. Kassell, T. Germanson, L. Truskowski, and W. Alves. (1993). Plasma glucose levels and outcome after aneurysmal subarachnoid hemorrhage. *J.Neurosurg.* 79:885-891.

Mackenzie, I. M., T. Whitehouse, and P. G. Nightingale. (2011). The metrics of glycaemic control in critical care. *Intensive Care Med.* 37:435-443.

Marik, P. E. and J. C. Preiser. (2010). Toward understanding tight glycemic control in the ICU: a systematic review and metaanalysis. *Chest* 137:544-551.

McCowen, K. C., P. R. Ling, A. Ciccarone, Y. Mao, J. C. Chow, B. R. Bistrian, and R. J. Smith. (2001). Sustained endotoxemia leads to marked down-regulation of early steps in the insulin-signaling cascade. *Crit Care Med.* 29:839-846.

Meierhans, R., M. Bechir, S. Ludwig, J. Sommerfeld, G. Brandi, C. Haberthur, R. Stocker, and J. F. Stover. (2010). Brain metabolism is significantly impaired at blood glucose below 6 mM and brain glucose below 1 mM in patients with severe traumatic brain injury. *Crit Care* 14:R13.

Meyer, C., M. Stumvoll, J. Dostou, S. Welle, M. Haymond, and J. Gerich. (2002). Renal substrate exchange and gluconeogenesis in normal postabsorptive humans. *Am.J.Physiol Endocrinol.Metab* 282:E428-E434.

Meyer, C., M. Stumvoll, S. Welle, H. J. Woerle, M. Haymond, and J. Gerich. (2003). Relative importance of liver, kidney, and substrates in epinephrine-induced increased gluconeogenesis in humans. *Am.J.Physiol Endocrinol.Metab* 285:E819-E826.

Meyfroidt, G., D. M. Keenan, X. Wang, P. J. Wouters, J. D. Veldhuis, and Berghe G. Van den. (2010). Dynamic characteristics of blood glucose time series during the course of critical illness: effects of intensive insulin therapy and relative association with mortality. *Crit Care Med.* 38:1021-1029.

Mizock, B. A. (1995). Alterations in carbohydrate metabolism during stress: a review of the literature. *Am.J.Med.* 98:75-84.

Morohoshi, M., K. Fujisawa, I. Uchimura, and F. Numano. (1996). Glucose-dependent interleukin 6 and tumor necrosis factor production by human peripheral blood monocytes in vitro. *Diabetes* 45:954-959.

Offner, H., S. Subramanian, S. M. Parker, M. E. Afentoulis, A. A. Vandenbark, and P. D. Hurn. (2006). Experimental stroke induces massive, rapid activation of the peripheral immune system. *J.Cereb.Blood Flow Metab* 26:654-665.

Oksanen, T., M. B. Skrifvars, T. Varpula, A. Kuitunen, V. Pettila, J. Nurmi, and M. Castren. (2007). Strict versus moderate glucose control after resuscitation from ventricular fibrillation. *Intensive Care Med.* 33:2093-2100.

Parkin, M., S. Hopwood, D. A. Jones, P. Hashemi, H. Landolt, M. Fabricius, M. Lauritzen, M. G. Boutelle, and A. J. Strong. (2005). Dynamic changes in brain glucose and lactate in pericontusional areas of the human cerebral cortex, monitored with rapid sampling on-line microdialysis: relationship with depolarisation-like events. *J.Cereb.Blood Flow Metab* 25:402-413.

Passero, S., G. Ciacci, and M. Ulivelli. (2003). The influence of diabetes and hyperglycemia on clinical course after intracerebral hemorrhage. *Neurology* 61:1351-1356.

Pellerin, L., A. K. Bouzier-Sore, A. Aubert, S. Serres, M. Merle, R. Costalat, and P. J. Magistretti. (2007). Activity-dependent regulation of energy metabolism by astrocytes: an update. *Glia* 55:1251-1262.

Pellerin, L. and P. J. Magistretti. (2004). Neuroenergetics: calling upon astrocytes to satisfy hungry neurons. *Neuroscientist.* 10:53-62.

Preiser, J. C., P. Devos, S. Ruiz-Santana, C. Melot, D. Annane, J. Groeneveld, G. Iapichino, X. Leverve, G. Nitenberg, P. Singer, J. Wernerman, M. Joannidis, A. Stecher, and R. Chiolero. (2009). A prospective randomised multi-centre controlled trial on tight glucose control by intensive insulin therapy in adult intensive care units: the Glucontrol study. *Intensive Care Med.* 35:1738-1748.

Price, G. C., K. Stevenson, and T. S. Walsh. (2008). Evaluation of a continuous glucose monitor in an unselected general intensive care population. *Crit Care Resusc.* 10:209-216.

Rady, M. Y., D. J. Johnson, B. M. Patel, J. S. Larson, and R. A. Helmers. (2005). Influence of individual characteristics on outcome of glycemic control in intensive care unit patients with or without diabetes mellitus. *Mayo Clin.Proc.* 80:1558-1567.

Raichle, M. E. and M. A. Mintun. (2006). Brain work and brain imaging. *Annu.Rev.Neurosci.* 29:449-476.

Rothman, D. L., N. R. Sibson, F. Hyder, J. Shen, K. L. Behar, and R. G. Shulman. (1999). In vivo nuclear magnetic resonance spectroscopy studies of the relationship between the glutamate-glutamine neurotransmitter cycle and functional neuroenergetics. *Philos.Trans.R.Soc.Lond B Biol.Sci.* 354:1165-1177.

Rovlias, A. and S. Kotsou. (2000). The influence of hyperglycemia on neurological outcome in patients with severe head injury. *Neurosurgery* 46:335-342.

Salim, A., P. Hadjizacharia, J. Dubose, C. Brown, K. Inaba, L. S. Chan, and D. Margulies. (2009). Persistent hyperglycemia in severe traumatic brain injury: an independent predictor of outcome. *Am.Surg.* 75:25-29.

Schleis, T. G. (2007). Interference of maltose, icodextrin, galactose, or xylose with some blood glucose monitoring systems. *Pharmacotherapy* 27:1313-1321.

Simpson, I. A., A. Carruthers, and S. J. Vannucci. (2007). Supply and demand in cerebral energy metabolism: the role of nutrient transporters. *J.Cereb.Blood Flow Metab* 27:1766-1791.

Suh, S. W., A. M. Hamby, and R. A. Swanson. (2007). Hypoglycemia, brain energetics, and hypoglycemic neuronal death. *Glia* 55:1280-1286.

Turina, M., D. E. Fry, and H. C. Polk, Jr. (2005). Acute hyperglycemia and the innate immune system: clinical, cellular, and molecular aspects. *Crit Care Med.* 33:1624-1633.

Ueki, K., T. Kondo, and C. R. Kahn. (2004). Suppressor of cytokine signaling 1 (SOCS-1) and SOCS-3 cause insulin resistance through inhibition of tyrosine phosphorylation of insulin receptor substrate proteins by discrete mechanisms. *Mol.Cell Biol.* 24:5434-5446.

Van den, Berghe G., A. Wilmer, G. Hermans, W. Meersseman, P. J. Wouters, I. Milants, Wijngaerden E. Van, H. Bobbaers, and R. Bouillon. (2006a). Intensive insulin therapy in the medical ICU. *N.Engl.J.Med.* 354:449-461.

Van den, Berghe G., A. Wilmer, I. Milants, P. J. Wouters, B. Bouckaert, F. Bruyninckx, R. Bouillon, and M. Schetz. (2006b). Intensive insulin therapy in mixed medical/surgical intensive care units: benefit versus harm. *Diabetes* 55:3151-3159.

Van den, Berghe G., P. Wouters, F. Weekers, C. Verwaest, F. Bruyninckx, M. Schetz, D. Vlasselaers, P. Ferdinande, P. Lauwers, and R. Bouillon. (2001). Intensive insulin therapy in the critically ill patients. *N.Engl.J.Med.* 345:1359-1367.

Van den, Berghe G., P. J. Wouters, R. Bouillon, F. Weekers, C. Verwaest, M. Schetz, D. Vlasselaers, P. Ferdinande, and P. Lauwers. (2003). Outcome benefit of intensive insulin therapy in the critically ill: Insulin dose versus glycemic control. *Crit Care Med.* 31:359-366.

van, den Oever, I, H. G. Raterman, M. T. Nurmohamed, and S. Simsek. (2010). Endothelial dysfunction, inflammation, and apoptosis in diabetes mellitus. *Mediators.Inflamm.* 2010:792393.

Vriesendorp, T. M., Santen S. van, J. H. DeVries, Jonge E. de, F. R. Rosendaal, M. J. Schultz, and J. B. Hoekstra. (2006). Predisposing factors for hypoglycemia in the intensive care unit. *Crit Care Med.* 34:96-101.

Watts, A. G. and C. M. Donovan. (2010). Sweet talk in the brain: glucosensing, neural networks, and hypoglycemic counterregulation. *Front Neuroendocrinol.* 31:32-43.

Whitcomb, B. W., E. K. Pradhan, A. G. Pittas, M. C. Roghmann, and E. N. Perencevich. (2005). Impact of admission hyperglycemia on hospital mortality in various intensive care unit populations. *Crit Care Med.* 33:2772-2777.

Part 3

Section C

5

Inflammation and Hypoglycemia: The Lipid Connection

Oren Tirosh
*Institute of Biochemistry, Food Science and Nutrition,
The Robert H Smith Faculty of Agriculture, Food and Environment,
The Hebrew University of Jerusalem, Rehovot,
Israel*

1. Introduction

Patients can be exposed to a variety of potentially life threatening acute inflammations mainly sepsis, which accounts to 9% of all death in the US. The prevalence of non-alcoholic fatty liver disease (NAFLD) is about 30% in the general population. Fatty liver is known to be more sensitive to endotoxins. It has been reported that metabolic aspects of sepsis and endotoxemia are suppression of the fatty acid beta-oxidation pathway and severe hypoglycemia. This can be due to lipotoxic effects following accumulation of free fatty acids in the liver and suppression of gluconeogenesis. In this chapter we will review the published facts about the development of hypoglycemic effects during sepsis and the possible connection of such an effect to the dysregulation of lipid metabolism. Secondly a possible redox related antilipotoxic cellular mechanism will be suggested. Such mechanism can alleviate the endotoxic hypoglycemic effect and is related to nitric oxide signaling. Nitric oxide signaling has been demonstrated to regulate the metabolic status of cells including upregulation of mitochondrial biogenesis, promoting liver glucose production and depending on the biological setting to protect cells against accumulation of oxidative damage, all possibly protect against development of hypoglycemia following liver injury.

2. Non-alcoholic fatty liver disease

2.1 Introduction

Non-alcoholic fatty liver disease NAFLD comprises a spectrum of hepatic pathology, ranging from simple steatosis (SS), in which there is an increase of fat accumulation in hepatocytes, through steatohepatitis to cirrhosis (Farrell, GC et al., 2008). Primary NAFLD is associated with obesity, insulin resistance and metabolic syndrome, diabetes and dyslipidemia, while secondary NAFLD is associated with all forms of liver damage including viral infections autoimmune and heradetory disease, drugs, toxins and nutrition (parenteral nutrition , B12/folic acid deficiency etc.) (Musso, G et al., 2010) (Figure 1). Nonalcoholic steatohepatitis (NASH) is a progressive lesion in which steatosis is accompanied by hepatocyte injury and death, as well as hepatic infiltration by inflammatory cells. NASH-related liver damage often triggers liver fibrosis. In severe cases, NASH may progress to cirrhosis and possibly hepatocellular carcinoma (Lim, JH et al., 2006). NAFLD is one of the most common liver diseases worldwide, affecting all racial, ethnic, and age groups without sex predilection. The prevalence of NAFLD is around 30 % of the general population (Musso, G et al., 2009; Musso, G et al., 2010), NASH affects about 3 percent of the lean population (those weighing less than 110 percent of their ideal body weight), 19 percent of the obese population, and almost half of morbidly obese people. It is estimated about that 8.6 million obese adult Americans may have NASH and about 30.1 million may have the simple steatosis. Thus, the very high prevalence of fatty liver means that this disorder will contribute significantly to an increased burden of ill-health at the present and in the future (Farrell, GC et al., 2008).

NAFLD refers to the presence of hepatic stetosis not associated with a significant intake of alcohol (Adams, LA & KD Lindor, 2007) and its incidence is paralleling the increasing numbers of overweight and obese individuals worldwide (Yan, E et al., 2007). When fat accounts for more than 10% of liver's weight, then the condition is called fatty liver and it can develop more serious complications (American Liver Foundation). Fatty liver may cause no damage, but the excess fat leads to inflammation causing liver damage is refered to as steatohepatitis (American Liver Foundation). The term nonalcoholic steatohepatitis (NASH) was first coined by Ludwig et al at 1980 (Ludwig, J et al., 1980) describing the pathology of 20 patients histologically similar with alcoholic hepatitis but without the history of alcohol abuse. Sometimes, inflammation from a fatty liver is linked to alcohol abuse; this is known as alcoholic steatohepatitis (ASH). Otherwise the condition is called NASH (American Liver Foundation). NAFLD comprises a spectrum of liver pathology including bland steatosis, steatohepatitis, cirrhosis (Yang, L & A Diehl, 2007) and hepatocellular carcinoma (Angulo, P, 2007) where most liver related morbidity and mortality occur. The histological damage in NAFLD is very similar to that seen in patients with alcoholic liver disease (ALD), but NAFLD is by definition not alcohol induced (Angulo, P, 2007).

NAFLD is the most common chronic liver disease in the western world (Adams, LA & KD Lindor, 2007). Sedentary lifestyle and poor dietary choices are leading to a weight gain epidemic in westernized countries, subsequently increasing the risk for developing the metabolic syndrome and NAFLD (Rector, RS et al., 2008). Although, NAFLD may be categorized as primary and secondary depending on the underlying pathogenesis both type of NAFLD can be interrelated (Figure 1).

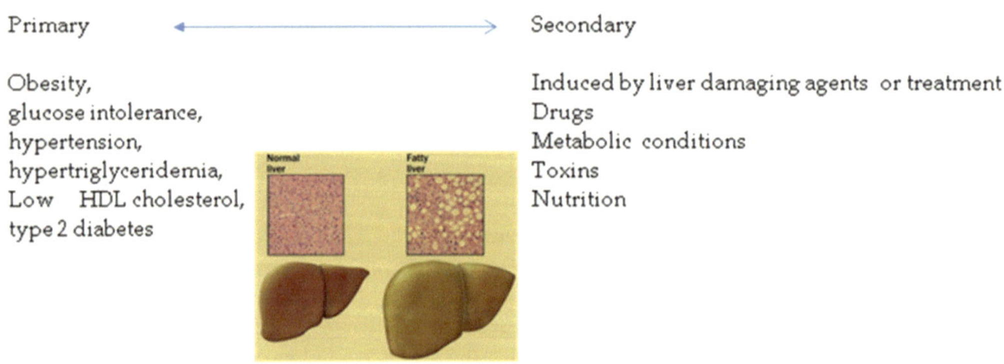

Fig. 1. Type and causes of NAFLD. Primary and secondary NAFLD may be interrelated. Induction of liver damage with may lead to fat accumulation in the liver may exacerbate primary NAFLD under conditions of hyperlipidemic, on the other hand primary NAFLD can increase the vulnerability of the liver to different kind of stressors and damaging agents.

2.2 Epidemiology

NAFLD is increasingly being recognized as an important and common condition, affecting approximately 20-45% of the general population (Joy, D et al., 2003) in different countries. It is estimated to affect approximately 30% of the general US population and is considered the hepatic manifestation of the metabolic syndrome (Rector, RS et al., 2008; Zivkovic, AM et al., 2007). According to (Angulo, P, 2007), NAFLD affects one in three adults and one in 10 children in the United States. Although NAFLD typically occurs between the fourth and six decades of life (Targher, G et al., 2007; Zhou, YJ et al., 2007), it is known to affect children as well as adults and is not considered discriminatory to age (Imhof, A et al., 2007; Zhou, YJ et al., 2007). Many studies have found a wide discrimination of NAFLD between the sexes (Amarapurkar, D et al., 2007; Zelber-Sagi, S et al., 2006).

Among different ethnic groups, however, the picture becomes a bit more complicated. Browning et al (Browning, JD et al., 2004) reported that the prevalence of fatty liver was highest in Hispanics (45%) compared to Caucasians (33%) or African Americans (24%) which introduced the possibility of race related variability in the susceptibility to NAFLD. Furthermore, within specific race, such as Caucasians, sex-related differences in the presence of fatty liver (42% in men and 24% in women) had been observed, which indicates the risk factors for NAFLD may vary depending on ethnicity and sex (Browning et al, 2004). Among 3543 peoples, surveyed in South China, 609 (17.2%) were diagnosed having fatty liver disease (FLD, 23.0% in urban and 14.5% in rural) out of which prevalence of NAFLD was 15.5% (Zhou, YJ et al., 2007). In the same study, prevalence of FLD among the children at the age of 7-18 years was 1.3% with all having NAFLD. The prevalence and incidence of NAFLD is expected to increase worldwide as the global obesity epidemic spreads and the trend in developing countries toward the western lifestyle continues (Angulo, P, 2007).

2.3 Clinical aspects of NAFLD

Most patients with NAFLD have no symptoms or signs of liver disease at the time of diagnosis (Angulo, P & KD Lindor, 2002). NAFLD has been characterized with asymptomatic elevation of aminotransferases, radiological findings of fatty liver or unexplained persistent hepatomegaly (Angulo, P & KD Lindor, 2002). NAFLD patients may be complaint of fatigue or a sensation of fullness or discomfort in the right upper abdomen . Hepatomegaly is one of the more consistent physical findings, described in up to 75% of patients with NAFLD (Yan, E et al., 2007). Other findings on physical examination that may suggest NAFLD as the cause of liver abnormalities include those characterizing insulin resistance and metabolic syndrome, such as central obesity, hypertriglyceridemia, and hypertension (Yan, E et al., 2007).

The most common and often the only laboratory abnormality found in NAFLD patients, is mild to moderate elevation of liver enzymes (Angulo, P, 2007; Angulo, P & KD Lindor, 2002) alanine aminotransferase (ALT) and aspartate aminotransferase (AST): defined as ALT>45 U/L, AST>45 U/L or γ Glutamyl transferase (GGT) >50 U/L (Hickman, I et al., 2008)In the patients with FLD, AST/ALT ratio is usually less than one, but this ratio increases as fibrosis advances (Angulo, P, 2007). A study on Japanese adults showed that triglycerides, total protein albumin, AST and ALT were all significantly higher while high density lipoprotein (HDL) cholesterol and AST/ALT ratio were significantly lower in subjects with NAFLD than those without fatty liver (Jimba, S et al., 2005).

3. Association of fatty liver with hypoglycemia

3.1 Fatty acid oxidation defects

Adipocytes have the unique capacity to store excess fatty acids in the form of TGs in lipid droplets. Non-adipose tissues, such as hepatocytes, cardiac myocytes and pancreatic beta-cells, have a limited capacity for lipid storage. In hyperlipidemic states, the accumulation of excess lipid in non-adipose tissues can lead to cellular dysfunction and/or cell death, a phenomenon known as lipotoxicity (Listenberger, LL et al., 2003; Unger, RH, 1995; Weinberg, JM, 2006). Most studies attribute strong lipiotoxic effects to free fatty acids (FFAs). Lipotoxic effects in the liver include disruption of liver-cell function (Alkhouri, N et al., 2009).

The connection between increased levels of fatty acids to hypoglycemia is known in genetic diseases of fatty acid oxidation defects (Figure 2). Inherited defects in mitochondrial fatty-acid beta-oxidation comprise a group of at least 12 diseases characterized by distinct enzyme or transporter deficiencies. Most of these diseases have a variable age of onset and clinical severity. Symptoms are often episodic and associated with mild viral illness, physiologic

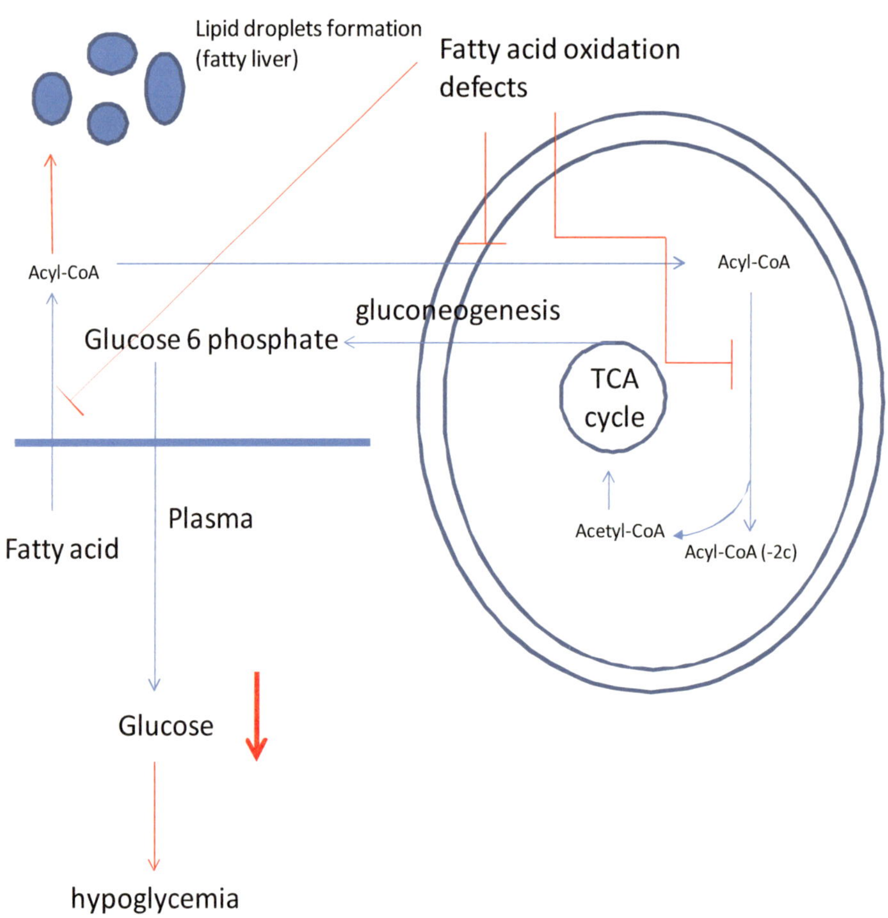

Fig. 2. Classical theory of how biochemical fatty acid oxidation defects generate hypoglycemic phenotype

stress, or prolonged exercise that overwhelms the ability of mitochondria to oxidize fatty acids. Depending on the specific genetic defect, patients develop fasting hypoketotic hypoglycemia, cardiomyopathy, rhabdomyolysis, liver dysfunction, or sudden death (Kompare, M & WB Rizzo, 2008). Medium-chain acyl-CoA deshydrogenase (MCAD) deficiency is the most frequent disorder of mitochondrial fatty acid oxidation (Baruteau, J et al., 2009), The pathophysiology of these diseases is still not completely understood, hampering optimal treatment (Houten, SM & RJ Wanders). Hypoglycemia as one major clinical sign in all fatty acid oxidation defects and occurs due to a reduced hepatic glucose output and an enhanced peripheral glucose uptake (Spiekerkoetter, U & PA Wood). A connection of such disorders-phenotype with metabolic derangement that are not necessarily related to genetic defected has been demonstrated recently via the Sirtuins. Sirtuin 3 (SIRT3) is localized in the mitochondrial matrix, where it regulates the acetylation levels of metabolic enzymes, including acetyl coenzyme A synthetase 2. Mice lacking SIRT3 exhibit hallmarks of fatty-acid oxidation disorders during fasting (Hirschey, MD et al.).

3.2 Liver regeneration

The liver is known for its regenerative capacity. It is now well accepted that there are two physiological forms of regeneration in the liver as responses to different types of liver injury. The first line for regeneration are mature, normally quiescent adult hepatocytes. During mild liver injury due to drugs, toxins, resection, or acute viral diseases, hepatocytes are the main cell type to proliferate and regenerate the liver. The mature hepatocytes have relatively low proliferative capacity. The second line of defense are the progenitor cell population, that are activated when injury is severe, or when the mature hepatocytes can no longer regenerate the liver due to senescence or arrest (Riehle, KJ et al., 2011). The metabolic requirements of the generating liver form Partial hepatectomy (PH) of from liver damage are impressive. There is a need to activate Kupffer cells in order to initiate the regenerating cascade. For these reasons increased accumulation of insulin independent glucose utilization is needed which may cause plasma glucose utilization due to the high metabolic demend. Impaired regenerative capacity of fatty livers might promote the progression of nonalcoholic fatty liver disease (NAFLD). Partial hepatectomy (PH) activats oxidant-sensitive, growth-regulatory kinase cascades which is abnormal in fatty hepatocytes. The normal coordinated induction of Jun N-terminal kinases (Jnks) and extracellular regulated kinases (Erks) does not occur after PH in ob/ob mice. This is associated with enhanced activation of Akt, which inhibits phosphoenolpyruvate carboxykinase (PEPCK) induction, causing severe hypoglycemia and increased lethality in the ob/ob group (Yang, SQ et al., 2001).

4. Alcoholic liver injury

4.1 Introduction

The liver breaks down alcohol so that it can be eliminated from our body. When alcohol is over consumed than the liver can process, the resulting imbalance can injure the liver by interfering with its normal breakdown of proteins, fats, and carbohydrates (American Liver Foundation). ALD is a common consequence of long term alcohol abuse (Zeng, MD et al., 2008) and represents a major cause of mortality and morbidity worldwide (Albano, E, 2008; Bergheim, I et al., 2005). ALD encompasses a broad spectrum of morphological features ranging from simple steatosis with minimal injury to more advanced stage liver injury, including alcoholic steatohepatitis, alcoholic fibrosis and alcoholic cirrhosis (Albano, E, 2008;

Zeng, MD et al., 2008). The risk of steatosis, inflammation and fibrosis are more common in alcoholics and increases with time and the amount of ethanol consumed (Vidali, M et al., 2008).

4.2 Clinical aspects of ALD

Fatty liver, the most common syndrome of ALD, is characterized by the excessive accumulation of fat inside hepatocytes (Adachi, M & DA Brenner, 2005). Indeed the excessive fat accumulation in the hepatocytes is the most common and earliest response of the liver to chronic alcohol consumption (Song, Z et al., 2008). Morphological criteria of steatohepatitis are steatosis, ballooning of hepatocytes, pericellular fibrosis and inflammation (Denk, H et al., 2005). In an animal model of ALD, rats exposed 4 weeks to alcohol exhibited a significant increase in liver to body weight ratio, serum ALT levels and hepatic TNF- α compared to control group (Song, Z et al., 2008). Tabassum, F et al. (Tabassum, F et al., 2001) found that the levels of alkaline phosphate, ALT, protein and globulin were significantly increased in alcoholic males compared to control subjects. The AST/ALT ratio is significantly higher in ALD patients sometimes even higher than two (Adachi, M & DA Brenner, 2005).

4.3 Ethanol metabolism and role of acetaldehyde

There are multiple mechanisms for the development and progression of ALD (Figure 3) and many of these mechanisms interact to each other (Barve, A et al., 2008).

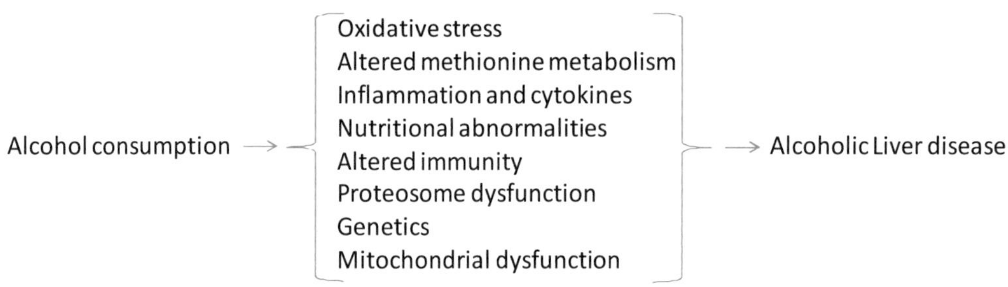

Fig. 3. Mechanisms for the development of non-alcoholic fatty liver disease

ALD has a complex pathogenesis, in which acetaldehyde; the major ethanol metabolite plays a central role (Lieber, CS, 1997). Alcohol is primarily metabolized by the successive oxidative activities of alcohol dehydrogenase (ADH) and acetaldehyde dehydrogenase (ALDH), Figure 4, (Hasse, J & L Matarese, 2004; Lumeng, L & DW Crabb, 2001). Ethanol is metabolized mainly in the hepatocytes in three different sites: cytosol, endoplasmic reticulum, peroxisome and mitochondria (De Minicis, S & DA Brenner, 2008). According to (Lieber, CS, 1997) the main pathway involves cytoplasmic ADH which catalyzes the oxidation of ethanol to acetaldehyde then oxidized to acetate by the mitochondrial ALDH. Most of acetate is released into the blood (Hasse, J & L Matarese, 2004). According to Novitskiy, G *et al* (Novitskiy, G et al., 2006) acetaldehyde enhances the formation of ROS.

According to (Lieber, CS, 1997), sever toxic manifestations are produced by an accessory inducible pathway, the microsomal ethanol-oxidizing system (MEOS) in endoplasmic reticulum involving an ethanol-inducible CYP2E1 in which the oxidation of ethanol to acetaldehyde and acetate also leads to generation of ROS [hydroxyethyl free radicals,

hydrogen peroxides (H_2O_2) and super oxide anion (O_2^-)]. High reduced nicotinamide adenine dinucleotide (NADH) is produced due to alcohol metabolism leading to high $NADH/NAD^+$ ratio which overrides the cell's ability to maintain normal redox state (Hasse, J & L Matarese, 2004).
The lactic acid cannot be converted into pyruvate due to lack of NAD^+ leading to hyperlacticacedemia (Hasse and Matarese, 2004). They also reported that tricarboxylic acid cycle (TCA) is also diminished because; in one hand it requires a lot of NAD^+ and on the other hand the excess NADH inhibits two regulatory enzymes isocitrate dehydrogenase and α-ketoglutarate dehydrogenase, as a consequence acetyl coenzyme A (CoA) is accumulated. The mitochondria in turn use hydrogen produced from the ethanol metabolism as a fuel source and all these activities lead to decreased fatty acid oxidation and accumulation of triglycerides in the hepatocytes (Hasse, J & L Matarese, 2004). They also reported that malnutrition can also occur in early alcoholic liver disease due to the suppression of TCA cycle coupled with decreased gluconeogenesis due to ethanol.

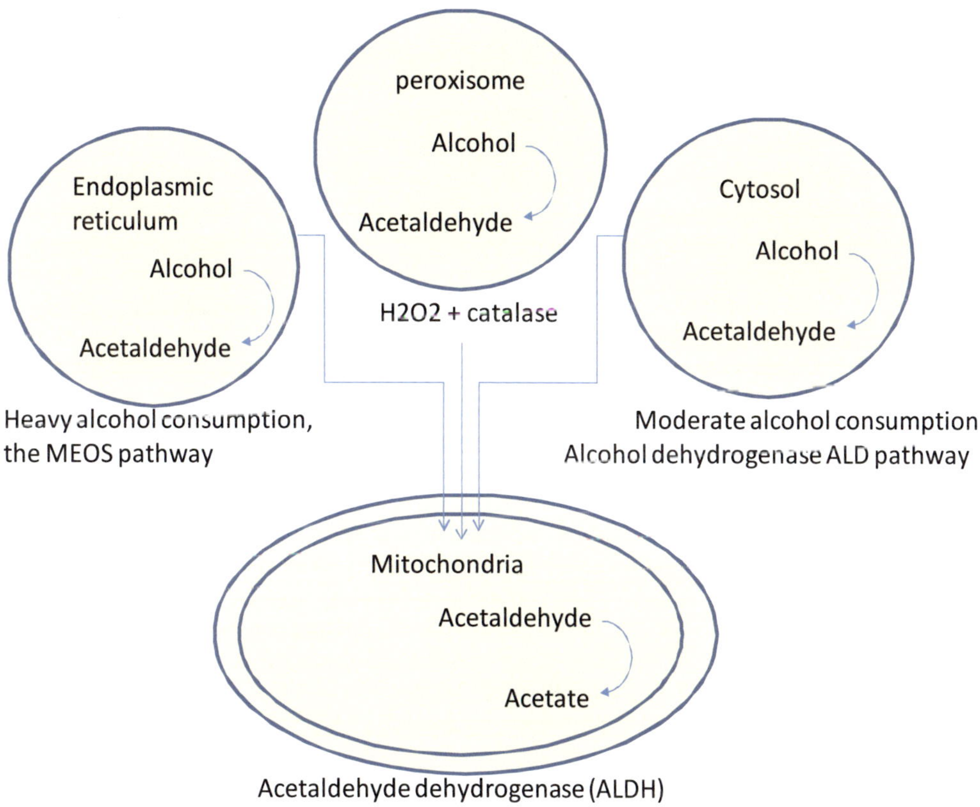

Fig. 4. Ethanol metabolism in hepatocytes. These mechanisms are potentially involved in oxidative stress production. Ethanol is metabolized in acetaldehyde and then transformed into acetate, as shown.

Chronic ethanol consumption increases fatty acid synthesis by inducing the expression of lipogenic enzymes which are regulated by transcription factor SREBP (Adachi, M & DA Brenner, 2005). Chronic ethanol consumption significantly inhibits mitochondrial ALDH activity while the rate of ethanol oxidation to acetaldehyde is even enhanced, resulting in striking increase in tissue and plasma levels of acetaldehyde which results in metabolic disturbances, such as hyperlactacidemia, acidosis, hyperglycemia, hyperuricemia and fatty liver (Lieber, CS, 1997). However, in many cases Alcohol consumption can generate a life threatening hypoglycemia.

5. ALD and hypoglycemia

Alcohol consumption may have beneficial as well as deadly consequences. It is generally considered that alcohol consumption interferes with all three glucose sources and with the actions of the regulatory hormones. Chronic heavy drinkers often have insufficient dietary intake of glucose. Without eating, glycogen stores are exhausted in a few hours (Gordon, GG & CS Lieber, 1992). In addition, the body's glucose production is inhibited while alcohol is being metabolized (Sneyd, JGT, 1989). The combination of these effects can cause severe hypoglycemia 6 to 36 hours after the drinking episode (1). Even in well-nourished people, alcohol can disturb blood sugar levels. Acute alcohol consumption, especially in combination with sugar, augments insulin secretion and causes temporary hypoglycemia (O'Keefe, SJ & V Marks, 1977). In addition, studies in healthy subjects and insulin-dependent diabetics have shown that acute alcohol consumption can impair the hormonal response to hypoglycemia. Alcohol consumption can be especially harmful in people with a predisposition to hypoglycemia, such as patients who are being treated for diabetes. Alcohol can interfere with the management of diabetes in different ways. Acute as well as chronic alcohol consumption can alter the effectiveness of hypoglycemic medications. Treatment of diabetes by tight control of blood glucose levels is difficult in alcoholics, and both hypoglycemic and hyperglycemic episodes are common. In a Japanese study, alcoholics with diabetes had a significantly lower survival rate than other alcoholics (Judith Fradkin, MD, 1994). A recent meta analysis indicated beneficial effect of moderate alcohol consumption reduces the incidence of type 2 diabetes (T2D), however, binge drinking seems to increase the incidence. Acute intake of alcohol does not increase risk of hypoglycemia in diet treated subjects with T2D, only when sulphonylurea is co-administered. Long-term alcohol use seems to be associated with improved glycemic control in T2D probably due to improved insulin sensitivity (Pietraszek, A et al., 2010). The capacity of alcohol to shift its activity from beneficial to deleterious could be related to other factors that are related to impairment in lipid metabolism.

ALD has been suspected known to generate the sudden death syndrome in alcoholic individuals. Two major factors have been considered contributory to ethanol-induced hypoglycaemia (Arky, RA & N Freinkel, 1966; Madison, LL, 1968) suppression of hepatic gluconeogenesis resulting from an increase in the NADH/NAD+ ratio accompanied by enhanced ethanol metabolism, and depletion of hepatic glycogen storage secondary to starvation. In cases of alcohol-related sudden deaths hydroxybutyrate levels are significantly elevated. Platia and Hsu (Platia, EV & TH Hsu, 1979)) described five non-diabetic alcohol abusers with hypoglycaemic coma and ketoacidosis and contended that the combination of alcohol-related hypoglycaemia and ketoacidosis may be common.

Part of the pathogenesis of the widely known syndrome of sudden death with hepatic fatty metamorphosis observed in alcohol abusers was described by Yuzuriha *et al.* (Yuzuriha, T et al., 1997), 11 subjects who died under such circumstances between 1987 and 1993 were scrutinized both for clinical and pathological data. Death occurred followed several days of uninterrupted drinking often with little dietary intake. Most of these individuals suffered from severe hypoglycemia. The common hepatic pathology was the extensive appearance of numerous microvesicular fatty droplets in the hepatocytes together with varying degrees of macrovesicular fatty change; four subjects had an underlying cirrhosis. Death undoubtedly results from a variety of metabolic disturbances triggered by the combination of massive ethanol intake and starvation. The appearance of extensive microvesicular fatty change superimposed on macrovesicular fatty change was considered to be an associated phenomenon. The most striking findings in the liver were extensive microvesicular fatty change within hepatocyte and the presence of megamitochondria.

6. Ischemic hepatitis

Ischemic hepatitis also known Hypoxic hepatitis or shock liver, can be characterized by necrosis of the zone 3 hepatocytes and significant increase in serum aminotransferase levels. It is the consequence of multiorgan injury. Outcome is influenced by the severity of liver impairment and the etiology and severity of the basic disease (Fuhrmann, V et al., 2009).The syndrome occurs under conditions of clinical setting of cardiac, circulatory or respiratory failure. It is recognized as the most frequent cause of acute liver injury with a reported prevalence of up to 10% in the intensive care unit (Fuhrmann, V et al., 2010). Patients with ischemic hepatitis and vasopressor therapy have a significantly increased mortality risk in the medical intensive care unit population. Ischemic hepatitis causes several complications including spontaneous hypoglycemia which can be considered secondary to impairment of gluconeogenic response in the exhausted liver (Fuhrmann, V et al., 2010; Fuhrmann, V et al., 2009; Nomura, T et al., 2009).

7. Sepsis

7.1 Introduction

Definition "Systemic Inflammatory Response Syndrome or **(SIRS)** is evidence of the body's ongoing inflammatory response. When SIRS is suspected or known to be caused by an infection, this is sepsis. Severe sepsis occurs when sepsis leads to organ dysfunction, such as trouble breathing, coagulation or other blood abnormalities, decreased urine production, or altered mental status. If the organ dysfunction of severe sepsis is low blood pressure (hypotension), or insufficient blood flow (hypoperfusion) to one or more organs (causing, for example, lactic acidosis), this is septic shock. Sepsis can lead to multiple organ dysfunction syndrome (MODS) (formerly known as multiple organ failure), and death. Organ dysfunction results from local changes in blood flow, from sepsis-induced hypotension (< 90 mmHg or a reduction of ≥ 40 mmHg from baseline) and from diffuse intravascular coagulation, among other things.

Sepsis can be defined as the body's response to an infection. An infection is caused by microorganisms or bacteria invading the body and can be limited to a particular body region or can be widespread in the bloodstream. Sepsis is acquired quickest with infections developed in surgery and physical contact with someone with sepsis.

Bacteremia is the presence of viable bacteria in the bloodstream. Likewise, the terms viremia and fungemia simply refer to viruses and fungi in the bloodstream. These terms say nothing about the consequences this has on the body. For example, bacteria can be introduced into the bloodstream during toothbrushing. This form of bacteremia almost never causes problems in normal individuals. However, bacteremia associated with certain dental

procedures can cause bacterial infection of the heart valves (known as endocarditis) in high-risk patients. Conversely, a systemic inflammatory response syndrome can occur in patients without the presence of infection, for example in those with burns, polytrauma, or the initial state in pancreatitis and chemical pneumonitis" (wikipedia).
Severe sepsis is a significant cause of mortality worldwide. Current research estimates that more than 9% of all deaths in the US can be attributed to severe sepsis. Experimental evidence shows that the liver is an important target organ in the development of multiple organ dysfunction during sepsis (Koo, DJ et al., 1999; Koo, DJ et al., 2000). Due to its major role in metabolism and host-defense mechanisms, the liver is pivotal in participating in the systemic response to severe infection, because it contains the largest mass of resident macrophage Kupffer cells (KC) in the body, making up approximately 15% of the liver cells (Szabo, G et al., 2002). KC are highly relevant in the inflammatory response to bacterial infection and non-bacterial inflammation by 1) playing a major role in both clearance and detoxification, e.g. removal of LPS from the circulation (especially the portal vein) and 2) producing inflammatory mediators (Van Amersfoort, ES et al., 2003).

8. Sepsis and hypoglycemia

8.1 The use of intensive insulin therapy (IIT) to maintain normal blood glucose levels in septic patients

At 2001 van den Berghe and colleagues published the clinical implications of tight euglycemic control (van den Berghe, G et al., 2001). This observation significantly and rapidly changed intensive care unit (ICU) practice. It has been suggested that insulin administered to maintain glucose at levels below 110 mg/dl decreased mortality, the incidence of infections, sepsis, and sepsis-associated multiorgan failure in surgical patients, reduced kidney injury, and accelerated weaning from mechanical ventilation and discharge from the ICU in medical patients. However, current evidences suggest that the tight euglycemic control which is implemented in intensive care units around the world could be detrimental. Increasing evidence suggest that tight euglycemic control is which is associated with development of hypoglycemia has detrimental outcomes (Brunkhorst, FM et al., 2008; Jeschke, MG et al., 2010).Therefore, In practice regulating blood glucose levels is recommended to target glucose level below 8.3 mmol/L. This is indicated for the management of severe sepsis by the Surviving Sepsis guidelines (Orford, NR, 2006)
The main problem with IIT is the risk of development of hypoglycemia. The recent trials reporting reduced morbidity and mortality in critically ill patients treated with IIT require careful examination, including the subsequent post-hoc analyses. An understanding of the molecular and metabolic mechanisms by which IIT may be beneficial and the evidence that it benefits patients with severe sepsis, and a review of the risks of hypoglycaemia are also necessary when deciding whether to implement IIT in severe sepsis. Patients with severe sepsis are likely to benefit from IIT based on metabolic effects and their prolonged stays in the intensive care unit. All together, The current evidence suggests IIT should be implemented, aiming for the lowest glycaemic range that can be safely achieved while avoiding hypoglycaemia.

8.2 Development of hypoglycemia in septic patients without IIT

The severity of sepsis is shown to correlate with the risk of sustaining hyperglycemia as well as critical hypoglycemia (Krinsley, JS, 2008). Hypoglycemia during hospitalization occurs in patients with and without diabetes. In elderly hospitalized patients a predicted increase in-hospital 3- and 6-month cumulative mortality has been documented (Kagansky, N et al., 2003). In addition, sepsis is 10 times more common in these patients than in non-hypoglycemic patients. Previously, it has been shown that features of hepatitis and steatosis are the primary histological findings in the liver of patients dying from sepsis (Koskinas, J et al., 2008). The hypoglycemic effect due to fatty liver is also a known phenomenon in alcoholic patients and is related to the fatty liver sudden death syndrome (Denmark, LN, 1993; Randall, B, 1980; Yuzuriha, T et al., 1997). Altogether, the accumulated data suggest that although fatty liver and inflammation can generate a phenotype of insulin resistance, it can also lead to severe hypoglycemic life-threatening situations in patients with steatosis and acute inflammation due to an increase in hepatic insulin sensitivity (Thompson, BT, 2008; van der Crabben, SN et al., 2009). The mechanism(s) for hypoglycemia with sepsis is not well defined. Depleted glycogen stores, impaired gluconeogenesis and increased peripheral glucose utilization may all be contributing factors. Incubation of bacteria in fresh blood at room temperature does not increase the normal rate of breakdown of glucose suggesting that the hypoglycemia occurs in vivo by increased glucose utilization or by a decrease in glucose production. Hypoglycemia is an important sign of overwhelming sepsis (Miller, SI et al., 1980). Fischer et al" have reported that hypoglycemic episodes in nondiabetics were associated with infection and septic shock. The majority of cases of hypoglycemia reported in their study were related to liver disease, infections, shock, pregnancy, neoplasia, or burns. Hypoglycemia was not the apparent cause of death in any patient, but the overall hospital mortality was 27 percent and was related to the degree of hypoglycemia and the number of risk factors for hypoglycemia (Fischer, KF et al., 1986).

In 1991 Charles et al have studied the mechanism by which infection can lead to hypoglycemia. A hypermetabolic septic state was produced in rats by subcutaneous injections of live Escherichia coli. Sepsis increased whole body glucose disposal by 53% under basal euglycemic conditions and this increase resulted from an enhanced rate of glucose removal by liver, spleen, lung, ileum, and skin. In sepsis, the rate of non-insulin-mediated glucose uptake (NIMGU) was46% higher than in nonseptic animals. Severe hypoglycemia (2 mmol/L) produced a relative insulin deficiency and decreased whole body glucose disposal in both septic and nonseptic animals by 53% to 56%. Compared with euglycemic insulinopenic animals. The decrease in blood glucose decreased glucose uptake by all tissues examined, except brain and heart. However, sepsis still increased glucose uptake by liver, spleen, lung, ileum, and skin (25% to SO%), compared with hypoglycemic nonseptic rats. Therefore, the conclusion of the study was that sepsis increases NIMGU under basal conditions due to an increased glucose uptake by macrophage-rich tissues, and that this enhanced rate is maintained during hypoglycemia (Lang, CH & C Dobrescu, 1991).

It is therefore suggested that during sepsis there is increased glucose utilization by macrophages-rich tissues, which may lead to hypoglycemia. However, there is also a strong connection between the liver capacity to generate glucose and the development of hypoglycemia. A case report which connect hypoglycemia with sepsis and liver disease was reported at 1994 in Japan. A 78-year-old woman that was admitted to a hospital because of disturbance of consciousness. On admission, the body temperature was 35.5 degrees C and systolic blood pressure was 50 mmHg. Ascites and semicomatose consciousness were detected. Laboratory evaluation demonstrated the following values: leukocyte count 38800/microliters, blood sugar 3 mg/l and arterial blood pH 6.9. Therapy with catecholamine and antibiotics was started, but she expired 10 hours after admission. Bacteroides ovatus was detected from her blood. Autopsy findings disclosed the connection to advance liver disease and indicated abscess and perforation of the uterus, and liver cirrhosis (Suzuki, A et al., 1994). It is known that Sepsis suppresses fatty acid oxidation, It has been reported that fatty acid oxidation is significantly suppressed under conditions of sepsis and endotoxemia. During the acute-phase response, fatty acid oxidation decrease is associated with hypertriglyceridemia. LPS was demonstrated to suppress FFAs oxidation, and consequently contributes to elevated plasma levels of FFAs and TGs. LPS suppresses FFAs oxidation through decreasing the expression levels of key FFA oxidative genes including CPT-1 and MCAD in both liver and kidney tissues. LPS has been shown to selectively suppress the levels of PPARalpha and PGC-1alpha in tissues (Maitra, U et al., 2009). The decrease was rapid and occurred at very low doses of LPS. Similar decreases in levels of these genes occurred during zymosan- and turpentine-induced inflammation, indicating that suppression of the PGC-1alpha, and medium chain acyl coA dehydrogenase pathway is a general response during infection and inflammation (Kim, MS et al., 2005). We have demonstrated in a model of liver steatosis and endotoxemia that the expression of gluconeogenic enzymes and gluconeogenesis are strongly suppressed. This was accompanied with lowered blood glucose levels. The treated mice had a phenotype of insulin sensitivity with decreased blood insulin levels (Tirosh, O et al., 2010). Therefore, the effect of free fatty acids and triglycerids on expression of key gluconeogenic enzymes was studied. The effect of exposing hepatocytes to free fatty acids was to suppress the inducible expression of gluconeogenic enzymes Figure 5 and Figure 6.

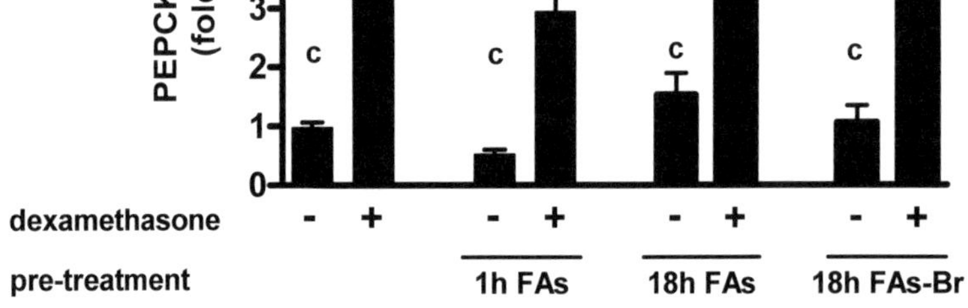

Fig. 5. **Inhibition of gluconeogenic response by free FAs in FaO cells.** FaO cells were cultured and pre-treated with FAs mixture (2:1 oleate/palmitate with 1% BSA) or with FAs-Br mixture (2:1 oleate/2-Bromopalmitate with 1% BSA) to final concentration of 1mM FAs. After that, dexamethasone (1μM) was added to cells media for 6 hours. mRNA expression levels of PEPCK was measured by quantitative real-time RT-PCR. Means with different letters differ at $P<0.05$.

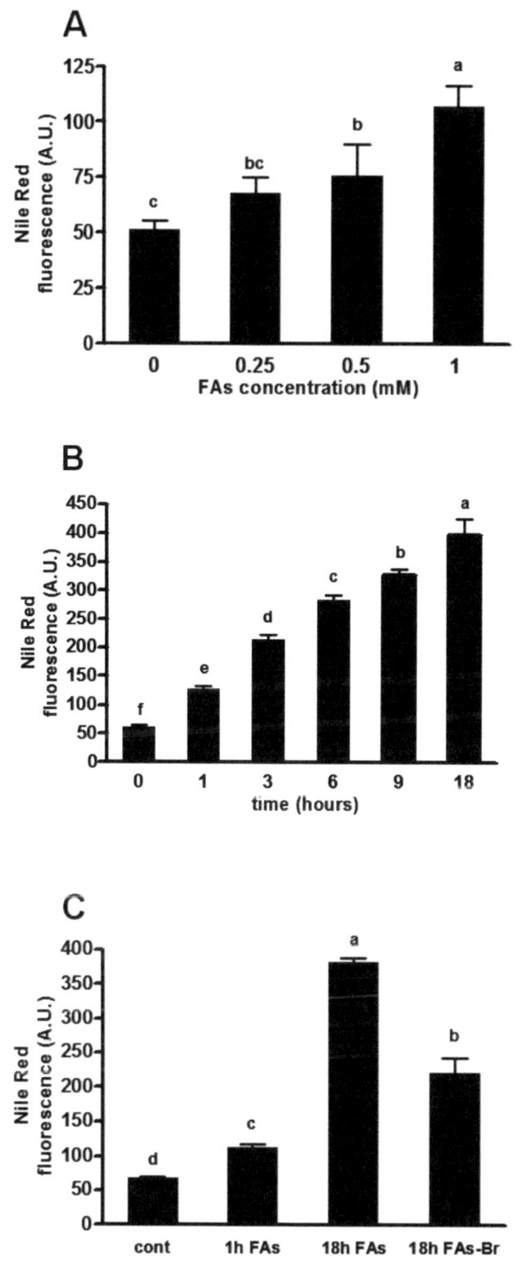

Fig. 6. **Fat accumulation in FaO cultures.** FaO cells were cultured and exposed to FAs mixture (2:1 oleate/palmitate with 1% BSA) at different concentrations for 18 hours (A) or to final concentration of 1mM FAs for different times (B). Alternatively, FaO cells were cultured and exposed to FAs mixture (2:1 oleate/palmitate with 1% BSA) or to FAs-Br mixture (2:1 oleate/2-Bromopalmitate with 1% BSA) to final concentration of 1mM FAs (C). After that, cells were stained with Nile-Red and fluorescence was examined by FACS analysis. Means with different letters differ at $P<0.05$.

The mechanism for the development of hypoglycemia during sepsis and the lipid connection can be therefore explained by the following figure 7:

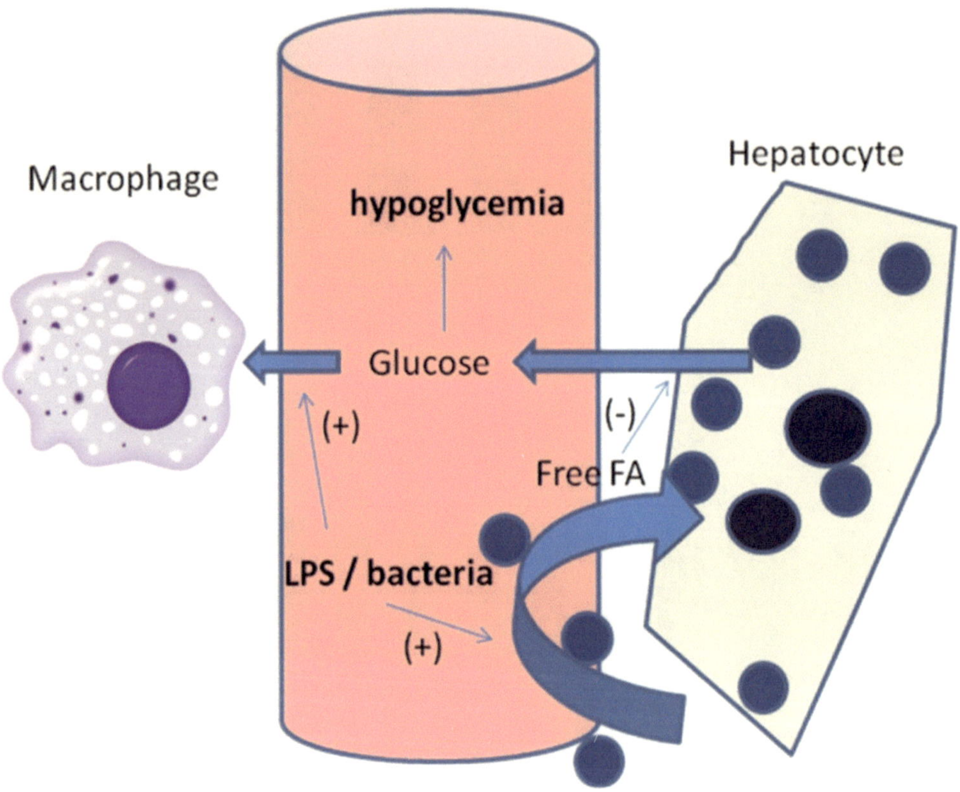

Fig. 7. LPS and bacteria facilitate 1) non-insulin-mediated glucose uptake 2) release of triglycerides and suppression of beta-oxidation in hepatocytes therefore elevating the FFA levels. This results in suppression of liver glucose output capacity. The results is hypoglycemia.

9. Nitric oxide as a potential antihypoglycemic agent

9.1 Nitric oxide involvement in liver damage and sepsis

One of the main effects of the inflammatory response in the liver is an increase in the levels of inducible nitric oxide synthase (iNOS). Therefore, it has been postulated that nitric oxide (NO) would contribute to hepatotoxicity through inhibition of ATP synthesis, increased reactive oxygen species (ROS), and the inability to adapt to hypoxic stress (Mantena, SK et al., 2008). Other studies imply that decreased production of NO from endothelial nitric oxide synthase (eNOS) contributes to liver pathology via dysregulation of blood flow and oxygen delivery (Liu, J & MP Waalkes, 2005). Furthermore, in iNOS knockout mice, hepatocytes undergo necrosis and apoptosis after PH, indicating that the production of NO is essential to protect hepatocytes from death after liver resection (Rai, RM et al., 1998). We have demonstrated that a decreased in eNOS expression precedes formation of liver damage following intensive blood infusion of triglycerides (TGs) in rats (Tirosh, O et al., 2009). Thus, it appears that NO can be both toxic or protective, depending on the acute physicological environment in the liver.

In the case of sepsis, there are also contractory reports concerning the role of NO. Although it has been suggested that NO is a mediator of organ dysfunction, different opinions suggest a protective role of NO in sepsis. Indeed, numerous reports of benefits associated with NO donor administration in clinical and preclinical studies of sepsis have been published (Lamontagne, F et al., 2008). Obesity increases sensitivity to endotoxin liver injury. It is known that fatty liver sensitivity to acute inflammation injury is much higher compared to normal livers (Yang, SQ et al., 1997). Our published studies in a mouse model of fatty liver and endotoxemia demonstrated a significant protective role for iNOS expression. iNOS(-/-) mice were found to be more sensitive to liver damage thereby supporting the hypothesis that iNOS has a protective effect. Additionally, iNOS(-/-) mice with fatty liver suffered from severe fatal hypoglycemia after endotoxic treatment (Tirosh, O et al., 2010).

9.2 Hyperglycemia or hypoglycemia: A paradox of inflammation, and the involvement of nitric oxide

Along with a rising prevalence of non-alcoholic fatty liver disease (NAFLD), there is a marked increase in individuals suffering from metabolic impairments. One widespread imbalance is the insulin resistance syndrome or metabolic syndrome which refers to a constellation of symptoms, including glucose intolerance, obesity, dyslipidemia, and hypertension. This syndrome is known to promote the development of type 2 diabetes, cardiovascular disease, cancer, and other disorders. The liver plays a major role in the regulation of glucose, lipid and energy metabolism, which are tightly regulated by insulin (Leclercq, IA et al., 2007; Raddatz, D & G Ramadori, 2007). In addition, insulin resistance is now recognized as a pathological factor in the development of NAFLD (Leclercq, IA et al., 2007; Raddatz, D & G Ramadori, 2007). It has been suggested that prolonged elevation of the levels of sterol regulatory element binding proteins (SREBPs) is responsible for inhibition of insulin signaling in fatty liver (Shimano, H, 2007) and that the intracellular accumulation of lipids-namely, diacylglycerol-triggers activation of novel protein kinases C(PKCε) with subsequent impairments in insulin signaling (Samuel, VT et al.). Hepatic insulin resistance can be defined as the failure of insulin to adequately suppress hepatic glucose production (Weickert, MO & AF Pfeiffer, 2006).

Several studies indicate the involvement of inflammatory activation in the development of hepatic and peripheral insulin resistance (Cai, D et al., 2005). On the other hand, acute inflammation induced by lipopolysaccharides (LPS) facilitates a hypoglycemic effect and impairment of hepatic Glucose-6 phosphatase (G6Pase) expression (Lo, YC et al., 2004; Maitra, SR et al., 1999; Oguri, S et al., 2002). Indeed, as metioned above in critically ill patients, sepsis-induced hypoglycemia is a well known event (van der Crabben, SN et al., 2009). We showed by temporal kinetics that the rapid induction of iNOS played a role in counteracting hypoglycemic effect of LPS and lipids rather than exacerbating it (Tirosh, O et al.). NO had a direct stimulatory effect promoting liver glucose production, making iNOS expression necessary for survival. Experiments performed with the NO donor DETA-NONOate in cultured hepatocytes showed a positive effect of NO on expression of gluconeogenic enzymes. Our data indicate that NO generated by the iNOS protein can support the expression of PGC 1alpha and liver gluconeogenic genes during acute inflammation. We believe that this effect is mediated by NO's capacity to promote the removal of free fatty acids (FFAs). Indeed, NO was found to act as a signaling molecule that can activate the transcription factor co-activator PGC 1alpha facilitating mitochondrial biogenesis (Nisoli, E & MO Carruba, 2006; Nisoli, E et al., 2007).

Our results that nitric oxide produced during the acute inflammatory process in fatty liver promotes PGC1 expression and liver glucose production supports the hypothesis that it acts as an antihypoglycemic factor. The lipotoxicity during acute inflammation in the fatty liver is manifested by increased oxidative stress and lipid peroxidation and therefore NO also function as an antioxidant (Kanner, J et al., 1991; Kanner, J et al., 1992; Volk, J et al., 2009) protecting the liver. Therefore, NO derived from inducible nitric oxide synthase (iNOS) may paradoxically function as an antioxidant protecting fatty liver during acute inflammation. This phenomenon is probably quite the reverse of the reactive nitrogen species and ROS effect in long term chronic inflammation which leads to liver cirrhosis (Wei, CL et al., 2005).

10. Acknowledgment

I would like to thank My Ph.D. Student Noga Budick-Harmelin for performing the experiments with FaO hepatocytes treated with fatty acid mix (Fig. 5 and 6). I thank also my student khem Bahadur Adhikari for his writing help.

11. References

Adachi, M., & Brenner, D.A. 2005. Clinical syndromes of alcoholic liver disease. *Dig Dis.* 23:255-63.

Adams, L.A., & Lindor, K.D. 2007. Nonalcoholic fatty liver disease. *Ann Epidemiol.* 17:863-9.

Albano, E. 2008. Oxidative mechanisms in the pathogenesis of alcoholic liver disease. *Mol Aspects Med.* 29:9-16.

Alkhouri, N., Dixon, L.J., & Feldstein, A.E. 2009. Lipotoxicity in nonalcoholic fatty liver disease: not all lipids are created equal. *Expert Rev Gastroenterol Hepatol.* 3:445-51.

Amarapurkar, D., Kamani, P., Patel, N., Gupte, P., Kumar, P., Agal, S., Baijal, R., Lala, S., Chaudhary, D., & Deshpande, A. 2007. Prevalence of non-alcoholic fatty liver disease: population based study. *Ann Hepatol.* 6:161-3.

Angulo, P. 2007. Obesity and nonalcoholic fatty liver disease. *Nutr Rev.* 65:S57-63.

Angulo, P., & Lindor, K.D. 2002. Non-alcoholic fatty liver disease. *J Gastroenterol Hepatol.* 17 Suppl:S186-90.

Arky, R.A., & Freinkel, N. 1966. Alcohol hypoglycemia. V. Alcohol infusion to test gluconeogenesis in starvation, with special reference to obesity. *N Engl J Med.* 274:426-33.

Baruteau, J., Levade, T., Redonnet-Vernhet, I., Mesli, S., Bloom, M.C., & Broue, P. 2009. Hypoketotic hypoglycemia with myolysis and hypoparathyroidism: an unusual association in medium chain acyl-CoA desydrogenase deficiency (MCADD). *J Pediatr Endocrinol Metab.* 22:1175-7.

Barve, A., Khan, R., Marsano, L., Ravindra, K.V., & McClain, C. 2008. Treatment of alcoholic liver disease. *Ann Hepatol.* 7:5-15.

Bergheim, I., McClain, C.J., & Arteel, G.E. 2005. Treatment of alcoholic liver disease. *Dig Dis.* 23:275-84.

Browning, J.D., Szczepaniak, L.S., Dobbins, R., Nuremberg, P., Horton, J.D., Cohen, J.C., Grundy, S.M., & Hobbs, H.H. 2004. Prevalence of hepatic steatosis in an urban population in the United States: impact of ethnicity. *Hepatology*. 40:1387-95.

Brunkhorst, F.M., Engel, C., Bloos, F., Meier-Hellmann, A., Ragaller, M., Weiler, N., Moerer, O., Gruendling, M., Oppert, M., Grond, S., Olthoff, D., Jaschinski, U., John, S., Rossaint, R., Welte, T., Schaefer, M., Kern, P., Kuhnt, E., Kiehntopf, M., Hartog, C., Natanson, C., Loeffler, M., & Reinhart, K. 2008. Intensive insulin therapy and pentastarch resuscitation in severe sepsis. *N Engl J Med*. 358:125-39.

Cai, D., Yuan, M., Frantz, D.F., Melendez, P.A., Hansen, L., Lee, J., & Shoelson, S.E. 2005. Local and systemic insulin resistance resulting from hepatic activation of IKK-beta and NF-kappaB. *Nat Med*. 11:183-90.

De Minicis, S., & Brenner, D.A. 2008. Oxidative stress in alcoholic liver disease: role of NADPH oxidase complex. *J Gastroenterol Hepatol*. 23 Suppl 1:S98-103.

Denk, H., Stumptner, C., Fuchsbichler, A., & Zatloukal, K. 2005. [Alcoholic and non-alcoholic steatohepatitis]. *Verh Dtsch Ges Pathol*. 89:137-43.

Denmark, L.N. 1993. The investigation of beta-hydroxybutyrate as a marker for sudden death due to hypoglycemia in alcoholics. *Forensic Sci Int*. 62:225-32.

Farrell, G.C., Teoh, N.C., & McCuskey, R.S. 2008. Hepatic microcirculation in fatty liver disease. *Anat Rec (Hoboken)*. 291:684-92.

Fischer, K.F., Lees, J.A., & Newman, J.H. 1986. Hypoglycemia in hospitalized patients. Causes and outcomes. *N Engl J Med*. 315:1245-50.

Fuhrmann, V., Jager, B., Zubkova, A., & Drolz, A. 2010. Hypoxic hepatitis - epidemiology, pathophysiology and clinical management. *Wien Klin Wochenschr*. 122:129-39.

Fuhrmann, V., Kneidinger, N., Herkner, H., Heinz, G., Nikfardjam, M., Bojic, A., Schellongowski, P., Angermayr, B., Kitzberger, R., Warszawska, J., Holzinger, U., Schenk, P., & Madl, C. 2009. Hypoxic hepatitis: underlying conditions and risk factors for mortality in critically ill patients. *Intensive Care Med*. 35:1397-405.

Gordon, G.G., & Lieber, C.S. 1992. Alcohol, hormones, and metabolism. New York: Plenum Publishing Corp. 55-90 pp.

Hasse, J., & Matarese, L. 2004. Medical nutrition therapy for liver, biliary system, and exocrine pancreas disorders. Elsevier, Philadelphia, . 738-67 pp.

Hickman, I., Russell, A., Prins, J., Macdonald, G., & 2008. Should patient with type 2 diabetes and raised liver enzymes be referred for further evaluation of liver disease? Diabetes. *In* Res and Clin Prac [serial online]. Vol. .Available at www.sciencedirect.com . ;80:e10-e12.

Hirschey, M.D., Shimazu, T., Goetzman, E., Jing, E., Schwer, B., Lombard, D.B., Grueter, C.A., Harris, C., Biddinger, S., Ilkayeva, O.R., Stevens, R.D., Li, Y., Saha, A.K., Ruderman, N.B., Bain, J.R., Newgard, C.B., Farese, R.V., Jr., Alt, F.W., Kahn, C.R., & Verdin, E. 2010. SIRT3 regulates mitochondrial fatty-acid oxidation by reversible enzyme deacetylation. *Nature*. 464:121-5.

Houten, S.M., & Wanders, R.J. 2010. A general introduction to the biochemistry of mitochondrial fatty acid beta-oxidation. *J Inherit Metab Dis*.

Imhof, A., Kratzer, W., Boehm, B., Meitinger, K., Trischler, G., Steinbach, G., Piechotowski, I., & Koenig, W. 2007. Prevalence of non-alcoholic fatty liver and characteristics in overweight adolescents in the general population. *Eur J Epidemiol.* 22:889-97.

Jeschke, M.G., Kraft, R., Emdad, F., Kulp, G.A., Williams, F.N., & Herndon, D.N. 2010. Glucose control in severely thermally injured pediatric patients: what glucose range should be the target? *Ann Surg.* 252:521-7; discussion 527-8.

Jimba, S., Nakagami, T., Takahashi, M., Wakamatsu, T., Hirota, Y., Iwamoto, Y., & Wasada, T. 2005. Prevalence of non-alcoholic fatty liver disease and its association with impaired glucose metabolism in Japanese adults. *Diabet Med.* 22:1141-5.

Joy, D., Thava, V.R., & Scott, B.B. 2003. Diagnosis of fatty liver disease: is biopsy necessary? *Eur J Gastroenterol Hepatol.* 15:539-43.

Judith Fradkin, M.D. 1994. Alcohol Alert. Vol. (National Institute on Alcohol Abuse and Alcoholism Health, N.I.o.A.A.a.A.o.t.N.I.o., editor.

Kagansky, N., Levy, S., Rimon, E., Cojocaru, L., Fridman, A., Ozer, Z., & Knobler, H. 2003. Hypoglycemia as a predictor of mortality in hospitalized elderly patients. *Arch Intern Med.* 163:1825-9.

Kanner, J., Harel, S., & Granit, R. 1991. Nitric oxide as an antioxidant. *Arch Biochem Biophys.* 289:130-6.

Kanner, J., Harel, S., & Granit, R. 1992. Nitric oxide, an inhibitor of lipid oxidation by lipoxygenase, cyclooxygenase and hemoglobin. *Lipids.* 27:46-9.

Kim, M.S., Shigenaga, J.K., Moser, A.H., Feingold, K.R., & Grunfeld, C. 2005. Suppression of estrogen-related receptor alpha and medium-chain acyl-coenzyme A dehydrogenase in the acute-phase response. *J Lipid Res.* 46:2282-8.

Kompare, M., & Rizzo, W.B. 2008. Mitochondrial fatty-acid oxidation disorders. *Semin Pediatr Neurol.* 15:140-9.

Koo, D.J., Chaudry, I.H., & Wang, P. 1999. Kupffer cells are responsible for producing inflammatory cytokines and hepatocellular dysfunction during early sepsis. *J Surg Res.* 83:151-7.

Koo, D.J., Chaudry, I.H., & Wang, P. 2000. Mechanism of hepatocellular dysfunction during sepsis: the role of gut-derived norepinephrine (review). *Int J Mol Med.* 5:457-65.

Koskinas, J., Gomatos, I.P., Tiniakos, D.G., Memos, N., Boutsikou, M., Garatzioti, A., Archimandritis, A., & Betrosian, A. 2008. Liver histology in ICU patients dying from sepsis: a clinico-pathological study. *World J Gastroenterol.* 14:1389-93.

Krinsley, J.S. 2008. The severity of sepsis: yet another factor influencing glycemic control. *Crit Care.* 12:194.

Lamontagne, F., Meade, M., Ondiveeran, H.K., Lesur, O., & Robichaud, A.E. 2008. Nitric oxide donors in sepsis: a systematic review of clinical and in vivo preclinical data. *Shock.* 30:653-9.

Lang, C.H., & Dobrescu, C. 1991. Sepsis-induced increases in glucose uptake by macrophage-rich tissues persist during hypoglycemia. *Metabolism.* 40:585-93.

Leclercq, I.A., Da Silva Morais, A., Schroyen, B., Van Hul, N., & Geerts, A. 2007. Insulin resistance in hepatocytes and sinusoidal liver cells: Mechanisms and consequences>. *J Hepatol.* 47:142-56.

Lieber, C.S. 1997. Ethanol metabolism, cirrhosis and alcoholism. *Clin Chim Acta.* 257:59-84.

Lim, J.H., Lee, J.C., Lee, Y.H., Choi, I.Y., Oh, Y.K., Kim, H.S., Park, J.S., & Kim, W.K. 2006. Simvastatin prevents oxygen and glucose deprivation/reoxygenation-induced death of cortical neurons by reducing the production and toxicity of 4-hydroxy-2E-nonenal. *J Neurochem*. 97:140-50.

Listenberger, L.L., Han, X., Lewis, S.E., Cases, S., Farese, R.V., Jr., Ory, D.S., & Schaffer, J.E. 2003. Triglyceride accumulation protects against fatty acid-induced lipotoxicity. *Proc Natl Acad Sci U S A*. 100:3077-82.

Liu, J., & Waalkes, M.P. 2005. Nitric oxide and chemically induced hepatotoxicity: beneficial effects of the liver-selective nitric oxide donor, V-PYRRO/NO. *Toxicology*. 208:289-97.

Lo, Y.C., Wang, C.C., Shen, K.P., Wu, B.N., Yu, K.L., & Chen, I.J. 2004. Urgosedin inhibits hypotension, hypoglycemia, and pro-inflammatory mediators induced by lipopolysaccharide. *J Cardiovasc Pharmacol*. 44:363-71.

Ludwig, J., Viggiano, T.R., McGill, D.B., & Oh, B.J. 1980. Nonalcoholic steatohepatitis: Mayo Clinic experiences with a hitherto unnamed disease. *Mayo Clin Proc*. 55:434-8.

Lumeng, L., & Crabb, D.W. 2001. Alcoholic liver disease. *Curr Opin Gastroenterol*. 17:211-20.

Madison, L.L. 1968. Ethanol-induced hypoglycemia. *Adv Metab Disord*. 3:85-109.

Maitra, S.R., Gestring, M.L., El-Maghrabi, M.R., Lang, C.H., & Henry, M.C. 1999. Endotoxin-induced alterations in hepatic glucose-6-phosphatase activity and gene expression. *Mol Cell Biochem*. 196:79-83.

Maitra, U., Chang, S., Singh, N., & Li, L. 2009. Molecular mechanism underlying the suppression of lipid oxidation during endotoxemia. *Mol Immunol*. 47:420-5.

Mantena, S.K., King, A.L., Andringa, K.K., Eccleston, H.B., & Bailey, S.M. 2008. Mitochondrial dysfunction and oxidative stress in the pathogenesis of alcohol- and obesity-induced fatty liver diseases. *Free Radic Biol Med*. 44:1259-72.

Miller, S.I., Wallace, R.J., Jr., Musher, D.M., Septimus, E.J., Kohl, S., & Baughn, R.E. 1980. Hypoglycemia as a manifestation of sepsis. *Am J Med*. 68:649-54.

Musso, G., Gambino, R., & Cassader, M. 2009. Non-alcoholic fatty liver disease from pathogenesis to management: an update. *Obes Rev*.

Musso, G., Gambino, R., & Cassader, M. 2010. Non-alcoholic fatty liver disease from pathogenesis to management: an update. *Obes Rev*. 11:430-45.

Nisoli, E., & Carruba, M.O. 2006. Nitric oxide and mitochondrial biogenesis. *J Cell Sci*. 119:2855-62.

Nisoli, E., Clementi, E., Carruba, M.O., & Moncada, S. 2007. Defective mitochondrial biogenesis: a hallmark of the high cardiovascular risk in the metabolic syndrome? *Circ Res*. 100:795-806.

Nomura, T., Keira, N., Urakabe, Y., Naito, D., Nakayama, M., Kido, A., Kanemasa, H., Matsubara, H., & Tatsumi, T. 2009. Chronic pericardial constriction induced severe ischemic hepatitis manifesting as hypoglycemic attack. *Circ J*. 73:183-6.

Novitskiy, G., Traore, K., Wang, L., Trush, M.A., & Mezey, E. 2006. Effects of ethanol and acetaldehyde on reactive oxygen species production in rat hepatic stellate cells. *Alcohol Clin Exp Res*. 30:1429-35.

O'Keefe, S.J., & Marks, V. 1977. Lunchtime gin and tonic a cause of reactive hypoglycaemia. *Lancet*. 1:1286-8.

Oguri, S., Motegi, K., Iwakura, Y., & Endo, Y. 2002. Primary role of interleukin-1 alpha and interleukin-1 beta in lipopolysaccharide-induced hypoglycemia in mice. *Clin Diagn Lab Immunol*. 9:1307-12.

Orford, N.R. 2006. Intensive insulin therapy in septic shock. *Crit Care Resusc*. 8:230-4.

Pietraszek, A., Gregersen, S., & Hermansen, K. 2010. Alcohol and type 2 diabetes. A review. *Nutr Metab Cardiovasc Dis*.

Platia, E.V., & Hsu, T.H. 1979. Hypoglycemic coma with ketoacidosis in nondiabetic alcoholics. *West J Med*. 131:270-6.

Raddatz, D., & Ramadori, G. 2007. Carbohydrate metabolism and the liver: actual aspects from physiology and disease. *Z Gastroenterol*. 45:51-62.

Rai, R.M., Lee, F.Y., Rosen, A., Yang, S.Q., Lin, H.Z., Koteish, A., Liew, F.Y., Zaragoza, C., Lowenstein, C., & Diehl, A.M. 1998. Impaired liver regeneration in inducible nitric oxide synthasedeficient mice. *Proc Natl Acad Sci U S A*. 95:13829-34.

Randall, B. 1980. Fatty liver and sudden death. A review. *Hum Pathol*. 11:147-53.

Rector, R.S., Thyfault, J.P., Wei, Y., & Ibdah, J.A. 2008. Non-alcoholic fatty liver disease and the metabolic syndrome: an update. *World J Gastroenterol*. 14:185-92.

Riehle, K.J., Dan, Y.Y., Campbell, J.S., & Fausto, N. 2011. New concepts in liver regeneration. *J Gastroenterol Hepatol*. 26 Suppl 1:203-12.

Samuel, V.T., Petersen, K.F., & Shulman, G.I. 2010. Lipid-induced insulin resistance: unravelling the mechanism. *Lancet*. 375:2267-77.

Shimano, H. 2007. SREBP-1c and TFE3, energy transcription factors that regulate hepatic insulin signaling. *J Mol Med*. 85:437-44.

Sneyd, J.G.T. 1989. Interactions of ethanol and carbohydrate metabolism. Boca Raton, FL: CRC Press, . 115-124 pp.

Song, Z., Zhou, Z., Deaciuc, I., Chen, T., & McClain, C.J. 2008. Inhibition of adiponectin production by homocysteine: a potential mechanism for alcoholic liver disease. *Hepatology*. 47:867-79.

Spiekerkoetter, U., & Wood, P.A. 2010. Mitochondrial fatty acid oxidation disorders: pathophysiological studies in mouse models. *J Inherit Metab Dis*.

Suzuki, A., Uno, M., Arima, K., Obana, M., Matsuoka, Y., Irimajiri, S., & Fukuda, J. 1994. [A case report: sepsis associated with hypoglycemia]. Kansenshogaku Zasshi. 68:986-9.

Szabo, G., Romics, L., Jr., & Frendl, G. 2002. Liver in sepsis and systemic inflammatory response syndrome. *Clin Liver Dis*. 6:1045-66, x.

Tabassum, F., Khurshid, R., Karim, S., & Akhtar, M.S. 2001. Metabolic effects of alcoholism and its relationship with alcoholic liver disease. *J Ayub Med Coll Abbottabad*. 13:19-21.

Targher, G., Bertolini, L., Padovani, R., Rodella, S., Tessari, R., Zenari, L., Day, C., & Arcaro, G. 2007. Prevalence of nonalcoholic fatty liver disease and its association with cardiovascular disease among type 2 diabetic patients. Diabetes Care. 30:1212-8.

Thompson, B.T. 2008. Glucose control in sepsis. *Clin Chest Med*. 29:713-20, x.

Tirosh, O., Artan, A., Aharoni-Simon, M., Ramadori, G., & Madar, Z. 2010. Impaired liver glucose production in a murine model of steatosis and endotoxemia: protection by inducible nitric oxide synthase. *Antioxid Redox Signal*. 13:13-26.

Tirosh, O., Ilan, E., Budick-harmelin, N., Ramadori, G., & Madar, Z. 2009. Down regulation of eNOS in a nutritional model of fatty liver. *e-SPEN.* 4(2):e101-e104.

Unger, R.H. 1995. Lipotoxicity in the pathogenesis of obesity-dependent NIDDM. Genetic and clinical implications. *Diabetes.* 44:863-70.

Van Amersfoort, E.S., Van Berkel, T.J., & Kuiper, J. 2003. Receptors, mediators, and mechanisms involved in bacterial sepsis and septic shock. *Clin Microbiol Rev.* 16:379-414.

van den Berghe, G., Wouters, P., Weekers, F., Verwaest, C., Bruyninckx, F., Schetz, M., Vlasselaers, D., Ferdinande, P., Lauwers, P., & Bouillon, R. 2001. Intensive insulin therapy in the critically ill patients. *N Engl J Med.* 345:1359-67.

van der Crabben, S.N., Blumer, R.M., Stegenga, M.E., Ackermans, M.T., Endert, E., Tanck, M.W., Serlie, M.J., van der Poll, T., & Sauerwein, H.P. 2009. Early endotoxemia increases peripheral and hepatic insulin sensitivity in healthy humans. *J Clin Endocrinol Metab.* 94:463-8.

Vidali, M., Stewart, S.F., & Albano, E. 2008. Interplay between oxidative stress and immunity in the progression of alcohol-mediated liver injury. *Trends Mol Med.* 14:63-71.

Volk, J., Gorelik, S., Granit, R., Kohen, R., & Kanner, J. 2009. The dual function of nitrite under stomach conditions is modulated by reducing compounds. *Free Radic Biol Med.* 47:496-502.

Wei, C.L., Hon, W.M., Lee, K.H., & Khoo, H.E. 2005. Temporal expression of hepatic inducible nitric oxide synthase in liver cirrhosis. *World J Gastroenterol.* 11:362-7.

Weickert, M.O., & Pfeiffer, A.F. 2006. Signalling mechanisms linking hepatic glucose and lipid metabolism. *Diabetologia.* 49:1732-41.

Weinberg, J.M. 2006. Lipotoxicity. *Kidney Int.* 70:1560-6.

Yan, E., Durazo, F., Tong, M., & Hong, K. 2007. Nonalcoholic fatty liver disease: pathogenesis, identification, progression, and management. *Nutr Rev.* 65:376-84.

Yang, L., & Diehl, A. 2007. Role of immune response in nonalcoholic fatty liver disease: evidence in human and animal studies. Totowa: Humana Press. 337-45 pp.

Yang, S.Q., Lin, H.Z., Lane, M.D., Clemens, M., & Diehl, A.M. 1997. Obesity increases sensitivity to endotoxin liver injury: implications for the pathogenesis of steatohepatitis. *Proc Natl Acad Sci U S A.* 94:2557-62.

Yang, S.Q., Lin, H.Z., Mandal, A.K., Huang, J., & Diehl, A.M. 2001. Disrupted signaling and inhibited regeneration in obese mice with fatty livers: implications for nonalcoholic fatty liver disease pathophysiology. *Hepatology.* 34:694-706.

Yuzuriha, T., Okudaira, M., Tominaga, I., Hori, S., Suzuki, H., Matsuo, Y., Shoji, M., Yokoyama, A., Takagi, S., & Hayashida, M. 1997. Alcohol-related sudden death with hepatic fatty metamorphosis: a comprehensive clinicopathological inquiry into its pathogenesis. *Alcohol Alcohol.* 32:745-52.

Zelber-Sagi, S., Nitzan-Kaluski, D., Halpern, Z., & Oren, R. 2006. Prevalence of primary non-alcoholic fatty liver disease in a population-based study and its association with biochemical and anthropometric measures. *Liver Int.* 26:856-63.

Zeng, M.D., Li, Y.M., Chen, C.W., Lu, L.G., Fan, J.G., Wang, B.Y., & Mao, Y.M. 2008. Guidelines for the diagnosis and treatment of alcoholic liver disease. *J Dig Dis.* 9:113-6.

Zhou, Y.J., Li, Y.Y., Nie, Y.Q., Ma, J.X., Lu, L.G., Shi, S.L., Chen, M.H., & Hu, P.J. 2007. Prevalence of fatty liver disease and its risk factors in the population of South China. *World J Gastroenterol*. 13:6419-24.

Zivkovic, A.M., German, J.B., & Sanyal, A.J. 2007. Comparative review of diets for the metabolic syndrome: implications for nonalcoholic fatty liver disease. *Am J Clin Nutr*. 86:285-300.

6

Postprandial Hypoglycemia

Mubeen Khan[1] and Udaya M. Kabadi[2,3,4]
[1]*University of Iowa-Des Moines Internal Medicine Residency Program at Iowa Methodist Medical Center, Des Moines, Iowa*
[2]*Veterans Affairs Medical Center, Iowa Methodist Medical Center,*
[3]*Des Moines University of Osteopathic Medicine, Des Moines, Iowa,*
[4]*University of Iowa Carver College of Medicine, Iowa City, Iowa, USA*

1. Introduction

Postprandial hypoglycemia is a syndrome secondary to disorders in which hypoglycemia is manifested within 5 hours after a meal (1). It is classified into two types depending on the time of occurrence, i.e., 'early,' with onset within 2 hours, and 'late,' occurring between 3 and 5 hours after a meal. The early variety is thought to be secondary to abnormally rapid gastric emptying, whereas late postprandial hypoglycemia is frequently deemed to be a precursor to the onset of type 2 diabetes mellitus (1-14). Causes of late postprandial hypoglycemia also include disorders manifesting as fasting hypoglycemia, such as factitious hypoglycemia due to exogenous insulin administration or surreptitious use of insulin secretogogues, e.g, sulfonylureas, glinides, or other hypoglycemic agents, insulinoma, islet cell hyperplasia, autoimmune hyperinsulinemia, hyperinsulinemia caused by drugs and toxins, excess of circulating IGF2 secreted by non-pancreatic tumors, adrenal or pituitary hypofunction, advanced liver dysfunction, and end-stage renal disease(15-29) Several rare disorders, including some congenital syndromes, e.g., glycogen storage disorders, can also cause late postprandial hypoglycemia(30). In contrast, early postprandial hypoglycemia occurs only postprandially and usually is noted in subjects following upper gastrointestinal surgery, including bariatric procedures, hyperthyroidism, etc (1,21,26,31,32). In some subjects, it occurs without an obvious apparent cause and is therefore termed 'idiopathic reactive hypoglycemia.' Arguably, many endocrinologists approve of this syndrome, whereas others question its existence and call it 'postprandial syndrome,' probably because of the debate over the diagnosis of hypoglycemia itself (8,21,29).

Hypoglycemia presents with manifestations of increased sympathetic activity, i.e., anxiety, jitters, palpitations, dizziness, tremor, weakness, drenching perspiration, hunger, systolic hypertension, mydriasis, etc., attributed to prompt release of catecholamines, which is documented to occur with a fall of blood sugar to lower than 70 mg /dl (29,34,35). Manifestations more seriously detrimental to life, i.e., of a neuroglycopenic nature, include convulsion, confusion, coma, or other altered states of consciousness, and transient CNS manifestations, including hemiparesis. Cardiac manifestations include symptomatic coronary artery disease, i.e., angina pectoris, arrhythmias, or even myocardial infarction following extreme lowering of blood sugars, usually to concentrations below 50 mg/dl (35).

Few authorities still believe that the onset of manifestations of exaggerated sympathetic activity may be dependent on the rapidity of rate of fall in blood glucose irrespective of the exact concentration, although several studies have refuted this hypothesis.
Therefore, in subjects with diabetes, hypoglycemia is deemed to occur with the onset of symptoms even when the blood sugar is between 50 and 70 mg/dl. Moreover, blood sugars lower than 70 mg/dl in the absence of manifestations of sympathetic overactivity are also defined as hypoglycemia and the subject is deemed to manifest hypoglycemia unawareness (36-38). Finally, all efforts are made to prevent 'hypoglycemia' in both these circumstances frequently by altering the treatment plan. In contrast, several authorities promote that the diagnosis of hypoglycemia should be made in the presence of blood sugar <50 mg/dl and that too only if criteria for Whipple's triad are fulfilled (39). The triad consists of documentation of a blood sugar <50 mg/dl accompanied by symptoms of hypoglycemia, and resolution of symptoms by inducing a rise in blood sugar by either ingestion of sugar or a meal, or iv administration of glucose.
Thus, according to these authors, subjects with documentation of a blood sugar < 50 mg/dl, after an overnight fast, postprandially, or randomly, deserve evaluation in the absence of diabetes mellitus only if the low blood sugar is accompanied by symptoms (21,26,29),. The recommendation is totally different in the presence of diabetes. In subjects with diabetes, a thorough assessment of hypoglycemic symptoms and even asymptomatic low blood sugar is recommended. Therefore, in the absence of symptoms, in non-diabetic subjects, a blood sugar < 50 mg/dl is not defined as a syndrome of 'hypoglycemia' by these authors. However, this concept is in stark contrast to the tenet of ethical medical practice to define and treat disorders with definite documentation of metabolic abnormalities despite the absence of symptoms, e.g., hyperglycemia, hypercalcemia, changes in sodium and potassium concentrations, and many other medical disorders, including subclinical hypo and hyperthyroidism. This practice is obviously prudent in the light of clear documentation of increased morbidity and even mortality of subclinical disorders, especially with lack of restoration of the normal state. Furthermore, restoring and preserving the normal state with appropriate treatment is also documented to improve the quality of life in these subjects manifesting subclinical disorders. Therefore, it is difficult to fathom why the same principle is not applied in the management of well documented postprandial hypoglycemia in the absence of typical symptoms or frequently even in the presence of characteristic manifestations.
We firmly believe that postprandial hypoglycemia is a 'true' disorder with a distinct deterioration in quality of life, including attention deficit and loss of productivity (1,9 - 14,40),. Moreover, a cause of the abnormality is easily determined by a detailed history, a thorough physical examination, and simple laboratory testing. A history of upper gastrointestinal surgery for esophageal and gastric diseases, bariatric procedures, symptoms of hyperthyroidism, the timing of the occurrence of symptoms following a meal, i.e., 'early' or 'late' onset, dietary pattern provoking symptoms, i.e., high carbohydrate content or ingestion of simple sugars, changes in body weight, use of certain drugs, history of gestational diabetes; all provide clues to indicate a specific diagnosis. Family history of type 2 diabetes mellitus is important information as well. Similarly, a thorough physical examination may indicate the presence of a specific disorder. Finally, the determination of appropriate laboratory tests after an overnight fast and at frequent (30 minute) intervals, up

to 5 hours or at the onset of symptoms of hypoglycemia following ingestion of a mixed meal or glucose (OGGT) often clinches the diagnosis.

The occurrence of postprandial hypoglycemia within 2 hours is attributed to an exaggerated insulin response to markedly elevated plasma glucose levels within 15-30 minutes caused by a prompt absorption of carbohydrate content, especially the simple variety due to a super fast transit of an ingested meal across the stomach as initially documented in subjects undergoing gastric surgery e.g. partial or total gastrectomy for several decades and more recently in morbidly obese subjects undergoing gastric bypass surgery(1,54,8,20,21,26) In fact ,we believe that persistent occurrence of hypoglycemia irrespective of timing of the meal during the later years following gastric bypass surgery may attributed to repeated frequent postprandial stimulation of pancreatic beta cells ultimately leading to autonomous beta cell hyperplasia requiring excision (26) .Surgery may be prevented by appropriate dietary changes as well as a prompt therapy with medications during the initial period following a bariatric procedure (42-47)

In the absence of documentation of a known disorder, early postprandial hypoglycemia is also termed 'Idiopathic reactive hypoglycemia' by some and 'postprandial syndrome' by others. We firmly believe that 'Idiopathic reactive hypoglycemia' is a genuine disorder, since several pathophysiologic mechanisms have been implicated (2-14).The occurrence of hypoglycemia in this disorder has been attributed to rapid gastric emptying secondary to lack of rise in Gastric Inhibitory Polypeptide following an ingestion of a meal or altered secretion of other gastrointestinal motility factors,e.g.Motilin, Bombesin etc(1-4) Remission of hypoglycemia by inhibition of gastric emptying by use of drugs with ability to induce cholinergic blockade enhances this hypothesis. Alternatively, altered function of both pancreatic alpha and beta cells has also been invoked. We have documented enhanced 1st or early phase insulin secretion within 30-60 minutes in response to glucose ingestion as well as aberrant pancreatic alpha cell function in this syndrome (Table 1). plasma glucagon is elevated after an overnight fast in comparison to normal subjects despite presence of normal glucose concentration indicating glucagon insensitivity (Table1). However, inhibited glucagon decline with initial hyperglycemia and a blunted rise following onset of hypoglycemia documents altered glucagon secretion in this syndrome.(Figure1) Impaired regulation of glucagon in this syndrome is further confirmed by decline in glucagon response following oral administration of a protein meal (figure 2), a well established stimulus for facilitating glucagon secretion and release by pancreatic alpha cells(41).This altered pancreatic alpha and beta cell function is also documented in several other studies (7,9,1,33,40). Finally, the presence of the disorder is further enhanced by documentation of remission of symptoms and hypoglycemia by appropriate intervention with several protocols, including lifestyle changes with use of a diet with tolerated amount of fiber as well as high protein, low carbohydrate contents, avoidance of ingestion of simple or free sugars, and frequent small feedings (1,5,14). Moreover, in the absence of total remission with these lifestyle changes, several drugs have been successfully used. These include agents, e.g. atropine derivatives which delay gastric emptying by cholinergic blockade as mentioned earlier, drugs inhibiting conversion of complex to simple carbohydrates,e.g.alpha-glucosidase inhibitors, medications altering insulin secretion e.g.calcium channel blockers, or drugs possessing all of these properties, e.g. octreotide (3,42-47). In contrast, 'late reactive or postrprandial hypoglycemia'documented in 'impaired glucose tolerance', a prediabetic state is induced by exaggerated 2nd or late phase insulin secretion occurring between 90 -120 minutes induced by marked elevated plasma glucose concentration at 60-90 minutes due to inhibition of 1`st phase insulin secretion following a meal or oral administration of glucose (48-52)).Moreover, hypoglycemia in this disorder also is remediable by appropriate lifestyle changes and certain drugs (53).

Therefore, A subject manifesting symptoms of hypoglycemia following a meal must be evaluated by a detailed history, a thorough physical examination and appropriate laboratory testing. First and foremost, the presence of low blood sugar level, e.g $\leq$ 6O mg/dl must be documented with accompanying hypoglycemic symptoms. The diagnosis could be further established by assessment of blood sugars following ingestion of a mixed meal or oral administration of glucose. Once the diagnosis is confirmed, the appropriate treatment should be provided as it distinctly improves quality of life. Early postprandial hypoglycemia with onset within 2 hours may be treated with life style dietary changes initially. The drugs may be used later as an adjunctive therapy if dietary manipulations fail to attain and maintain remission. The documentation of late reactive hypoglycemia indicates a presence of 'Prediabetes' which also may be managed with lifestyle changes, e.g. diet and exercise, to achieve weight loss especially in the obese subjects as well as with drugs, e.g. Metformin in subjects with increased risk for progression to Diabetes as recommended by American Diabetes Association(48),

Therefore, in the final analysis, it is imperative to consider the presence of postprandial hypoglycemia as a disorder and conduct an appropriate evaluation and provide suitable therapeutic strategies.

Group	Age (yr)	Body Weight (kg)	Fasting Plasma Glucose (mmol/L)*	Fasting Plasma Insulin (mU/L)*	Fasting Plasma Glucagon (ng/L)*
IHR	37±6	59±8	4.9±0.2	7±2	347±83†
Normal	34±5	62±7	5.2±0.1	6±1	135±20

* The average of 2 values in individual subjects, 1 during the OGTT and the other during the protein meal study, was used for calculation.

† P< .025, IRH v normal.

Reprinted from reference 12, with permission

Table 1. Fasting Plasma Glucose, Insulin,and Glucagon Levels in Five Subjects With IRH and Six Normal Subjects.

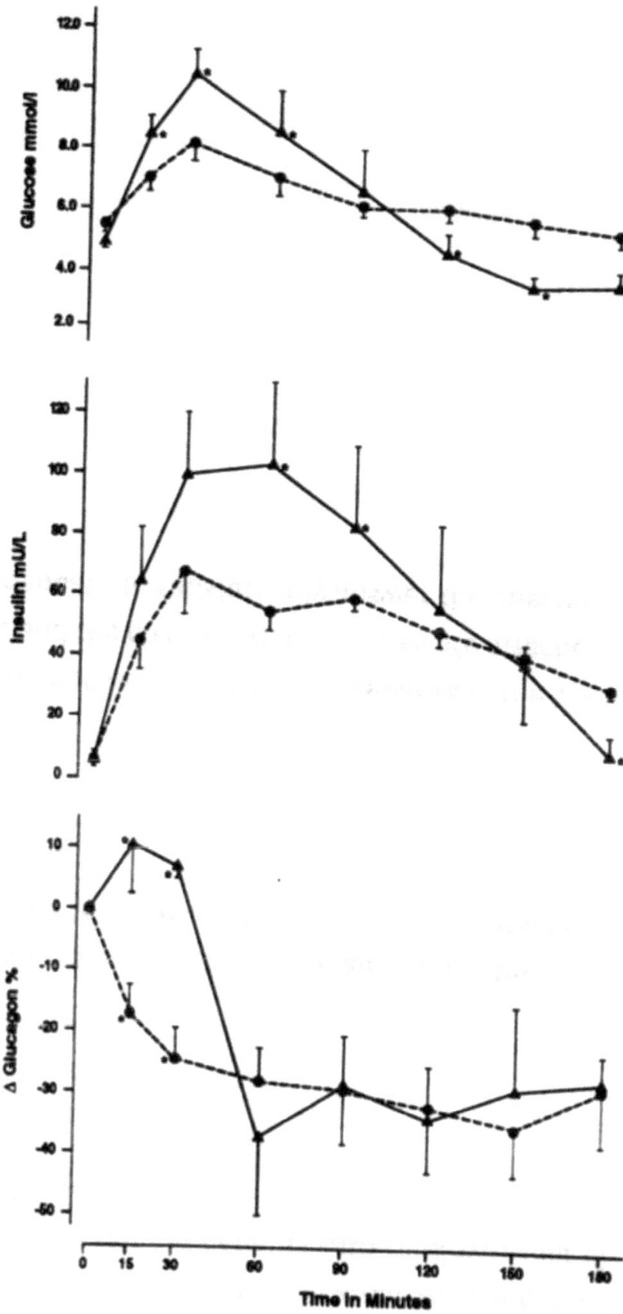

Fig. 1. Glucose, insulin, and glucagon responses to oral ingestion of 100 g glucose(OGTT) in 5 subjects with IRH (▲) and 6 normal subjects (●) * P< .01 v normal. Reprinted from reference 12, with permission

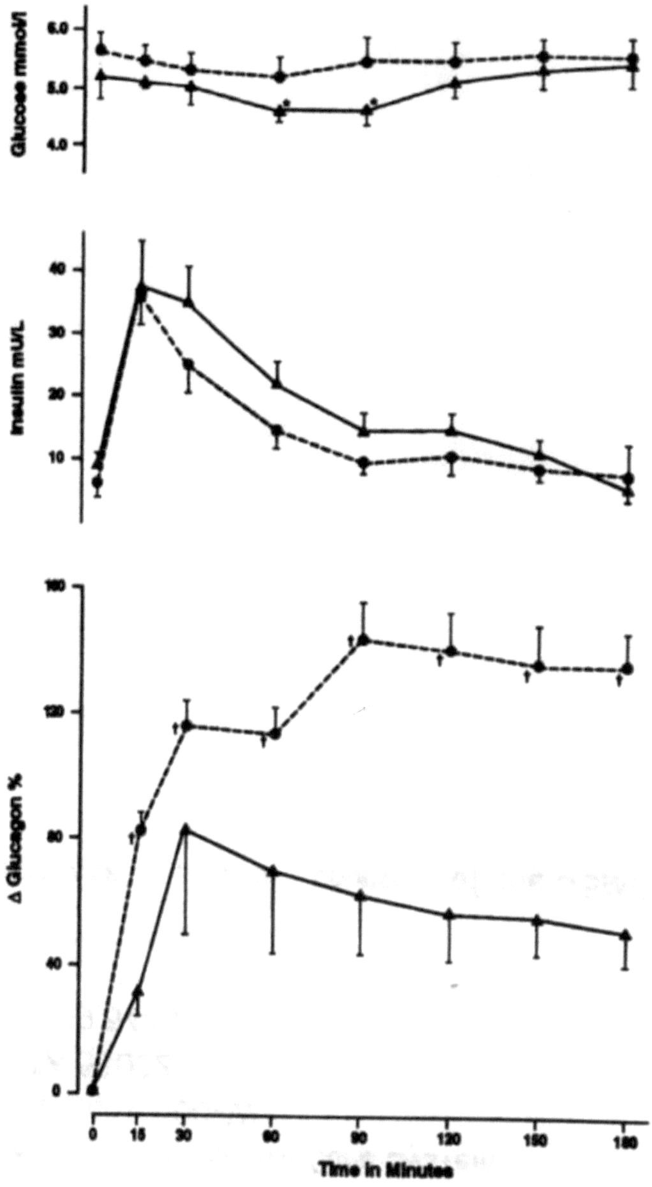

Fig. 2. Glucose, insulin, and glucagon responses to oral ingestion of a protein meal in 5 subjects with IRH (▲) and 6 normal subjects (●). * < .05 v normal. † P< .01 IRH. Reprinted from reference 12, with permission

2. References

[1] Kunkel S, Kabadi,U Non-diabetic hypoglycemia BMJ Point of Care,2011

[2] O'Keefe SJ, Marks V. Lunchtime gin and tonic as a cause of reactive hypoglycemia. Lancet. 1977;1:1286-1288

[3] Permutt MA, Keller D, Santiago J.Cholinergic blockade in reactive hypoglycemia. Diabetes. 1977 Feb;26(2):121-7.

[4] Lev-Ran A, Anderson RW The diagnosis of postprandial hypoglycemia. Diabetes. 1981 Dec;30(12):996-9.

[5] Betteridge DJ Reactive hypoglycaemia. Br Med J (Clin Res Ed). 1987 Aug 1;295:286-7.

[6] Palardy J, Havrankova J, Lepage R, et al. Blood glucose measurements during symptomatic episodes in patients with suspected postprandial hypoglycemia. N Engl J Med. 1989;321:1421-1425

[7] Tamburrano G, Leonetti F, Sbraccia P, Giaccari A, Locuratolo N, Lala A Increased insulin sensitivity in patients with idiopathic reactive hypoglycemia. J Clin Endocrinol Metab. 1989 Oct;69(4):885-90.

[8] Hofeldt FD.Reactive hypoglycemia. Endocrinol Metab Clin North Am. 1989 Mar;18(1):185-201

[9] Leonetti F, Morviducci L, Giaccari A, Sbraccia P, Caiola S, Zorretta D, Lostia O, Tamburrano G Idiopathic reactive hypoglycemia: a role for glucagon? J Endocrinol Invest. 1992 Apr;15(4):273-8.

[10] Berlin I, Grimaldi A, Landault C, Cesselin F, Puech AJ Suspected postprandial hypoglycemia is associated with beta-adrenergic hypersensitivity and emotional distress. J Clin Endocrinol Metab. 1994 Nov;79(5):1428-33.

[11] Leonetti F, Foniciello M, Iozzo P, Riggio O, Merli M, Giovannetti P, Sbraccia P, Giaccari A, Tamburrano G Increased nonoxidative glucose metabolism in idiopathic reactive hypoglycemia. Metabolism. 1996 May;45(5):606-10.

[12] Ahmadpour S, Kabadi UM.Pancreatic alpha-cell function in idiopathic reactive hypoglycemia. Metabolism. 1997 Jun;46(6):639-43.

[13] Altuntas Y, Bilir M, Ucak S, Gundogdu S. Reactive hypoglycemia in lean young women with PCOS and correlations with insulin sensitivity and with beta cell function. Eur J Obstet Gynecol Reprod Biol. 2005 Apr 1;119(2):198-205.

[14] Sørensen M, Johansen OE Idiopathic reactive hypoglycaemia - prevalence and effect of fibre on glucose excursions.Scand J Clin Lab Invest. 2010 Oct;70(6):385-91

[15] Kogut MD, Blaskovics M, Donnell GN, et al. Idiopathic hypoglycemia: a study of twenty-six children. J Pediatr. 1969;74:853-871

[16] Bressler R, Corredor C, Brendel K. Hypoglycin and hypoglycin-like compounds. Pharmacol Rev. 1969;21:105-130

[17] Merimee TJ, Felif P, Marliss E, et al. Glucose and lipid homeostasis in the absence of human growth hormone. J Clin Invest. 1971;50:574-582

[18] Service FJ. Factitial hypoglycemia. Endocrinologist. 1992;2:173- 176.

[19] Cryer PE. Glucose counterregulation: prevention and correction of hypoglycemia in humans. Am J Physiol. 1993;264:E149-E155

[20] Marks V, Teale JD Hypoglycaemia in the adult. Baillieres Clin Endocrinol Metab. 1993 Jul;7(3):705-29.

[21] Service FJ.Hypoglycemic disorders. N Engl J Med. 1995;332:1144-1152

[22] Fischer KF, Lees JA, Newman JH, et al. Hypoglycemia in hospitalized patients: causes and outcomes. N Engl J Med. 1996;315:1245-1250

[23] Hizuka N, Fukuda I, Takano K, et al. Serum insulin-like growth factor II in 44 patients with non-islet cell tumor hypoglycemia. Endocr J. 1998;45:S61-S65

[24] Cavaco B, Uchigata Y, Porto T, Amparo-Santos M, Sobrinho L, Leite V Hypoglycaemia due to insulin autoimmune syndrome: report of two cases with characterisation of HLA alleles and insulin autoantibodies. Eur J Endocrinol. 2001 Sep;145(3):311-6.

[25] Kim CH, Park JH, Park TS, et al. Autoimmune hypoglycemia in a type 2 diabetic patient with anti-insulin and insulin receptor antibodies. Diabetes Care. 2004;27:288-289

[26] Service GJ, Thompson GB, Service FJ, et al. Hyperinsulinemic hypoglycemia with nesidioblastosis after gastric-bypass surgery. N Engl J Med. 2005;353: 249-254

[27] Karachaliou R, Vlachopapadopoulou E, Kaldrymidis P, et al. Malignant insulinoma in childhood. J Pediatr Endocrinol Metab. 2006;19:757-760

[28] Murad MH, Coto-Yglesias F, Wang AT, et al. Clinical review: drug-induced hypoglycemia: a systematic review. J Clin Endocrinol Metab. 2009;94: 741-745.

[29] Cryer PE, Axelrod L, Grossman AB, et al. Evaluation and management of adult hypoglycemic disorders: an Endocrine Society clinical practice guideline. J Clin Endocrinol Metab. 2009;94:709-728.

[30] Talente GM, Coleman RA, Alter C, et al. Glycogen storage disease in adults. Ann Intern Med. 1994;120:218-226

[31] Kabadi UM and Eisenstein AB Glucose Intolerance in Hyperthyroidism:Role of Glucagon J Clin Endocrinol Metab50:392-396,1980

[32] Kabadi UM, Eisenstein AB. Impaired pancreatic @-cell response in hyperthyroidism. J Clin Endo Metab 51:478, 1980.

[33] Kabadi UM Hepatic regulation of pancreatic alpha-cell function. Metabolism. 1993 May;42(5):535-43.

[34] Cryer PE Mechanisms of hypoglycemia-associated autonomic failure and its component syndromes in diabetes. Diabetes. 2005 Dec;54(12):3592-601.

[35] Cryer PE Hypoglycemia, functional brain failure, and brain death.J Clin Invest. 2007 Apr;117(4):868-70

[36] Arbelaez AM, Powers WJ, Videen TO, Price JL,Cryer PE Attenuation of counterregulatory responses to recurrent hypoglycemia by active thalamic inhibition: a mechanism for hypoglycemia-associated autonomic failure. Diabetes. 2008 Feb;57(2):470-5.

[37] Akram K, Pedersen-Bjergaard U, Carstensen B, Borch-Johnsen K, Thorsteinsson B Frequency and risk factors of severe hypoglycaemia in insulin-treated

Type 2 diabetes: a cross-sectional survey. Diabet Med. 2006 Jul;23(7): 750-6.

[38] Weber KK, Lohmann T, Busch K, Donati-Hirsch I, Riel R. High frequency of unrecognized hypoglycaemias in patients with Type 2 diabetes is discovered by continuous glucose monitoring. Exp Clin Endocrinol Diabetes. 2007 Sep;115(8): 491-4

[39] Whipple AOThe Surgical Therapy of Hyperinsulinoma J.Int Chir 3:237, 1938

[40] Kabadi UM and Kabadi MU Idiopathic Reactive Hypoglycemia: Resolution on Increased Protein Intake secondary to Decreased Insulin Response with Enhanced Glucagon Rise. Endocrine Society Annual Meeting ,Page 540,Absract no P2-568,June 2006

[41] Kabadi UM.Dose-kinetics of pancreatic alpha- and beta-cell responses to a protein meal in normal subjects. Metabolism. 1991 Mar;40(3):236-40

[42] Richard JL, Rodier M, Monnier L, Orsetti A, Mirouze J Effect of acarbose on glucose and insulin response to sucrose load in reactive hypoglycemia. Diabete Metab. 1988 ,14(2):114-8.

[43] Peter S. Acarbose and idiopathic reactive hypoglycemia. Horm Res, 2003;60(4):166-7.

[44] Renard E, Parer-Richard C, Richard JL, Jureidini S, Orsetti A, Mirouze J.Effect of Miglitol (Bay m1099), a new alpha-glucosidase inhibitor, on glucose, insulin, C-peptide and GIP responses to an oral sucrose load in patients with post-prandial hypoglycaemic symptoms. Diabete Metab. 1991 May-Jun;17(3):355-62.

[45] Sanke T, Nanjo K, Kondo M, Ni M, Moriyama Y Effect of calcium antagonists on reactive hypoglycemia associated with hyperinsulinemia. MetabolismJun;38(6):568-71.

[46] Baschieri L, Antonelli A, del Guerra P, Fialdini A, Gasperini L. Somatostatin effect in postprandial hypoglycemia. Metabolism. 1989 Jun;38(6):568-71.

[47] Weyer C., Bogardus C., Mott D.M., Pratley R.E. (1999) The natural history of insulin secretory dysfunction and insulin resistance in the pathogenesis of type 2 diabetes mellitus. *The Journal of Clinical Investigation*, 104, 787-794.

[48] Kabadi MU, Kabadi, UM. Effects of glimepiride on insulin secretion and sensitivity in patients with recently diagnosed type 2 diabetes mellitus. Clinical Therapeutics 26(1) 2004

[49] Ferrannini E., Gastaldelli A., Miyazaki Y., Matsuda M., Mari A., DeFronzo R.A.B-cell function in subjects spanning the range from normal glucose Tolerance to overt diabetes: A new analysis. *The Journal of Clinical Endocrinology & Metabolism*. 90, 493-500. 2005

[50] Abdul-Ghani M.A., Tripathy D., Jenckinson C., Ritchardson D., DeFronzo R.A.Insulin secretion and insulin action in subjects with impaired fasting glucose and impaired glucose tolerance: results from the Veterans Administration Genetic Epidemiology Study (VEGAS). *Diabetes*, 55, 1430-1435. 2006

[51] Kabadi UM ,Kabadi MU Early Postprandial Insulin Secretion:Its Relation to Insulin Sensitivity J Diabetes Mellitus1(1),1-5,2011.

[52] American Diabetes association. Standard of Medical Care in Diabetes Diabetes Care : 34,S11-S61,2011

7

The Role of the Pituitary-Growth Hormone-IGF Axis in Glucose Homeostasis

Stephen F. Kemp
University of Arkansas for Medical Sciences
Arkansas Children's Hospital
U. S. A.

1. Introduction

Hypoglycemia results when either carbohydrate intake is low, tissue use is high (glycolysis or glucagons synthesis), or endogenous production of glucose is low (glycogenolysis and glyuconeogenesis)(Berry, Nathan et al. 2009). Glucose levels are controlled by the hormone insulin, and also by the counterregulatory hormones glucagons, cortisol, growth hormone (GH), epinephrine, and norepinephrine. The counterregulatory hormones stimulate production and release of glucose. Hypoglycemia is the most common metabolic problem in neonates, and is also seen in children and adults.

2. The pituitary-growth hormone-IGF axis

2.1 Embryology of the pituitary gland

The pituitary gland develops from invagination of the oral ectoderm (Rathke's pouch)(Frohnert and Miller 2009). Nearby neuroectoderm becomes the posterior pituitary, which secretes the hormones oxytocin and vasopressin. Signalling factors involved in the initial differentiation of the anterior pituitary (thickening of the oral ectoderm) include the transcription factors HESX1, PITX1, LHX3, and LHX4. Under the influence of the transcription factor TPIT some of the cells develop into corticotrophs which secrete ACTH. When influenced by transcription factors PROP1, PIT1 (now called POU1F1), PITX1 and PITX2 the remaining cells differentiate into gonadotrophs (which secrete FSH and LH), thyrotrophs (which secrete TSH), somatotrophs (which secrete GH), and lactotrophs (which secrete PRL). During this process the oral ectoderm and the neuroectoderm remain in contact with each other, and both migrate together to form the pituitary with distinct anterior and posterior lobes. All of the hormones of the anterior pituitary are influenced by secretions from the hypothalamus and are regulated through specific feedback loops. Two hormones of the anterior pituitary protect against hypoglycemia— GH and ACTH. ACTH stimulates secretion of cortisol by the adrenal gland. Both GH and cortisol protect against hypoglycemia by countering the effects of insulin.

2.2 The GH-IGF system

The GH/IGF axis is shown in Figure 1. It is regulated by three peptides, two from the hypothalamus (that part of the brain closest to the pituitary gland) (Growth Hormone

Transcription Factor	Function
HESX1	Involved in formation of Rathke's pouch
PITX1	Formation of pituitary. Involved in differentiation of pituitary cell into a corticotroph (secreting ACTH) or a gonadotroph (LH/FSH)
PITX2	Formation of pituitary. Differentiation of pituitary cell into a somatotroph (GH) or a lactotroph (PRL)
LHX3	Formation of pituitary. Differentiation of pituitary cell into precursor for gonadotrophs, thyrotrophs, samatotrophs, and lactotrophs.
LHX4	Formation of pituitary. Differentiation of pituitary cell into precursor for gonadotrophs, thyrotrophs, samatotrophs, and lactotrophs.
SF1	Differentiation of gonadotrophs.
TPIT	Differentiation of corticotrophs.
NEUROD1	Differentiation of corticotrophs
POU1F1 (PIT1)	Differentiation of cells into precursors of thyrotrophs, somatotrophs, and lactotrophs.
PROP1	Differentiation of cells into precursors of gonadotrophs, thyrotrophs, somatotrophs, and lactotrophs.

Table 1. Transcription factors involved in the differentiation of the anterior pituitary.

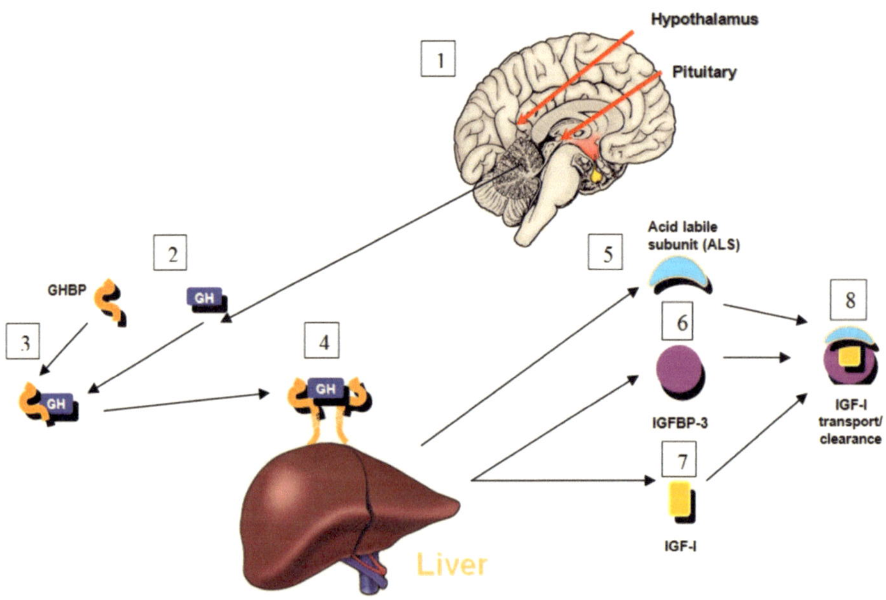

Fig. 1. The Hypothalamic-GH-IGF system 1. The hypothalamus secretes GHRH and somatostatin. 2. GH is secreted into the general circulation. 3. GH circulates bound to its binding protein, GHBP. 4. GH binds to the GH receptor. 5. ALS, 6. IGFBP-3, and 7. IGF-I circulate together in a 140 kDa complex. 8. IGF-I acts at the growth plate.

Releasing Hormone (GHRH) and somatostatin), and one from the gastrointestinal tract (ghrelin). Growth hormone releasing hormone (GHRH), signals the pituitary to secrete GH into the general circulation. The other hypothalamic signal is somatostatin, which inhibits GH secretion. These two signals alternate in their expression, so that when GHRH is high, somatostatin is low, and vice versa. The third factor, ghrelin, also stimulates GH secretion. GH is secreted in discrete bursts, and, once secreted, remains in circulation for about 20 mintues.

GH circulates bound to GH binding protein (GHBP), which in humans is identical to the extracellular portion of the GH receptor. GHBP is produced as a result of cleavage of the extracellular portion of the GH receptor. In order for GH to act two GH molecules bind to adjacent GH receptors, resulting in a conformational shift in the GH receptor, which activates the JAK-STAT pathway in the cell. Activation of the JAK-STAT pathway initiates a cascade of intracellular events, ultimately increasing production of Insulin-like Growth Factor I (IGF-I). GH stimulates statural growth by action directly at the growth plate and indirectly through the production of IGF-I. The name growth hormone is somewhat unfortunate, in that it suggests that its only function is to stimulate growth. In addition to its involvement in the growth process, GH has many metabolic functions, such as increasing muscle mass and bone mineral density. Generally, the effects of GH are anabolic.

There are two GH genes, located on chromosome 17 in the human, GH-1 and GH-2. The GH-1 (or GH-N) gene encodes for GH. It consists of five exons separated by four introns (Parks, Nielson et al. 1985). The most abundant hormone of the pituitary gland, GH is a single chain α-helical non-glycosylated polypeptide consisting of 191 amino acids with two intramolecular disulphide bonds between amino acid 52-165 and 282-189. Different forms of GH exist with the most common form of GH being the one with a molecular weight of 22-kD, which accounts for about 75% of the GH produced in the pituitary gland. Alternative splicing of the second codon results in a 20-kD form that make up about 5-10% of the total GH. There is structural homology between the GH molecule and prolactin and human placental lactogen (human chorionic somatotropin), suggesting that they may all have descended from a common ancestral gene.

GH acts by binding to its receptor primarily at two sites, the liver and the growth plate. In the liver activation of the GH receptor stimulates production of IGF-I, its binding protein IGFBP-3, and the acid labile subunit (ALS). Growth hormone circulates at least 50% bound to its binding protein, GHBP (Rosenfeld 2005). It binds specifically with high affinity and low capacity. In humans the circulating GHBP is actually the extracellular domain of the GH receptor; it is thought that GHBP is shed or cleaved from intact receptors. The physiological significance of GH binding by GHBP is not completely understood; it may act to prolong the half-life of GH in the serum or it may compete with the GH receptor for binding.

Insulin-like growth factors (IGF-I and IGF-II) are small peptide hormones (~7.5 kDa) which share a high degree of homology with proinsulin (Rinderknecht and Humbel 1978; Rinderknecht and Humbel 1978). Almost ubiquitously produced, they circulate at high concentrations in serum. Beyond their insulin-like effects, these growth-promoting peptides influence cellular proliferation and differentiation in numerous tissues, including at the growth plate (Nilsson, Marino et al. 2005). For IGFs to exert their effects at the cell surface, they must first bind specific, high affinity cell-surface receptors, principally the type I IGF receptor. The interaction of IGFs with cell-surface receptors, however, is tightly regulated by at least six distinct high affinity carrier proteins, the IGF- binding proteins (IGFBPs).

IGF-I is the IGF most directly under GH control. It circulates in serum as part of a 140-kDa complex consisting of IGF-I, IGFBP3, and a third 85 KDa factor named acid-labile subunit (ALS) (Baxter 1994). It is probably binding of free (unbound) IGF-I to receptors on chondrocytes in the epiphyseal growth plates that stimulates linear growth. Although the primary site of synthesis of IGF binding proteins is the liver, it has been shown that most tissues produce IGFBPs locally. They may act as part of paracrine and autocrine functions of the IGFs. Functions that the IGFBPs may perform include; 1) increasing the half-life of IGF-I in serum; 2) decreasing binding of IGF-I with the insulin receptor reducing the risk of IGF-induced hypoglycemia; 3) being involved in the transport of IGF-I between the intravascular and the extravascular space ; 4) blocking the local effects of IGF-I; 5) enhancing IGF-I action by keeping the IGF-I in a slowly-releasing pool and 6) modulating cellular proliferation and apoptosis through interaction with receptors other than the IGF-I receptor. Disruption of the IGF:IGFBP:ALS complex is probably a prerequisite for IGFs to exert mitogenic and metabolic effects through the type I IGF receptor.

IGF-I, IGFBP3 and ALS all appear to be regulated by GH, since they are all low in GH deficiency and are restored with GH treatment (Jorgensen, Blum et al. 1991). About 80% of circulating IGF-I is produced the in the liver (IGF-I and ALS are produced by hepatocytes, while ALS is produced by Kupffer cells and sinusoidal endothelial cells), although locally produced IGF-I may be important for skeletal growth (Sjogren, Liu et al. 1999; Yakar, J. et al. 2002). It is not clear whether GH regulates all components of the 140-kDa complex directly, or whether one of the components may be regulated by GH, which, in turn, regulates synthesis of the others (Binoux 1997). Transcription of the rat ALS gene and ALS promoter activity has been shown to be stimulated by GH (Ooi, Cohen et al. 1997). In Growth Hormone Insensitivity Syndrome (GHIS) the patient is unresponsive to growth hormone; that is, the GHIS patient has high circulating levels of growth hormone, but low circulating levels of IGF-I and IGFBP3. In the case of a patient described with the IGF-I gene deletion (Woods, Camacho-Hubner et al. 1996), there are high circulating levels of growth hormone and low circulating levels of IGF-I, but normal circulating levels of IGFBP3.

2.3 GH receptor/signaling

The GH receptor is a member of the cytokine family of receptors. The gene for the human growth hormone receptor is located on chromosome 5p13.1-p12, and spans a region that is greater than 87 kb. The receptor consists of 620 amino acids (molecular weight 70 kD before glycosylation). It is highly homologous with the prolactin receptor, as well as receptors for interleukins 2,3,4,6, and 7, erythropoietin, granulocyte-macrophage colony-stimulating factor, and interferon. The GH receptor has extracellular, transmembrane, and intracellular domains, but it lacks intrinsic tyrosine kinase activity. Similar to other members of the cytokine family of receptors, it uses the JAK-STAT pathway for signal transduction (see Figure 2). Initially GH binds one GH receptor and then recruits a second GH receptor. This dimerization is followed by a conformational shift, which initiates the JAK-STAT cascade. Janus kinase (JAK2) is activated (it is a receptor-associated kinase which both autophosphorylates and phosphorylates the GH receptor). Once phosphorylated, these sites act as docking sites for molecules which undergo phosphorylation by JAK2, resulting in activation of STAT1, STAT3, and STAT5 (STAT stands for Signal Transducers and Activators of Transcription proteins). Once phosphorylated, cytoplasmic proteins form homodimers and heterodimers, travel to the nucleus, and bind specific DNA sequences, which activate gene transcription.

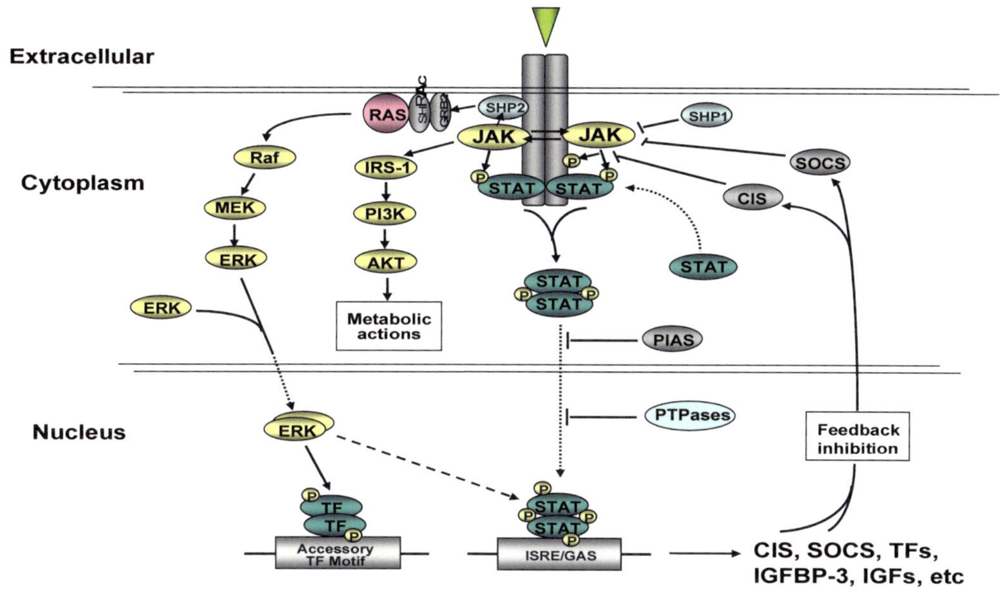

Fig. 2. The JAK-STAT Signalling System: The GH Receptor

3. GH action

3.1 IGF-I

In 1957 Salmon and Daughaday (Salmon and Daughaday 1957) described a "sulfation factor" to explain the observation that while normal serum stimulated sulfate incorporation into cartilage tissue (a marker for synthesis of glycosaminoglycan, a component of cartilage), this effect was reduced using serum from growth hormone deficient patients, and could not be restored by treating cartilage directly with GH. Sulfation factor was re-named somatomedin, and became the basis of the classical somatomedin hypothesis (Rosenfeld 2005); namely, that most of the actions of growth hormone are carried out by factors originally named somatomedins. At the same time others were studying a compound in the serum which they called "non-suppressible insulin-like activity" (NSILA), whose insulin-like action persisted even after removing insulin by the addition of anti-insulin antibodies. Rinderknecht and Humbel (Rinderknecht and Humbel 1978; Rinderknecht and Humbel 1978) identified and sequenced two proteins, NSILA-I and NSILA-II, which were structurally similar to proinsulin. In the early 1980's it became apparent that NSILA-I and somatomedin C were identical, which led to the renaming of NSILA-I and NSILA-II to the insulin-like growth factors IGF-I and IGF-II. Of these two proteins IGF-I is the most growth hormone dependent. It is also now apparent that there are distinct cell membrane receptors for insulin, IGF-I and IGF-II. Even though each receptor binds most strongly to its own ligand, there is cross-reactivity among these ligands for all the receptors (see 3.3, below) .

3.2 IGF proteins

There are three peptide hormones in the IGF family—insulin, IGF-I and IGF-II (Rosenfeld 2005). Insulin-like growth factors (IGF-I and IGF-II) are small peptide hormones (~7.5 kDa) which share a high degree of homology with proinsulin. As with insulin, the IGFs have A and

B chains connected by disulfide bonds, and a C-peptide region that bears no homology with that of proinsulin. IGF-I and IGF-II have a carboxy-terminal extension of variable amino acid lengths. Almost ubiquitously produced, compared with insulin which circulates at picomolar concentrations and has a half-life of minutes, IGF-I and IGF-II circulate at much higher (i. e., nanomolar) concentrations in serum and have much longer half-lives, primarily because they are part of a complex with IGF binding proteins. Beyond their insulin-like effects, these growth-promoting peptides influence cellular proliferation and differentiation in numerous tissues. For IGFs to exert their effects at the cell surface, they first must bind specific, high affinity cell-surface receptors, principally the type I IGF receptor. The interaction of IGFs with cell-surface receptors, however, is tightly regulated by at least six distinct high affinity carrier proteins, the IGF- binding proteins (IGFBPs), and possibly by several low-affinity IGFBP-like molecules. IGFBPs 1-6, which are present in serum and many biologic fluids, have similar or higher affinities for IGF-I and IGF-II than does the type I IGF receptor. Therefore, the interaction of IGFs with IGFBPs can prevent untoward IGF effects, such as uncontrolled cellular proliferation or hypoglycemia. Conversely, disruption of the IGF;IGFBP complex is probably a prerequisite for IGFs to exert their mitogenic and metabolic effects through the type I IGF receptor. It is probably binding of unbound IGF-I to receptors on chondrocytes in the epiphyseal growth plate that stimulates linear growth.

3.3 IGF receptors

The IGF-I receptor is similar in molecular structure to the insulin receptor (Rosenfeld 2005); in fact, it has approximately 60% homology in amino acid composition. There are two membrane-spanning alpha subunits connected by disulfide bonds, which form a pocket that mediates binding of IGF-I. There are two intracellular beta subunits which contain a transmembrane domain, an ATP binding site, and a tyrosine kinase domain that accounts for the presumed signal transduction mechanism for the receptor. The type I IGF receptor binds IGF-I, IGF-II, and insulin with high affinity and mediates the actions of IGF on all tissue specific cell types. Likewise, the insulin receptor can also be bound by IGF-I and IGF-II, which means that if either of these growth factors is in abundance in the serum without being part of a larger complex, it can bind the insulin receptor and cause hypoglycemia. IGF-II also binds to a second receptor that has neither an intrinsic tyrosine kinase domain nor a known signal transduction mechanism. This receptor was first called the mannose-6-phosphate receptor that binds lysomal enzymes at binding sites distinct from that of IGF-II. Given that this receptor binds mannose-6-phosphate-containing enzymes and to transport them between intracellular compartments, it may serve as a biological sink which would remove IGF-II as well as enzymes such as cathepsin and urokinase from the cellular environment.

4. Disorders of the pituitary-growth hormone-IGF axis

4.1 Congenital hypopituitarism

Children who are born with lack of pituitary function are at risk for hypoglycemia because they lack ACTH (and, thus, do not produce adequate cortisol) and GH. Male infants with hypopituitarism often present in the newborn period with hypoglycemia and micropenis (because of the inability to secrete the gonadotropins LH and FSH; LH is necessary for testosterone production, which is required for penile growth). In an analysis of a large GH registry (all patients in the registry were being treated with growth hormone) 169 infants were identified who presented with hypoglycemia. Of these 148 had hypopituitarism. There were 12 patients with isolated GH deficiency (GHD), and 9 were without hypothalamic or pituitary pathology. Structural central nervous system (CNS) lesions and/or midline facial defects were present in 39%. Of the males 55% had micropenis. Eighty-nine percent of the infants required multiple hormone replacement therapy (Bell, August et al. 2004).

A number of developmental occurrences may cause hypopituitarism. These include failure of LHX3 or LHX4. In mice the absence of LHX3 results in Rathke's pouch not growing or differentiating. Three patients were studied from a family with a mutation in LHX3. In humans LHX3 deletion has presented with severe growth failure. Other clinical features have included elevated and anteverted shoulders and a severe restriction of neck rotation, although vertebrae were not abnormal on MRI. The neck conformation appeared to be muscular in origin. One patient with an LHX3 deletion had severe pituitary hypoplasia, one had an enlarged anterior pituitary on MRI, and the third had a pituitary adenoma (Netchine, Sobrier et al. 2000). Individuals with LHX4 deficiency have been shown to be deficient in GH, TSH, and ACTH, and therefore, had short stature at the time of investigation. MRI findings include a small sella turcica with a hypoplastic anterior pituitary, a persistant craniopharyngeal canal, and a Chiari I malformation, as well as an ectopic posterior pituitary ("ectopic bright spot") on MRI. Deletions of LHX4 appear to be transmitted in an autosomal dominant fashion (Machinis, Pantel et al. 2001). Deficiencies in PROP1 ("Prophet of PIT1") may have a small pituitary on MRI, they can present with a large pituitary. They usually have deficiencies in GH, TSH, prolactin, FSH, and LH (Deladoëy, Flück et al. 1999). Mutations in the POU1F1 (formerly PIT1) gene result in deficiencies in GH, prolactin, and the β-subunit of TSH, but ACTH, FSH, and LH are not affected (Hendriks-Stegeman, Augustijn et al. 2001). At least 14 distinct mutations (some dominant and some recessive) in *POU1F1* have been described (Dattani and C. 2000; Hendriks-Stegeman, Augustijn et al. 2001; Malvagia, Poggi et al. 2003; Salemi, Besson et al. 2003) . Both dominant and recessive mutations have been reported. A mutation in the gene HESX1 is associated with hypopituitarism as part of a De Morsier syndrome, also known as Septo-optic Dysplasia (Dattani, Martinez-Barbera et al. 1999). Septo-optic Dysplasia includes optic nerve hypoplasia, midline anomolies (especially absence of the septum pellucidum and occasionally the corpus collosum), and varying degrees of hypopituitarism (usually of the anterior pituitary, but may also include the posterior pituitary) (Brickman, Clements et al. 2001).

Even children born with severe isolated GH deficiency also frequently have hypoglycemia, which usually resolves with GH therapy. A part of the work-up of hypoglycemia is to measure insulin, ketones, free fatty acids, GH, and cortisol levels on a specimen when the blood sugar is hypoglycemic (in children and adults, usually a specimen with a glucose < 50 mg/dl) (Berry, Nathan et al. 2009). A normal GH response should be a GH level >10 ng/ml, and a normal cortisol response should be >15 mg/dl. Elevated free fatty acids and ketones, along with a normal GH and cortisol response suggests hyperinsulinism, which can be further suspected if the insulin level is high. Either low GH or low cortisol alone suggests isolated GH deficiency or cortisol (or ACTH) deficiency. If GH and cortisol are both low, hypopituitarism is suspected. Binder et al.(G., Weidenkeller et al. 2010) have recently suggested that it is possible to diagnose severe congenital GH deficiency in neonates using a random blood sample in which the GH level is less than 7 mg/L. This test identified infants with GHD with 100% sensitivity and 98% specificity.

4.2 Idiopathic isolated GH deficiency

Idiopathic isolated GH deficiency is the most common form of GH deficiency, accounting for as many as 44% of patients treated with growth hormone (Root, Kemp et al. 1998). Because GH is secreted episodically and GH is present in the serum for only about 20 minutes after it is secreted, random assessment of serum GH levels is rarely helpful. In addition to measuring serum IGF-I and IGFBP3 levels, provocative testing of the GH axis is a means of evaluating a patient suspected of having GH deficiency. Provocative agents which stimulate GH secretion include dopaminergic agents (L-dOPA and clonidine), glucagon, the amino acid arginine, and insulin-induced hypoglycemia. When the pituitary gland was visualized using MRI, as many as 15% of patients diagnosed as having idiopathic isolated GH deficiency had abnormal findings (Frindik 2001). These abnormalities included small pituitary glands, empty sella tursicas and ectopic posterior pituitaries (i.e., the posterior pituitary had never descended into the sella tursica, but remained near its origin in the brain).

4.3 Growth hormone insensitivity syndrome

Growth hormone insensitivity syndrome (GHIS) is a rare autosomal recessive condition characterized by a failure to synthesize insulin-like growth factor-I (IGF-I) in spite of elevated levels of growth hormone. It was first described in 1966 (Laron, Pertzelan et al. 1966), and there have been a variety of different mutations described which account for this condition (Rosenfeld, Rosenbloom et al. 1994), most involving mutations in the growth hormone receptor. GHIS is characterized by growth failure starting in infancy which is unresponsive to GH administration, associated with elevated levels of GH and decreased levels of IGF-I and IGFBP3 (Laron, Lillos et al. 1993; Rosenbloom 2000; Savage, Burren et al. 2001). There has been a patient described who had a normal GH receptor, but a mutation in STAT5 (Kofoed, Hwa et al. 2003). A patient has also been described with a similar presentation who has a deletion of the gene for IGF-I (Woods, Camacho-Hubner et al. 1996). Patients with GHIS have frequently reported hypoglycemia without being treated with IGF-I. Because there is a GH receptor which is not fully functional, it may be that the hypoglycemia in this condition results from an inability of GH to function as a glucose counterregulatory hormone, independent of its function in stimulating production of IGF-I.

5. Treatment of disorders of the pituitary-growth hormone-IGF axis

5.1 Treatment of GH deficiency

Therapy for GH deficiency dates to 1958 when Rabin (Raben 1958) reported using growth hormone isolated from human pituitary glands to treat a patient who was growth hormone deficient. Between 1960 and 1985 human-derived growth hormone was available to treat this population. Because of limited supply, treatment was limited to the most GH deficient patients; in fact, as the supply became more plentiful the criteria for growth hormone deficiency gradually rose from peak GH responses to provocative stimuli of 5 ng/ml to allow treatment of patients who had peak GH responses to provocative stimuli of 10 ng/ml in the early 1980's. In 1985 the distribution of human-derived growth hormone was abruptly stopped with the discovery of Creutzfeld-Jacob disease in recipients of these preparations (Brown 1988; Hintz 1995), with the exception of GH deficient patients who experienced hypoglycemia in the absence of GH therapy. At about the same time a recombinant source of growth hormone was approved for use by the FDA, which allowed an almost limitless supply, albeit at a rather expensive cost. Since that time the use of growth hormone in treating growth hormone deficiency has expanded and at the same time the number of approved indications for growth hormone therapy has also increased. When GH therapy is used in a patient with GH deficiency who has hypoglycemia, the hypoglycemia usually resolves as soon as treatment is started. The etiology of this effect is somewhat complicated; GH administration reduces insulin sensitivity, which corrects the hypoglycemia. GH also increases insulin secretion. With GH excess these effects can lead to carbohydrate intolerance, and with GH deficiency they may result in hypoglycemia(Allen, Johanson et al. 1996).

5.2 Administration of IGF-I

For populations where treatment with growth hormone is not possible, such as in the case of GH Insenstivity Syndrome, STAT5b deficiency, or IGF-I Deficiency (Woods, Camacho-Hübner et al. 2000), treatment with IGF-I is now possible. Patents with GHIS or (Laron Syndrome) also frequently report problems with hypoglycemia. Because GH cannot activate the receptor, these individuals have very low concentrations of GH, GHBP-3, and ALS. It is not clear why this situation leads to hypoglycemia. There have been two compounds which have IGF-I as the major component. One, mecasermin, which is rhIGF-I alone (Increlex™, Tercica, Inc., Brisbane, CA), received approval from the FDA for treatment of severe growth hormone resistance in August, 2005 and approval from the European Agency for the Evaluation of Medical Products (EMEA) in 2007 (Collett-Solberg and Misra 2008). The second compound is mecasermin rinfabate (iPlex™, Insmed, Richmond, VA). It is a complex of equimolar amounts of rhIGF-I and its most abundant binding protein Insulin-like Growth Factor I binding protein 3 (rhIGFBP-3). The combination of IGF-I and IGFBP-3 was postulated to have the advantage and an increased serum half-life and protection against hypoglycemia, although there was never a head-to-head comparison of the two preparations which compared the propensity for hypoglycemia. Mecaserin rinfabate received approval from the FDA in December 2005, but is no longer available for the treatment of short stature due to a legal agreement (Collett-Solberg and Misra 2008).
Since hypoglycemia risk appears to be dose dependent, hypoglycemia risk has been reduced by dividing the IGF-I dose into two daily injections, twelve hours apart, and it is recommended to give the injection of IGF-I along with a meal. In a recent report, hypoglycemia was reported by 49% of subjects treated with recombinant IGF-I (Chernausek, Backeljauw et al. 2007). Most hypoglycemic events occurred during the first month of treatment. Seven of the events were reported as severe, and four resulted in seizures. Of the subjects reporting hypoglycemia, 32% had a history of hypoglycemia before starting treatment with IGF-I. It seemed to occur in younger, shorter subjects who had already had problems with hypoglycemia. This observation seems to be consistent with an earlier report, in which hypoglycemia occurred in some of the patients receiving IGF-I, but at the same rate as in those receiving placebo injections (Guevara-Aguirre, Vasconez et al. 1995), only rarely resulting in seizures (Backeljauw, Underwood et al. 2001). Hypoglycemia was lessened by giving the IGF-I dose with meals, and hypoglycemia was usually a problem when there was an intercurrent illness resulting in loss of appetite.

6. Summary

The GH-IGF axis plays an import role in glucose homeostasis, which is somewhat complicated. Growth hormone decreases insulin sensitivity and stimulates insulin secretion.

Most of the actions of growth hormone take place through Insulin-like Growth Factor-I. IGF-I can bind with the insulin receptor, but under normal circumstances is protected from direct contact insulin receptors, since this 6000 Kda protein circulates bound to Binding Protein 3 and acid labile subunit in a 140,000 Kda complex. With GH deficiency many patients experience hypoglycemia, which is corrected with GH treatment. Growth hormone resistant states also may present with hypoglycemia, but are not sensitive to growth hormone. Treatment of GH resistant states with IGF-I does cause an increase in the linear growth velocity, but IGF-I treatment carries a risk for hypoglycemia, presumably because its similarity to proinsulin allows it to bind the insulin receptor, and it is not protected by its binding protein or ALS.

7. References

Allen DB, Johanson AJ, Blizzard RM.. (1996). Growth Hormone Treatment. In: *Pediatric Endocrinology*, F. Lifshitz, pp. 61-81, Marcel Decker, 0-8247-9369-2 New York

Backeljauw PF, Underwood LE, the GHIS Collaborative Group. (2001). Therapy for 6.5-7.5 years with recombinant insulin-like growth factor I in children with growth hormone insensitivity syndrome: a clinical research center study. *Journal of Clinical Endocrinology and Metabolism*, 86, 4 (April, 2001), 1504-1510

Baxter RC. (1994). Insulin-like growth factor binding proteins in the human circulation: a review. *Hormone Research*, 42, 140-144

Bell JJ, August GP, Blethen SL, et al.. (2004). Neonatal hypoglycemia in a growth hormone registry: incidence and pathogenesis. *J Pediatr Endocrinol Metab*, 17, 4 (April, 2004), 629-35.

Berry SA, Nathan B, Hoffman GF, et al.. (2009). Emergency assessment and management of suspected inborn errors of metabolism and endocrine disorders. In: *Pediatric Endocrinology and Inborn Errors of Metabolism*. Sarafoglou K, Hoffman GF, Roth KS. pp. 3-16, McGraw Hill Medical, 978-0-07-143915-2, New York

Binoux M. (1997). GH, IGFs, IGF-binding protein-3 and acid-labile subunit: What is the pecking order? *European Journal of Endocrinology*, 137, 6, (December, 1997), pp 605-609

Brickman JM, Clements M, Tyrell R. et al. (2001). Molecular effects of novel mutations in Hesx1/HESX1 associated with human pituitary disorders. *Development*, 128, 24 (December, 2001), pp. 5189-99

Brown P. (1988). Human growth hormone therapy and Creutzfeldt-Jacob disease: a drama in three acts. *Pediatrics* , 8, (January, 1988), pp. 85-92

Chernausek SD, Backeljauw PF, Frank GR. (2007). Long-term treatment with recombinant insulin-like growth factor (IGF)-I in children with severe IGF-I deficiency due to growth hormone insensitivity. *J Clin Endocrinol Metab*, 92, 5, (May, 2007), pp. 902-910

Collett-Solberg PF, Misra M. (2008). The role of recombinant human insulin-like growth factor-I in treating children with short stature. *J Clin Endocrinol Metab*, 93, 1 (January, 2008), pp. 10-18

Dattani MT, Robinson IC. (2000). The molecular basis for developmental disorders of the pituitary gland in man. *Clin Genet*, 57, 5, (May, 2000), pp. 337-46

Dattani MT, Martinez-Barbera JP, Thomas PQ et al. (1999). HESX1: a novel gene implicated in a familial form of septo-optic dysplasia. *Acta Paediatr*, 88(Suppl), 433 (May, 1999), pp. 49-54

Deladoëy J, Flück C, Büyükgebiz A et al. (1999). Hot spot" in the PROP1 gene responsible for combined pituitary hormone deficiency. *J Clin Endocrinol Metab,* 84, 5 (May, 1999), pp. 1645-50

Frindik JP. (2001). Pituitary morphologic anomalies and magnetic resonance imaging in pediatric growth hormone deficiency. *The Endocrinologist* , 11, 4 (July/August, 2004 pp. 289-295

Frohnert B. Miller BS. (2009). Developmental Disorders of the Anterior Pituitary, *Pediatric Endocrinology and Inborn Errors of Metabolism,* K. Sarafoglou, GF Hoffman, KS Roth, pp. 487-494, McGraw Hill Medical, 978-0-07-143915-2, New York

Binder G, Weidenkeller M, Blumenstock G et al. (2010). Rational approach to the diagnosis of severe growth hormone deficiency in the newborn. *J Clin Endocrinol Metab* , 95, 5, (May, 2010), pp. 2219-26

Guevara-Aguirre J, Vasconez O, Martinez V et al. (1995). A randomized double-blind, placebo controlled trial on safety and efficacy of recombinant human insulin-like growth factor-I in children with growth hormone receptor deficiency. *J Clin Endocrinol Metab,* 80, 4, (April, 1995), pp. 1393-1398

Hendriks-Stegeman, B I, Augustijn KD, Bakker B et al. (2001). Combined pituitary hormone deficiency caused by compound heterozygosity for two novel mutations in the POU domain of the Pit1/POU1F1 gene. *J Clin Endocrinol Metab,* 86, 4, (April, 2001), pp. 1545-50

Hintz RL. (1995). The prismatic case of Creutzfeldt-Jacob disease associated with pituitary growth hormone treatment. *J Clin Endocrinol Metab,* 80, 8, (August, 1995), pp. 2298-2301

Jorgensen JOL, Blum WF, Moller N et al. (1991). Short-term changes in insulin-like growth factors (IGF's) and IGF-binding protein-3 after different modes of intravenous growth hormoen (GH) exposure to GH -deficient patients. *J Clinical Endocrinol Metab,* 72, 3, (March, 1991), pp. 582-587

Kofoed EM, Hwa V, Little B et al. (2003). Growth hormone insensitivity associated with a STAT5b mutation. *New England Journal of Medicine,* 349, 12, (September, 2003), pp. 1110-1112

Laron Z, Lillos P, Klinger B (1993). Growth curves for Laron syndrome. *Arch Dis Child,* 68, 6, (June, 1993), pp. 768-770

Laron Z, Pertzelan A, Mannheimer S. (1966). Genetic pituitary dwarfism with high serum concentrations of growth hormone--a new inborn error of metabolism? *Israel Journal of Medical Science,* 2, 2, (March/April, 1966), pp. 152-155

Machinis, K., J. Pantel, Netchine I et al. (2001). Syndromic short stature in patients with a germline mutation in the LIM homeobox LHX4. *Am J Hum Genet,* 69, 5, November, 2001), pp. 961-8

Malvagia S, Poggi GM, Pasquini E et al. (2003). The de novo Q167K mutation in the POU1F1 gene leads to combined pituitary hormone deficiency in an Italian patient. *Pediatr Res,* 54, 5, (November, 2003), pp. 635-40

Netchine I, Sobrier ML, Krude H et al. (2000). Mutations in LHX3 result in a new syndrome revealed by combined pituitary hormone deficiency. *Nat. Genet.* 25, 2, (June, 2000), pp. 182-6

Nilsson O, Marino R, De Luca F et al. (2005). Endocrine regulation of the growth plate. *Hormone Research,* 64, 4, (April, 2005), pp. 157-165

Ooi GT, Cohen FJ, Tseng LY et al. (1997). Growth hormone stimulates transcription of the gene encoding the acid-labile subunit (ALS) of the circulating insulin-like growth factor-binding protein complex and ALS promoter activity in rat liver. *Mol Endocrinol* 11, 7. (June, 1997), pp. 997-1007

Parks JS, Nielson PV, Sexton LA et al. (1985). An effect of gene dosage on production of human chorionic somatomammotropin. *J Clin Endocrinol Metab* 50, 5, (May, 1985), pp. 994-997

Raben MS. (1958). Treatment of a pituitary dwarf with human growth hormone. *J Clin Endocrinol Metab,* 18, 8, (August, 1958), pp. 901-903

Rinderknecht E, Humbel RE. (1978). The amino acid sequence of human insulin-like growth factor I and its strucutral homology with proinsulin. *J. Biol. Chem,* 253, 8, (April, 1978), pp. 2769-2776

Rinderknecht E, Humbel RE. (1978). Primary structure of human insulin-like growth factor II. *FEBS Lett,* 89, 2, (May, 1978), pp. 283-286

Root AW, Kemp SF, Rundle AC et al. (1998). Effect of long-term recombinant growth hormone therapy in children National Cooperative Growth Study, USA, 1985-1994. *J Pediatr Endocrinol Metab,* 11, 3, (March, 1998), pp. 403-412

Rosenbloom AL. (2000). IGF-I treatment of growth hormone insensitivity. In: *IGF in Health and Disease,* R. G. Rosenfeld and C. T. Roberts. pp. 739-770, Humana Press, Inc., Totowa, NJ

Rosenfeld RG (2005). The IGF system: new developments relevant to pediatric practice. *Endocr Dev, 9,1,* (January, 2005), pp. 1-10

Rosenfeld RG, Rosenbloom RL, Guevara-Aguirre J. (1994). Growth hormone (GH) insensitivity due to pituitary GH receptor deficiency. *Endocr Rev,* 15, 3, (June, 1994), pp. 369-390

Salemi S, Besson A, Eblé A et al. (2003). New N-terminal located mutation (Q4ter) within the POU1F1-gene (PIT-1) causes recessive combined pituitary hormone deficiency and variable phenotype. *Growth Horm IGF Res,* 13, 5, (October, 2003), pp. 264-8

Salmon WD, Daughaday WH. (1957). A hormonally controlled serum factor which stimulates sulfate incorporation by cartilage in vitro. *J. Lab. Clin. Med,* 49, 6, (June, 1957), pp. 825-836

Savage MO, Burren CP, Blair JC et al. (2001). Growth hormone insensitivity: Pathophysiology, diagnosis, clincal variation and future perspective. *Hormone Research* , 55, Suppl 2, pp. 32-5

Sjogren K, Liu JL, Blad K et al. (1999). Liver-derived insulin-like growth factor-I (IGF-I) is the principle source of IGF-I in blood but is not required for postnatal growth in mice. *Proc Natl Acad Sci, USA,* 96, 12, (June, 1999), pp. 7088-7092

Woods KA, Camacho-Hübner C, Bergman RN et al. (2000). Effects of insulin-like growth factor I (IGF-I) therapy on body composition and insulin resistance in IGF-I gene deletion, *J Clin Endocrinol Metab,* 85, 4. (April, 2000), pp. 1407-11

Woods KA, Camacho-Hubner C, Savage MO et al. (1996). Intrauterine growth retardation and postnatal growth failure associated with deletion of the insulin-like growth factor I gene. *N. Engl. J. Med.,* 335, 18 (October, 1996), pp. 1363-1367

Yakar S, Rosen CJ, Beamer WG et al. (2002). Circulating levels of IGF-I directly regulate bone growth and density. *J Clin Invest,* 110, 6, (September, 2002), pp. 771-781

8

Molecular Mechanism Underlying the Intra-Islet Regulation of Glucagon Secretion

Dan Kawamori[1,2] and Rohit N. Kulkarni[1]
[1]*Section of Islet Cell Biology and Regenerative Medicine, Joslin Diabetes Center and Department of Medicine, Harvard Medical School, Boston, MA,*
[2]*Medical Education Center and Department of Metabolic Medicine, Osaka University Graduate School of Medicine, Osaka,*
[1]*U.S.A.*
[2]*Japan*

1. Introduction

Glucagon secreted from pancreatic α-cells plays central roles for counteracting hypoglycemia by modulating hepatic glucose metabolism (Gromada et al., 2007). In addition, glucagon also contributes to the maintenance of glucose homeostasis together with insulin from β-cells. During hyperglycemia such as post-prandial state, insulin secretion from β-cells is stimulated while glucagon secretion from α-cells is suppressed, leading to a lowering of blood glucose levels due to enhanced hepatic- and adipo- glucose uptake and suppressed hepatic glucose output. In contrast, in hypoglycemia such as starvation, glucagon secretion is promoted while insulin secretion is reduced, causing elevated blood glucose levels via the effects of glucagon, including enhanced hepatic glucose output and breakdown of lipids and proteins to provide glucose that is critical to the central nervous system. Thus, both glucagon and insulin are pivotal in systemic energy homeostasis, and the balance between these two hormones determines the metabolic state of various organs in response to changes in energy status.

In both type 1 and type 2 diabetes, both of which exhibit a global increase in incidence, an imbalance between the two hormones appears to significantly impact glucose homeostasis (Unger, 1978). Insufficient insulin secretion and systemic insulin resistance both contribute to hyperglycemia due to quantitative and qualitative insulin shortage. In addition, abnormal elevations in circulating glucagon, due to lack of normal suppression mechanisms, worsens the hyperglycemia via enhanced hepatic glucose output. On the other hand, in patients undergoing treatment for diabetes, an increased incidence of hypoglycemia likely occurs due to a poor glucagon response. Whether this poor glucagon response is a consequence of impaired effects of insulin due to repeated treatment with exogenous insulin or other factors is not fully understood (Gerich et al., 1973). Therefore, diabetes can be recognized as "state where adequate hormones cannot work appropriately" when intra-islet hormone balance is focused on. These observations have prompted consideration of glucagon in the overall therapeutic approach to treat patients with both type 1 and type 2 diabetes. Furthermore, novel therapeutic approaches targeting Glucagon-like peptide (GLP)-1 action in α-cells

(GLP-1 analogues and DPP-4 inhibitors) are also being considered given the potential for GLP-1 to have direct suppressive effects on α-cells, thus these enabled comprehensive control of islet hormone balance including improvement of both insulin and glucagon secretion.

Therefore, it becomes more important to understand the underlying molecular mechanisms for the regulation of glucagon secretion to apply new therapeutic approaches to diabetes targeting α-cell dysfunction.

2. Functions of glucagon

2.1 Functions of glucagon

Glucagon is a 29 amino acid peptide hormone, secreted by pancreatic α-cells mainly in hypoglycemic state, and exerts multiple biological effects on a wide range of organs (Kawamori et al., 2010). Glucagon has important functions *in vivo* for sustaining appropriate blood glucose level. In physiological states, glucagon is released into the bloodstream in response to hypoglycemia to oppose the action of insulin in peripheral tissues, and works as a counter-regulatory hormone to restore normoglycemia. Secreted glucagon works predominantly on the liver, and promotes hepatic gluconeogenesis, glycogenolysis, and simultaneously inhibits glycolysis and glycogenesis (Exton et al., 1966; Unger and Orci, 1977), thus contributing to restoring glucose homeostasis by counteracting the action of insulin. In contrast, insulin suppresses hepatic glucose output while enhancing hepatic glucose uptake and glycogenesis, indicating that a balance between these two hormones ath the hepatocyte determines hepatic glucose metabolism, thus systemic glycemic homeostasis.

In addition to countering hypoglycemia and opposing the effects of insulin in the liver, glucagon has impacts the function of several metabolic organs together favoring the maintenance of glucose homeostasis. For example, in the adipose tissue, glucagon enhances lipid decomposition, while, in contrast, the lack of detectable glucagon receptors in skeletal muscle indicates glucagon has little effect in regulating systemic glucose metabolism by acting on skeletal muscle (Christophe, 1996). Glucagon can also stimulate insulin secretion from pancreatic β-cells (Scheen et al., 1996) and indirectly impact hepatic glucose output. Taken together, these actions indicate an important role for glucagon in maintaining glucose homeostasis.

2.2 Molecular mechanism underlying glucagon action

The glucagon receptor is a G-protein (Gs/Gq) coupled type receptor (Jelinek et al., 1993) and is widely expressed in insulin target organs, such as liver, adipose, β-cells and brain, with the exception of skeletal muscle (Burcelin et al., 1995). Following binding and conformational changes of the receptor the activation of Gs leads to recruitment of adenylate cyclase to the cellular membrane, causing an increase in intracellular cyclic adenosine monophosphate (cAMP) levels and subsequent activation of protein kinase A (PKA) (Weinstein et al., 2001). On the other hand, activation of Gq induces activation of phospholipase C, upregulation of inositol 1,4,5-triphosphate, and the subsequent release of intracellular calcium (Ca^{2+}) (Wakelam et al., 1986). The action of glucagon is relatively complex and involves the coordinate regulation of transcription factors and signal transduction networks which converge to regulate amino acid, lipid and carbohydrate metabolism. For example, in the liver, elevated PKA activity activates various downstream targets leading to the suppression of glycolysis and glycogenesis, and the enhancement of gluconeogenesis and glycogenolysis (Jiang and Zhang, 2003). In islet cells, the elevation of cAMP by glucagon has been reported to stimulate insulin and glucagon secretion from β- and α-cells respectively (Huypens et al., 2000; Ma et al., 2005) by PKA dependent and independent mechanisms. Upregulation of cAMP activates cAMP-regulated guanine nucleotide exchange factors (cAMPGEFs / Epac), which modulates intracellular Ca^{2+}-ion mobilization, enhancing exocytosis (Holz et al., 2006; Ma et al., 2005).

2.3 Anatomical characteristics of pancreatic islets and α-cells

Pancreatic islets possess unique anatomical characteristics and are composed of five different endocrine cell types distributed as islands randomly within the exocrine pancreas. Among these five endocrine cells in islets, the α-cells account for approximately 20% of islet cells.

In adult rodents, β-cells are restricted mostly to the islet core, while α-cells, somatostatin-secreting δ-cells, pancreatic polypeptide-secreting PP-cells, and ghrelin-secreting ε-cells, are scattered along the periphery of the islet and surrounding β-cells. It is likely that this distribution and arrangement of different islet cell types is teleologically important for physiological regulation between the cells since the blood flows from the center of the islets toward periphery; i.e.β-cells to non-β-cells in the islet microcirculation system (Bonner-Weir and Orci, 1982; Stagner and Samols, 1986), suggesting that secreted insulin regulates hormone secretion from other islet cell types. This architecture is typically preserved in rodent islets, while in humans, non-β-cells are often observed both at the periphery and also seemingly in clusters within the center of islets (Cabrera et al., 2006). This implies several possibilities; 1) rodent cellular hierarchy in the islets does not apply to human islets, or 2) human islets consist of several clover-leaf like 'rosettes', with each rosette resembling the basic islet architecture observed in rodent islets (Bonner-Weir and O'Brien, 2008) suggesting

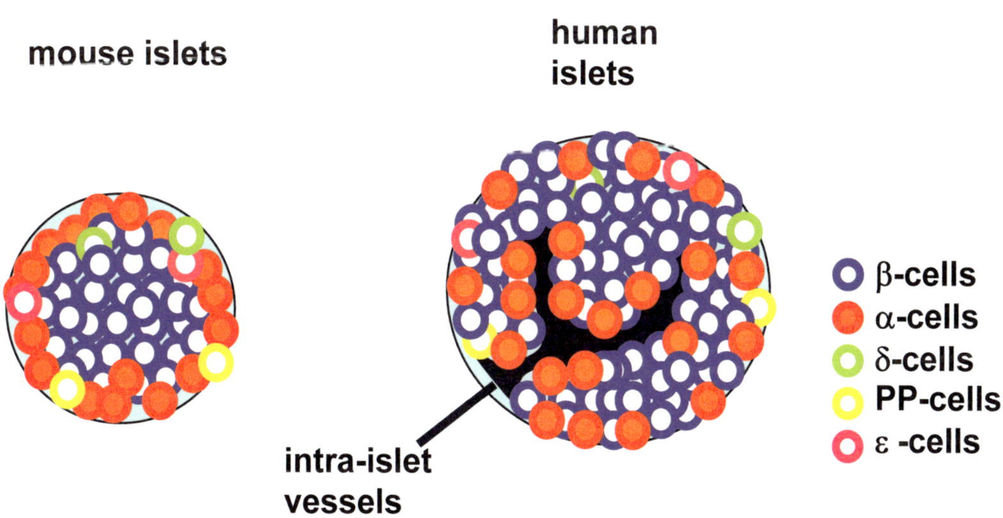

Schematic image for the structure of mouse and human islets adapted from the recent publication of (Bosco, 2010) (10).

the arrangement and interaction of the different cell types in human islets is similar to that in rodents. Recent studies report that in large human islets blood vessels penetrate and branch inside islets, and α-cells located within the core of islets are placed along these vessels and surrounded by β-cells (Bosco et al.). Thus, according to this report, in human islets, α-cells which appear to be placed in the islet core are still 'peripheral' in the islets since blood vessels are usually considered to be placed outside the islets. Given the direction of intraislet microcirculation described above, intraislet auto-/paracrine effects between islet cells especially from β- to non-β-cells can be applied to human islets.

2.4 Excessive glucagon secretion in diabetes

Glucagon plays critical roles in glucose homeostasis largely by regulating hepatic glucose metabolism. However, circulating glucagon levels are often elevated in both type 1 and type 2 diabetes, thus are suggested to contribute to the development of insulin resistance (e.g. hepatic insulin resistance) and exacerbation of diabetes (Ahren and Larsson, 2001; Dinneen et al., 1995; Larsson and Ahren, 2000; Unger, 1978). In addition, the absence of postprandial glucagon suppression in diabetes patients also contributes to postprandial hyperglycemia (Mitrakou et al., 1992; Raskin and Unger, 1978; Sherwin et al., 1976). Another potential contributor to the excess glucagon levels is a relative increase in α-cells compared to β-cells in pancreatic islets in both type 1 (Orci et al., 1976) and type 2 diabetes (Rahier et al., 1983; Yoon et al., 2003). Moreover, in type 1 diabetic islets, an increase in α-cell area and number, and dysregulated cell-type distribution in islets is due to specific β-cell destruction. Although the precise mechanism(s) of relative hyperglucagonemia in the diabetic state is still obscure, β-cell dysfunction is a possible candidate since β-cell secretory products, including insulin, are known to suppress glucagon secretion (see section 4.1.). Thus altered (impaired) β-cell function in diabetes can potentially induce inappropriately elevated glucagon in hyperglycemic states by impairing the intraislet influence of β-cells on glucagon regulation (Meier et al., 2006a).

2.5 Defective glucagon response to hypoglycemia in diabetes

Diabetes patients (both type 1 and type 2) frequently develop defective counter-regulatory responses to hypoglycemia that is associated with reduced or absent glucagon secretory responses. A defective glucagon secretory response to hypoglycemia in hyperinsulinemic states frequently exacerbates a hypoglycemic attack, and limits intensive glucose control by insulin therapy (Amiel et al., 1988; Gerich et al., 1973). Moreover, hypoglycemia associated autonomic failure is induced especially in patients with frequent exposure to hypoglycemia leading to a worsening phenotype (Cryer, 1994). This defective response to hypoglycemia includes sympathoadrenal and neurohormonal responses against hypoglycemia such as epinephrine, cortisol and growth hormone that act to decrease blood glucose further, finally leading to sudden states of hypoglycemia and hypoglycemia unawareness (Amiel et al., 1988; Gerich et al., 1973). How diabetes induces these defective responses to hypoglycemia is still under investigation and suggested theories include alteration in brain glucose transport and metabolism by frequent exposure to hypoglycemia (Criego et al., 2005) and/or defective intraislet β-cell effects on α-cell function, such as the "switch-off" of insulin (Hope et al., 2004; Zhou et al., 2004) or Zinc iron (Zhou et al., 2007) (see section 4.).

3. Regulation of glucagon secretion

3.1 Factors involved in glucagon secretion

The secretion of glucagon from α-cells is stimulated in response to hypoglycemia, and suppressed by hyperglycemia *in vivo*. However, the regulation of glucagon secretion is not simply determined only by glucose concentration, but is complex and finely controlled by additional contribution of neural, hormonal, and intra-islet interactions (Gromada et al., 2007). While it is still not conclusive whether α-cells can directly sense glucose concentration outside the cells and subsequently respond in glucagon secretion (section 3.2.), additional mechanisms which contribute to the secretion of glucagon have recently been revealed. For example, the central nervous system is reported to sense glucose concentration largely through the hypothalamus, and to modulate secretion of islet hormones via the autonomic nervous system (section 3.3.). In addition, circulating autonomic neurotransmitters such as γ-amino-butyric acid (GABA), epinephrine and norepinephrine can stimulate glucagon secretion from α-cells. As described above, various regulatory mechanisms for the glucagon secretion than glucose were uncovered. Among them, it is recently revealed that intra-islet regulation by neighboring β-cells plays critical roles in the physiology of glucagon secretion from α-cells (see section 4).

3.2 Regulation of glucagon secretion by glucose and other nutrients

The secretion of glucagon from α-cells is elevated in response to hypoglycemia and suppressed by hyperglycemia *in vivo*. While some studies suggest a direct suppressive effect of glucose on α-cell secretory function (Ravier and Rutter, 2005; Vieira et al., 2007), the paradoxical stimulation of glucagon secretion by high glucose in isolated islets and α-cell lines (Franklin et al., 2005; Olsen et al., 2005; Salehi et al., 2006) suggests that additional mechanisms contribute to the secretion of glucagon in response to glucose. Also, it is still not conclusive whether α-cells can directly sense glucose concentration outside the cells then respond in glucagon secretion or not.

Amino acids such as L-arginine are potent stimulators of glucagon secretion (Gerich et al., 1974). This is physiologically relevant to prevent hypoglycemia after protein intake since amino acids also stimulate insulin secretion. L-glutamate is produced, secreted by various cell types including neural cells, and acts as a neurotransmitter. In islet α-cells, glutamate is contained in glucagon secretory vesicles (Yamada et al., 2001). Interestingly, a recent study shows that glutamate secreted by α-cells functions as an autocrine positive feedback signal for glucagon secretion (Cabrera et al., 2008), as α-cells express glutamate transporters and receptors (Hayashi et al., 2001). Low glucose stimulates glutamate release from α-cells, which in turn acts on α-cells in an autocrine manner leading to membrane depolarization and glucagon secretion (Cabrera et al., 2008).

3.3 Involvement of nervous system and neurotransmitters

While glycemia might modulate glucagon secretion directly, several reports indicate the involvement of the central and/or autonomic nervous systems in the regulation of glucagon secretion (Ahren, 2000; Bloom et al., 1978; Evans et al., 2004; Marty et al., 2005). Hypoglycemia is a critical condition for body especially since glucose is an essential fuel for the central nervous system. Thus in response to hypoglycemia, the nervous response immediately triggers various counterregulatory mechanisms to protect the brain from energy deprivation, including the stimulation of glucagon secretion.

The dense innervations of the islets suggests that both α- and β-cells are regulated by the nervous system (Ahren, 2000). The autonomic nervous system (ANS) transmits stimuli to promote glucagon secretion especially under hypoglycemia when blood glucose must be increased to supply fuel for the body. The ANS can modulate all islet cells and regulate glucagon secretion directly via the parasympathetic pathway or indirectly by pathways that can modulate islet paracrine factors (see section 4.) (Ahren, 2000). In addition, circulating autonomic neurotransmitters epinephrine and norepinephrine have been reported to stimulate glucagon secretion from α-cells through adrenergic receptors (Schuit and Pipeleers, 1986; Vieira et al., 2004). Glucagon secretion is also modulated by other neurotransmitters including GABA (see section 4.2.) and glutamate (see section 3.2.).
The precise mechanism by which the central nervous system (CNS) senses blood glucose and affects glucagon secretion is not fully understood, although several possibilities have been suggested. Glucose sensing in the CNS is suggested to be an interaction between neurons and glial cells. For example, neurons in the ventro-medial hypothalamus (VMH) have been reported to play a role in sensing hypoglycemia in the brain and triggering the responses of counter-regulatory hormones to impact hypoglycemia (Borg et al., 1995), through AMPK (McCrimmon et al., 2004), K^{+}_{ATP} channels (Evans et al., 2004), and corticoptrophin releasing factor receptors (Cheng et al., 2007) in rat models. Moreover, it has also been reported that GLUT2 in cerebral astrocytes acts as a central glucose sensor in the modulation of glucagon secretion in mice (Marty et al., 2005).

4. Intra-islet regulation of glucagon secretion

In addition to glucose, various regulatory mechanisms for glucagon secretion have been detected. Among these mechanisms is the emerging concept that intra-islet regulation by secretory products from neighboring β-cells plays a critical role in determining α-cell function. This concept is supported, at least in the rodent, by the direction of the intraislet microcirculation which occurs from the core to the periphery and implicates α-cells as potential direct targets of β-cell secretory products such as insulin, (Asplin et al., 1981; Kawamori et al., 2009; Maruyama et al., 1984; Weir et al., 1976), GABA (Rorsman et al., 1989; Xu et al., 2006) and Zinc ions (Ishihara et al., 2003). In addition, another islet hormone somatostatin is reported to modulate glucagon secretion. Interestingly, glucagon itself is reported to regulate glucagon secretion. GLP-1 can suppress glucagon secretion directly and possibly indirectly by enhancing insulin secretion.

4.1 Insulin

Insulin, the major secretory product of β-cells, has been proposed as one of the intra-islet paracrine factors that can modulate the secretion of glucagon from neighboring α-cells (Asplin et al., 1981; Kawamori et al., 2009; Maruyama et al., 1984; Weir et al., 1976). Furthermore, proteins in the insulin signaling pathway are abundantly expressed in α-cells supporting an important role for insulin signaling in α-cells(Bhathena et al., 1982; Franklin et al., 2005; Patel et al., 1982).

4.1.1 Modulation of glucagon secretion by insulin

In clinical studies in human type 1 diabetes patients whose β-cell function is considered to be extinct (Asplin et al., 1981; Gerich et al., 1975), along with basic studies in insulinopenic animal models (Maruyama et al., 1984; Stagner and Samols, 1986; Weir et al., 1976), indicate

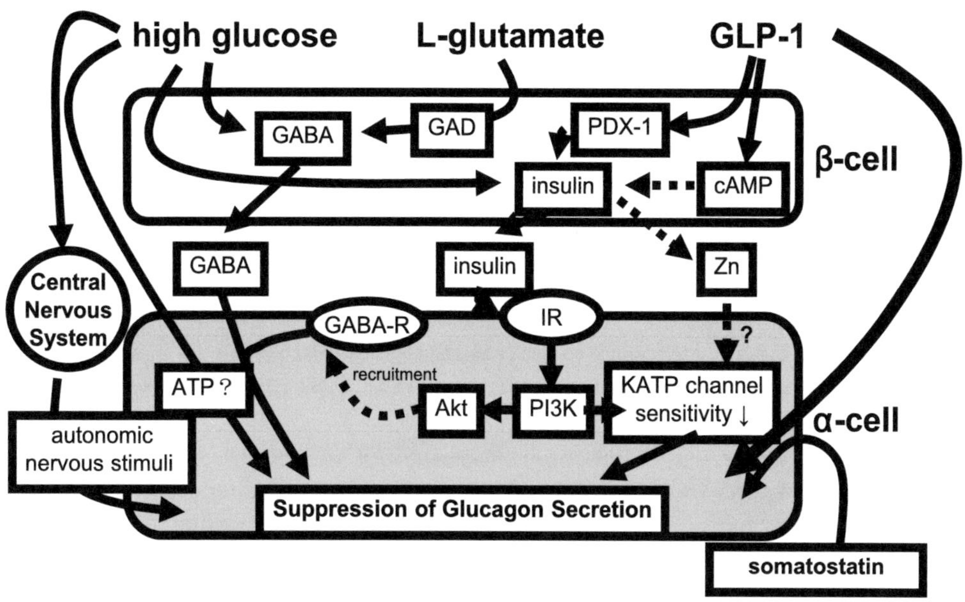

Schematic image for the β-cell-mediated suppression of glucagon secretion from α-cells via a paracrine mechanism. The β-cell secretes insulin, γ-amino-butyric acid (GABA), and zinc irons (Zn) which suppress glucagon secretion. High glucose/hyperglycaemia suppresses glucagon secretion through the nervous system and by stimulation of β-cell secretion. Somatostatin also suppresses glucagon secretion. GLP-1 suppresses glucagon secretion through β-cell mediated and direct pathways.

that insulin suppresses glucagon secretion *in vivo*. In insulinopenic animal models, exogenous insulin suppressed glucagon secretion (Greenbaum et al., 1991; Stagner and Samols, 1986; Weir et al., 1976). Conversely, suppression of insulin action by infusion of an anti-insulin antibody increased glucagon release (Maruyama et al., 1984). These studies clearly indicate the suppressive effect of insulin on glucagon secretion. Thus, it is conceivable that chronic and post-prandial hyperglucagonemia seen in diabetes patients (see section 2.4) is due to a lack of the direct suppression of insulin on glucagon secretion induced either by an absolute lack of insulin and/or α-cell insulin resistance(Meier et al., 2006a; Raju and Cryer, 2005).

In addition, insulin is reported to stimulate glucagon secretion through a "switch-off" mechanism (Hope et al., 2004; Zhou et al., 2004). During hypoglycemia, a decrease in intraislet insulin may act as a trigger for glucagon secretion as α-cells can sense the decrease in ambient insulin. This concept is proposed by studies wherein cessation of insulin administration in *in vivo* pancreas perfusion experiments in insulinopenic diabetic rats induces glucagon secretion in response to hypoglycemia (Hope et al., 2004; Zhou et al., 2004). It is also possible that the defective secretory response of glucagon to hypoglycemia in diabetes patients occurs secondary to a defect in insulin sensing in α-cells (see section 2.5). Thus, insulin is a center player not only in the suppression of glucagon secretion but also the stimulation of glucagon secretion.

4.1.2 Molecular mechanisms underlying the modulation of glucagon secretion by insulin signaling

These *in vivo* reports suggest a direct effect of insulin in modulating glucagon secretion. On the other hand, recent *in vitro* studies in α-cell lines using gene knock-down techniques indicate a role for the insulin receptor and its signaling pathway in suppressing glucagon secretion by high glucose (Ravier and Rutter, 2005), as well as in stimulating glucagon secretion by low glucose concentration (Diao et al., 2005).
The direct inhibitory effects of insulin to suppress glucagon secretion has been reported to occur either by 1) reducing the sensitivity of K^{+}_{ATP} channels (Franklin et al., 2005) which regulate glucagon secretion machinery via phosphatidyl inositol 3-kinase (PI3K) (Leung et al., 2006), or by 2) modulating Akt, a critical downstream effector of PI3K, leading to recruitment of the GABA-A receptor to the cellular membrane to allow its ligand, GABA, to inhibit glucagon secretion (see section 4.2) (Rorsman et al., 1989; Xu et al., 2006).

4.1.3 The α-cell specific insulin receptor knockout mouse model

While numerous reports indicate a pivotal role for insulin in the regulation of glucagon secretion, direct molecular evidence for the importance of insulin signaling in α-cells *in vivo* has been lacking until recently. The significance of systemic insulin signaling in glucose homeostasis is well known as insulin resistance is induced in insulin target organs including the liver, the skeletal muscle and the adipose tissues under diabetic state, and impacts on glycemic metabolism in these organs. Eventually, the genetic evidence of the *in vivo* significance of insulin signaling in α-cells in the regulation of glucagon secretion was provided by investigation of the α-cell specific insulin receptor knockout (αIRKO) mice (Kawamori et al., 2009).
The αIRKO mice exhibited glucose intolerance, hyperglycemia and hyperglucagonemia in the fed state together with enhanced glucagon secretion in response to L-arginine. These results indicate that disruption of insulin receptor in α-cells enhanced glucagon secretion by diminishing the glucagonostatic effect of insulin, and provided direct *in vivo* evidence for the suppression of glucagon secretion by insulin from β-cells through intra-islet paracrine manner. Interestingly, the mutant mice also displayed blunted glucagon response to hypoglycemia indicating a defective glucagon response through insulin "switch-off" mechanism (Hope et al., 2004; Zhou et al., 2004) by disruption of insulin signaling in α-cells. The results using αIRKO mice clearly demonstrate a critical role for insulin in the regulation of α-cell function in both normo- and hypoglycemic states *in vivo*.

4.1.4 Model for the intraislet regulation of glucagon secretion from α-cells by insulin

From these findings, a possible model for the intraislet regulation of glucagon secretion by insulin can be proposed. In states of hyperglycemia, the greater insulin secretion from β-cells is stimulated and would activate insulin signaling in α-cells via paracrine manner, and represses glucagon secretion. On the other hand, in hypoglycemic state, the consequent levels of low insulin would allow the α-cells to sense the reduction in ambient insulin leading to a lack of activation of insulin signaling that in turn leads to the stimulation of glucagon secretion. This would occur in addition to possible direct stimulation by low glucose itself. Indeed, a recent clinical study reported that this proposed mechanism is actually feasible in humans (Cooperberg and Cryer, 2010). In this report, patients with type 1 diabetes were subjected to normo- and hypoglycemic clamps and the effects of insulin analogue glulisine were evaluated. Continuous glulisine infusion suppressed glucagon secretion both under normo- and hypoglycemic states, while discontinuation of glulisine infusion stimulated glucagon secretion in hypoglycemic state. From these studies, it is proposed that insulin overrides the effects of glucose and suppresses glucagon secretion in the hyperglycemic state, and decreasing insulin levels triggers glucagon response to hypoglycemia and precedes the direct effect of low glucose.

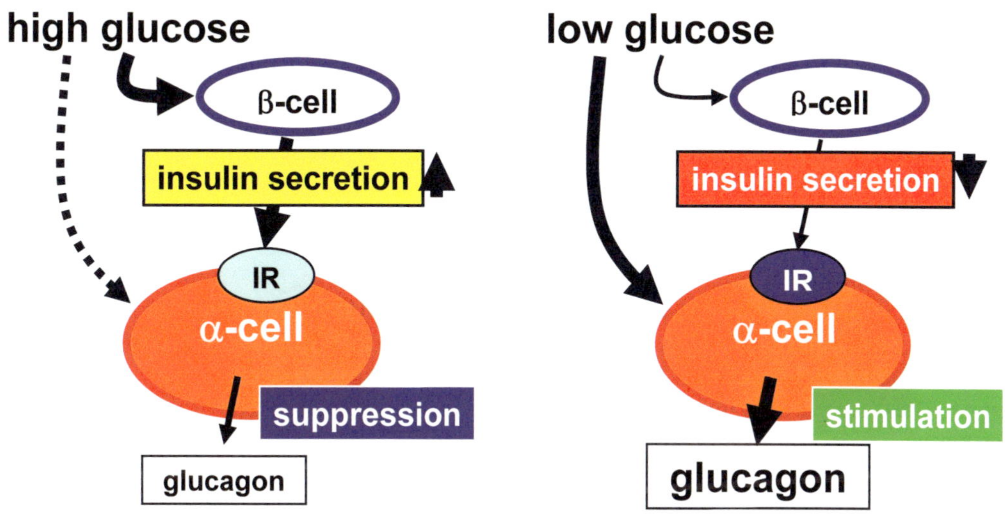

In high glucose state, stimulated insulin secretion from β-cells acts on insulin receptor on the surface of α-cells then suppresses glucagon secretion by paracrine manner. In low glucose state, decreased insulin secretion from β-cells is recognized by α-cells as a reduction of insulin signaling in α-cells through insulin receptor, then α-cells increase glucagon secretion in response.

4.2 GABA

γ-amino-butyric acid (GABA) is produced from the excitatory amino acid glutamate by glutamic acid decarboxylase (GAD) and works as an important inhibitory neurotransmitter in neural synapses, mainly in the central nervous system (Kittler and Moss, 2003). In neurons, GABA is released by the presynaptic terminal into synaptic junctions and binds to GABA receptors on the postsynaptic membrane, inhibiting cellular electrical firing through modulation of ion channels and consequent membrane hyperpolarization (Kittler and Moss, 2003). Islets are also innerved by GABA-ergic neurons (Sorenson et al., 1991), suggesting that GABA is a potential inhibitor of α-cell function.

In addition, GABA has also been reported to be secreted from β-cells and suppress glucagon secretion from α-cells in an intraislet paracrine manner (Rorsman et al., 1989; Wendt et al., 2004; Xu et al., 2006). High glucose or glutamate levels stimulate secretion of GABA from β-cells and the secreted GABA then binds to its receptor expressed on α-cells, inhibiting glucagon secretion through cellular membrane hyperpoloarization. Importantly, the GABA-A receptor is recruited to the cellular membrane by insulin-Akt signaling (Xu et al., 2006), and its activation suppresses glucagon secretion through desensitization of K^{+}_{ATP} channels. These observations suggest a cooperative role between insulin and GABA in the inhibition of glucagon secretion.

4.3 Zinc

Zinc ions (Zn^{2+}), co-released with insulin by β-cells in response to high glucose levels, have been reported to activate K^{+}_{ATP} channels on α-cells, desensitize the channels and suppress glucagon secretion (Ishihara et al., 2003). Zn^{2+} is also reported to stimulate glucagon secretion from α-cells when its concentration falls as part of a "switch-off" mechanism (Zhou et al., 2007). However, another study reports a lack of inhibitory effect of exogenous Zn^{2+} on glucagon secretion (Ravier and Rutter, 2005), indicating that the effects of Zn^{2+} on glucagon secretion are complex and require further investigation.

4.4 Somatostatin

Somatostatin, an inhibitory hormone, secreted by neuronal and pancreatic δ-cells in islets inhibits both insulin and glucagon in a paracrine manner in the islet (Barden et al., 1977; Gerich et al., 1974; Starke et al., 1987). Somatostatin is considered to exert its suppressive effect on glucagon secretion largely through interstitial communication between α- and δ-cells (Stagner and Samols, 1986). Following binding to its receptors on α-cells somatostatin inhibits glucagon secretion by inducing plasma membrane hyperpolarization (Yoshimoto et al., 1999), suppression of cAMP elevation (Schuit et al., 1989) and direct inhibition of the exocytotic machinery via a G-protein-dependent mechanism (Gromada et al., 2001).
Somatostatin secretion from islet δ-cells is stimulated by glucose (Gerber et al., 1981; Honey et al., 1980), consistent with the report that the suppressive effect of high glucose on glucagon secretion may be mediated by glucose-induced secretion of somatostatin (Hauge-Evans et al., 2009). Interestingly, global somatostatin knockout mice exhibit enhanced insulin and glucagon secretion *in vivo* and *ex vivo*. In addition the ability of exogenous glucose to suppress glucagon secretion is lost in islets isolated from somatostatin knockout mice (Hauge-Evans et al., 2009) and highlights the intra-islet interactions between somatostatin, glucagon, and insulin. These observations from a global knockout of somatostatin should be interpreted with caution since extra-pancreatic neuronal effects cannot be ruled out. It should also be noted that somatostatin involvement in glucagon suppression during hyperglycemia might be less important than the effects of β-cell secretion *in vivo* according to the direction of intraislet microcirculation, β-α-δ (Gerich, 1990; Stagner and Samols, 1986). Interestingly, somatostatin is also reported to be involved in GLP-1 mediated suppression of glucagon secretion (see section 4.6). Further investigation is thus necessary to clarify the intra-islet relationship of islet hormones.

4.5 Glucagon

Interestingly, glucagon which is secreted by α-cells is reported to stimulate glucagon secretion (Ma et al., 2005). Upregulation of cAMP by glucagon signaling is suggested to stimulate glucagon exocytosis via a mechanism that is similar to the stimulatory effects of glucagon on insulin and somatostatin secretion (Huypens et al., 2000; Stagner et al., 1989).

4.6 Glucagon like-peptide-1 (GLP-1)

The incretin hormone, glucagon-like peptide-1 (GLP-1), is secreted by intestinal L-cells in response to food intake and is a strong stimulator of insulin secretion and also regulates β-cell mass through modulation of cellular proliferation and death (Drucker, 2006). Therefore, GLP-1 contributes to glucose homeostasis acutely by enhancing β-cell secretory function and chronically by maintaining β-cell mass. In addition to these effects on β-cells, GLP-1 is reported to suppress glucagon secretion by directly acting on α-cells or indirectly by stimulating insulin secretion or modulating other non-β-cell hormones (e.g. somatostatin) which can in turn suppress glucagon secretion. However, the defects in GLP-1 secretion and action in type 2 diabetes likely impact the pathophysiology of the disease via abnormal regulation of both insulin and glucagon secretion (Holst et al., 2009).

Paradoxically, another incretin hormone, glucose-dependent insulinotropic polypeptide (GIP), can stimulate glucagon secretion despite stimulating insulin secretion from β-cells in a manner similar to GLP-1 (de Heer et al., 2008; Meier et al., 2003; Pederson and Brown, 1978). On the other hand, GLP-2, although derived from the same proglucagon gene as GLP-1, in intestinal L-cells, has not been reported to affect the secretory properties of β-cells but stimulates glucagon secretion in human subjects (Meier et al., 2006b), by activation of GLP-2 receptors on α-cells (de Heer et al., 2007).

4.6.1 Indirect suppression of glucagon secretion by GLP-1

GLP-1 is reported to suppress glucagon secretion directly and/or indirectly through other cell-types; β- and δ-cells. In this point, many studies were conducted and displayed pros and cons to both theories. However, considering these reports comprehensively, it is less possible that only one mechanism is working in the suppressive effect of GLP-1 on glucagon, and it is conceivable that these direct and indirect manners are both regulating glucagon secretion with interacting each other.

There are conflicting reports concerning the expression of GLP-1 receptors in α-cells (Heller et al., 1997; Moens et al., 1996). Previous studies investigating GLP-1 receptor expression in α-cells by RNA expression and immunohistochemical analyses indicate that GLP-1 receptors are not expressed in α-cells or if present are expressed at low levels (Tornehave et al., 2008), or by only a few α-cells (Heller et al., 1997). A recent study using *in situ* hybridization and immunofluorescence microscopy in mouse, rat, and human pancreas identified the islet cell types that express GLP-1 receptors (Tornehave et al., 2008) and concluded that GLP-1 receptors are not expressed in α-cells. Thus, it is unlikely that GLP-1 can exert its direct effects on α-cells to impact glucagon secretion. On the other hand, GLP-1 is a strong secretagogue for insulin from β-cells, and considering the central role for insulin in the regulation of glucagon secretion, it is reasonable to suggest that GLP-1 suppresses glucagon secretion by secreted insulin. GLP-1 is also reported to stimulate somatostatin secretion from δ-cells in response to high glucose (Orskov et al., 1988), and it is possible that the secreted somatostatin suppresses glucagon secretion (de Heer and Holst, 2007; Hauge-Evans et al., 2009). This suggestion is supported by the observation that expression of a highly specific somatostatin receptor subtype 2 (SSTR2) antagonist completely abolished the GLP-1 effect on glucagon secretion in isolated perfused rat pancreas (de Heer et al., 2008). However, considering that the direction of intra-islet microcirculation occurs from the core of islets to the mantle; from β-α-δ at least in rodents (Stagner and Samols, 1986), additional studies are necessary to explore these possibilities.

4.6.2 Direct suppression of glucagon secretion by GLP-1

In contrast, reports that GLP-1 (Creutzfeldt et al., 1996) and DPP-4 inhibitor (Foley et al., 2008) treatment suppressed excessive glucagon secretion in type 1 diabetes patients even in the absence of secretory products from β-cells, suggest a potential direct effect of GLP-1 on glucagon suppression. A recent study by De Marinis et al reported that the expression of

GLP-1 receptors in α-cells is less than 0.2 % of its expression in β-cells, and consequently GLP-1 can induce a small elevation in cAMP activating PKA followed by selective inhibition of N-type Ca^{2+} ion channels, thus suppressing glucagon exocytosis (De Marinis et al.). In contrast, receptors for epinephrine or GIP are expressed abundantly in α-cells, and these molecules stimulate electrical activity significantly leading to an increase in Ca^{2+} in α-cells, causing glucagon exocytosis to accelerate through activation of L-type Ca^{2+} ion channels (De Marinis et al.). Studies using isolated islets indicated that GLP-1 effect on glucagon suppression is independent of insulin and intra-islet paracrine effect.

4.6.3 Model for the GLP-1 mediated suppression of glucagon secretion

Considering these reports together, it is possible that GLP-1 suppresses glucagon secretion directly, but in postprandial state, GLP-1 enhances insulin secretion from β-cells together with another incretin GIP, and subsequently exerts suppressive effects on glucagon secretion. Further urgent investigations are necessary to understand the effects of GLP-1 on α-cell function. However, reports of GLP-1 induced suppression of glucagon secretion, in addition to its beneficial role on β-cells including augmentation of glucose-stimulated insulin secretion, promotion of β-cell proliferation, and protection of β-cells from various cytotoxicities, emphasizes the potential of GLP-1 therapy for the treatment of diabetes.

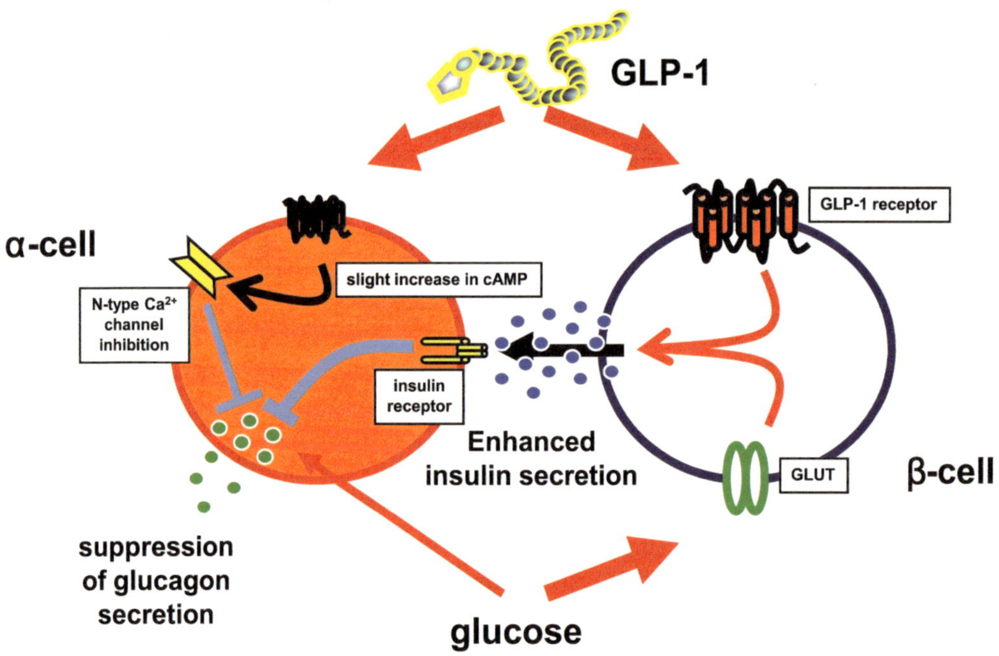

GLP-1 directly suppresses glucagon secretion from α-cells through slight increase of cAMP followed by inhibition of N-type Ca^{2+} channels (De Marinis, 2010) (57). GLP-1 also potentiates insulin secretion from β-cells then suppresses glucagon secretion through insulin effects on α-cells. Glucose stimulates insulin secretion from β-cells and suppresses glucagon from α-cells through insulin effects, while glucose can stimulate glucagon secretion from α-cells.

5. Conclusion and future perspectives

While glucagon was believed to elevate or decline simply in response to blood glucose levels, emerging work reveals a complex but sophisticated regulatory mechanism for the modulation of glucagon output from the α-cells with effects from pancreatic and endocrine hormones including insulin, somatostatin, epinephrine and incretins, nutrients and central and autonomic nervous pathways. The concept of intra-islet regulation of glucagon secretion that is mediated by insulin in a paracrine manner is now recognized as an important pathway that determines α-cell functions. Thus, disorder in intra-islet regulation of glucagon secretion is deeply involved in pathophysiology of diabetes. Considering that the diabetic state is characterized by systemic insulin resistance, that includes non-classical targets such as β-cells (Gunton et al., 2005; Kulkarni et al., 1999), it would be important to explore whether insulin resistance at the level of the α-cell underlies some of the early defects that lead to enhanced glucagon output and a consequent defect in glucose homeostasis.

Recently, new therapeutic approaches targeting excessive glucagon by suppression of glucagon secretion or inhibition of glucagon receptors and their function were tried in the treatment of diabetes, but simple inhibition of glucagon effect does not result in improvement of glucose homeostasis because of hypoglycemia by lack of glucagon effect. In future therapy in diabetes, we need to aim glucagon to work appropriately and rest properly, then improve its effects on other organs and hormonal balance between glucagon and insulin. Further studies are necessary to explore whether cells in the central and/or autonomic nervous systems can be targeted to modulate glucagon secretion for therapeutic purposes.

6. Acknowledgments

D.K. is the recipient of a Research Fellowship (Manpei Suzuki Diabetes Foundation, Japan) and a JDRF Postdoctoral Fellowship. The authors acknowledge support from the American Diabetes Association Research Grant (R.N.K.) and National Institutes of Health (R.N.K.).

7. References

Ahren, B. (2000). Autonomic regulation of islet hormone secretion--implications for health and disease. Diabetologia *43*, 393-410.

Ahren, B., and Larsson, H. (2001). Impaired glucose tolerance (IGT) is associated with reduced insulin-induced suppression of glucagon concentrations. Diabetologia *44*, 1998-2003.

Amiel, S. A., Sherwin, R. S., Simonson, D. C., and Tamborlane, W. V. (1988). Effect of intensive insulin therapy on glycemic thresholds for counterregulatory hormone release. Diabetes *37*, 901-907.

Asplin, C. M., Paquette, T. L., and Palmer, J. P. (1981). In vivo inhibition of glucagon secretion by paracrine beta cell activity in man. J Clin Invest *68*, 314-318.

Barden, N., Lavoie, M., Dupont, A., Cote, J., and Cote, J. P. (1977). Stimulation of glucagon release by addition of anti-stomatostatin serum to islets of Langerhans in vitro. Endocrinology *101*, 635-638.

Bhathena, S. J., Oie, H. K., Gazdar, A. F., Voyles, N. R., Wilkins, S. D., and Recant, L. (1982). Insulin, glucagon, and somatostatin receptors on cultured cells and clones from rat islet cell tumor. Diabetes *31*, 521-531.

Bloom, S. R., Edwards, A. V., and Hardy, R. N. (1978). The role of the autonomic nervous system in the control of glucagon, insulin and pancreatic polypeptide release from the pancreas. J Physiol *280*, 9-23.

Bonner-Weir, S., and O'Brien, T. D. (2008). Islets in type 2 diabetes: in honor of Dr. Robert C. Turner. Diabetes *57*, 2899-2904.

Bonner-Weir, S., and Orci, L. (1982). New perspectives on the microvasculature of the islets of Langerhans in the rat. Diabetes *31*, 883-889.

Borg, W. P., Sherwin, R. S., During, M. J., Borg, M. A., and Shulman, G. I. (1995). Local ventromedial hypothalamus glucopenia triggers counterregulatory hormone release. Diabetes *44*, 180-184.

Bosco, D., Armanet, M., Morel, P., Niclauss, N., Sgroi, A., Muller, Y. D., Giovannoni, L., Parnaud, G., and Berney, T. Unique arrangement of alpha- and beta-cells in human islets of Langerhans. Diabetes *59*, 1202-1210.

Burcelin, R., Li, J., and Charron, M. J. (1995). Cloning and sequence analysis of the murine glucagon receptor-encoding gene. Gene *164*, 305-310.

Cabrera, O., Berman, D. M., Kenyon, N. S., Ricordi, C., Berggren, P. O., and Caicedo, A. (2006). The unique cytoarchitecture of human pancreatic islets has implications for islet cell function. Proc Natl Acad Sci U S A *103*, 2334-2339.

Cabrera, O., Jacques-Silva, M. C., Speier, S., Yang, S. N., Kohler, M., Fachado, A., Vieira, E., Zierath, J. R., Kibbey, R., Berman, D. M., *et al.* (2008). Glutamate is a positive autocrine signal for glucagon release. Cell Metab *7*, 545-554.

Cheng, H., Zhou, L., Zhu, W., Wang, A., Tang, C., Chan, O., Sherwin, R. S., and McCrimmon, R. J. (2007). Type 1 corticotropin-releasing factor receptors in the ventromedial hypothalamus promote hypoglycemia-induced hormonal counterregulation. Am J Physiol Endocrinol Metab *293*, E705-712.

Christophe, J. (1996). Glucagon and its receptor in various tissues. Ann N Y Acad Sci *805*, 31-42; discussion 42-33.

Cooperberg, B. A., and Cryer, P. E. (2010). Insulin reciprocally regulates glucagon secretion in humans. Diabetes *59*, 2936-2940.

Creutzfeldt, W. O., Kleine, N., Willms, B., Orskov, C., Holst, J. J., and Nauck, M. A. (1996). Glucagonostatic actions and reduction of fasting hyperglycemia by exogenous glucagon-like peptide I(7-36) amide in type I diabetic patients. Diabetes Care *19*, 580-586.

Criego, A. B., Tkac, I., Kumar, A., Thomas, W., Gruetter, R., and Seaquist, E. R. (2005). Brain glucose concentrations in patients with type 1 diabetes and hypoglycemia unawareness. J Neurosci Res *79*, 42-47.

Cryer, P. E. (1994). Banting Lecture. Hypoglycemia: the limiting factor in the management of IDDM. Diabetes *43*, 1378-1389.

de Heer, J., and Holst, J. J. (2007). Sulfonylurea compounds uncouple the glucose dependence of the insulinotropic effect of glucagon-like peptide 1. Diabetes *56*, 438-443.

de Heer, J., Pedersen, J., Orskov, C., and Holst, J. J. (2007). The alpha cell expresses glucagon-like peptide-2 receptors and glucagon-like peptide-2 stimulates glucagon secretion from the rat pancreas. Diabetologia *50*, 2135-2142.

de Heer, J., Rasmussen, C., Coy, D. H., and Holst, J. J. (2008). Glucagon-like peptide-1, but not glucose-dependent insulinotropic peptide, inhibits glucagon secretion via somatostatin (receptor subtype 2) in the perfused rat pancreas. Diabetologia *51*, 2263-2270.

De Marinis, Y. Z., Salehi, A., Ward, C. E., Zhang, Q., Abdulkader, F., Bengtsson, M., Braha, O., Braun, M., Ramracheya, R., Amisten, S., *et al.* (2010). GLP-1 inhibits and adrenaline stimulates glucagon release by differential modulation of N- and L-type Ca2+ channel-dependent exocytosis. Cell Metab *11*, 543-553.

Diao, J., Asghar, Z., Chan, C. B., and Wheeler, M. B. (2005). Glucose-regulated glucagon secretion requires insulin receptor expression in pancreatic alpha-cells. J Biol Chem *280*, 33487-33496.

Dinneen, S., Alzaid, A., Turk, D., and Rizza, R. (1995). Failure of glucagon suppression contributes to postprandial hyperglycaemia in IDDM. Diabetologia *38*, 337-343.

Drucker, D. J. (2006). The biology of incretin hormones. Cell Metab *3*, 153-165.

Evans, M. L., McCrimmon, R. J., Flanagan, D. E., Keshavarz, T., Fan, X., McNay, E. C., Jacob, R. J., and Sherwin, R. S. (2004). Hypothalamic ATP-sensitive K + channels play a key role in sensing hypoglycemia and triggering counterregulatory epinephrine and glucagon responses. Diabetes *53*, 2542-2551.

Exton, J. H., Jefferson, L. S., Jr., Butcher, R. W., and Park, C. R. (1966). Gluconeogenesis in the perfused liver. The effects of fasting, alloxan diabetes, glucagon, epinephrine, adenosine 3',5'-monophosphate and insulin. Am J Med *40*, 709-715.

Foley, J. E., Ligueros-Saylan, M., He, Y. L., Holst, J. J., Deacon, C. F., Dunning, B. E., Leone-Jones, A., Yu, T., and Kelley, D. E. (2008). Effect of vildagliptin on glucagon concentration during meals in patients with type 1 diabetes. Horm Metab Res *40*, 727-730.

Franklin, I., Gromada, J., Gjinovci, A., Theander, S., and Wollheim, C. B. (2005). Beta-cell secretory products activate alpha-cell ATP-dependent potassium channels to inhibit glucagon release. Diabetes *54*, 1808-1815.

Gerber, P. P., Trimble, E. R., Wollheim, C. B., Renold, A. E., and Miller, R. E. (1981). Glucose and cyclic AMP as stimulators of somatostatin and insulin secretion from the isolated, perfused rat pancreas: a quantitative study. Diabetes *30*, 40-44.

Gerich, J. E. (1990). Role of somatostatin and its analogues in the pathogenesis and treatment of diabetes mellitus. Metabolism *39*, 52-54.

Gerich, J. E., Langlois, M., Noacco, C., Karam, J. H., and Forsham, P. H. (1973). Lack of glucagon response to hypoglycemia in diabetes: evidence for an intrinsic pancreatic alpha cell defect. Science *182*, 171-173.

Gerich, J. E., Lorenzi, M., Schneider, V., Kwan, C. W., Karam, J. H., Guillemin, R., and Forsham, P. H. (1974). Inhibition of pancreatic glucagon responses to arginine by somatostatin in normal man and in insulin-dependent diabetics. Diabetes *23*, 876-880.

Gerich, J. E., Tsalikian, E., Lorenzi, M., Schneider, V., Bohannon, N. V., Gustafson, G., and Karam, J. H. (1975). Normalization of fasting hyperglucagonemia and excessive glucagon responses to intravenous arginine in human diabetes mellitus by prolonged infusion of insulin. J Clin Endocrinol Metab *41*, 1178-1180.

Greenbaum, C. J., Havel, P. J., Taborsky, G. J., Jr., and Klaff, L. J. (1991). Intra-islet insulin permits glucose to directly suppress pancreatic A cell function. J Clin Invest *88*, 767-773.

Gromada, J., Franklin, I., and Wollheim, C. B. (2007). Alpha-cells of the endocrine pancreas: 35 years of research but the enigma remains. Endocr Rev *28*, 84-116.

Gromada, J., Hoy, M., Buschard, K., Salehi, A., and Rorsman, P. (2001). Somatostatin inhibits exocytosis in rat pancreatic alpha-cells by G(i2)-dependent activation of calcineurin and depriming of secretory granules. J Physiol *535*, 519-532.

Gunton, J. E., Kulkarni, R. N., Yim, S., Okada, T., Hawthorne, W. J., Tseng, Y. H., Roberson, R. S., Ricordi, C., O'Connell, P. J., Gonzalez, F. J., and Kahn, C. R. (2005). Loss of ARNT/HIF1beta mediates altered gene expression and pancreatic-islet dysfunction in human type 2 diabetes. Cell *122*, 337-349.

Hauge-Evans, A. C., King, A. J., Carmignac, D., Richardson, C. C., Robinson, I. C., Low, M. J., Christie, M. R., Persaud, S. J., and Jones, P. M. (2009). Somatostatin secreted by islet delta-cells fulfils multiple roles as a paracrine regulator of islet function. Diabetes *58*, 403-411.

Hayashi, M., Otsuka, M., Morimoto, R., Hirota, S., Yatsushiro, S., Takeda, J., Yamamoto, A., and Moriyama, Y. (2001). Differentiation-associated Na+-dependent inorganic phosphate cotransporter (DNPI) is a vesicular glutamate transporter in endocrine glutamatergic systems. J Biol Chem *276*, 43400-43406.

Heller, R. S., Kieffer, T. J., and Habener, J. F. (1997). Insulinotropic glucagon-like peptide I receptor expression in glucagon-producing alpha-cells of the rat endocrine pancreas. Diabetes *46*, 785-791.

Holst, J. J., Vilsboll, T., and Deacon, C. F. (2009). The incretin system and its role in type 2 diabetes mellitus. Mol Cell Endocrinol *297*, 127-136.

Holz, G. G., Kang, G., Harbeck, M., Roe, M. W., and Chepurny, O. G. (2006). Cell physiology of cAMP sensor Epac. J Physiol *577*, 5-15.

Honey, R. N., Schwarz, J. A., Mathe, C. J., and Weir, G. C. (1980). Insulin, glucagon, and somatostatin secretion from isolated perfused rat and chicken pancreas-duodenum. Am J Physiol *238*, E150-156.

Hope, K. M., Tran, P. O., Zhou, H., Oseid, E., Leroy, E., and Robertson, R. P. (2004). Regulation of alpha-cell function by the beta-cell in isolated human and rat islets deprived of glucose: the "switch-off" hypothesis. Diabetes *53*, 1488-1495.

Huypens, P., Ling, Z., Pipeleers, D., and Schuit, F. (2000). Glucagon receptors on human islet cells contribute to glucose competence of insulin release. Diabetologia *43*, 1012-1019.

Ishihara, H., Maechler, P., Gjinovci, A., Herrera, P. L., and Wollheim, C. B. (2003). Islet beta-cell secretion determines glucagon release from neighbouring alpha-cells. Nat Cell Biol *5*, 330-335.

Jelinek, L. J., Lok, S., Rosenberg, G. B., Smith, R. A., Grant, F. J., Biggs, S., Bensch, P. A., Kuijper, J. L., Sheppard, P. O., Sprecher, C. A., and et al. (1993). Expression cloning and signaling properties of the rat glucagon receptor. Science *259*, 1614-1616.

Jiang, G., and Zhang, B. B. (2003). Glucagon and regulation of glucose metabolism. Am J Physiol Endocrinol Metab *284*, E671-678.

Kawamori, D., Kurpad, A. J., Hu, J., Liew, C. W., Shih, J. L., Ford, E. L., Herrera, P. L., Polonsky, K. S., McGuinness, O. P., and Kulkarni, R. N. (2009). Insulin signaling in alpha cells modulates glucagon secretion in vivo. Cell Metab *9*, 350-361.

Kawamori, D., Welters, H. J., and Kulkarni, R. N. (2010). Molecular pathways underlying the pathogenesis of pancreatic alpha-cell dysfunction. Adv Exp Med Biol *654*, 421-445.

Kittler, J. T., and Moss, S. J. (2003). Modulation of GABAA receptor activity by phosphorylation and receptor trafficking: implications for the efficacy of synaptic inhibition. Curr Opin Neurobiol *13*, 341-347.

Kulkarni, R. N., Bruning, J. C., Winnay, J. N., Postic, C., Magnuson, M. A., and Kahn, C. R. (1999). Tissue-specific knockout of the insulin receptor in pancreatic beta cells creates an insulin secretory defect similar to that in type 2 diabetes. Cell *96*, 329-339.

Larsson, H., and Ahren, B. (2000). Islet dysfunction in insulin resistance involves impaired insulin secretion and increased glucagon secretion in postmenopausal women with impaired glucose tolerance. Diabetes Care *23*, 650-657.

Leung, Y. M., Ahmed, I., Sheu, L., Gao, X., Hara, M., Tsushima, R. G., Diamant, N. E., and Gaisano, H. Y. (2006). Insulin regulates islet alpha-cell function by reducing KATP channel sensitivity to adenosine 5'-triphosphate inhibition. Endocrinology *147*, 2155-2162.

Ma, X., Zhang, Y., Gromada, J., Sewing, S., Berggren, P. O., Buschard, K., Salehi, A., Vikman, J., Rorsman, P., and Eliasson, L. (2005). Glucagon stimulates exocytosis in mouse and rat pancreatic alpha-cells by binding to glucagon receptors. Mol Endocrinol *19*, 198-212.

Marty, N., Dallaporta, M., Foretz, M., Emery, M., Tarussio, D., Bady, I., Binnert, C., Beermann, F., and Thorens, B. (2005). Regulation of glucagon secretion by glucose transporter type 2 (glut2) and astrocyte-dependent glucose sensors. J Clin Invest *115*, 3545-3553.

Maruyama, H., Hisatomi, A., Orci, L., Grodsky, G. M., and Unger, R. H. (1984). Insulin within islets is a physiologic glucagon release inhibitor. J Clin Invest *74*, 2296-2299.

McCrimmon, R. J., Fan, X., Ding, Y., Zhu, W., Jacob, R. J., and Sherwin, R. S. (2004). Potential role for AMP-activated protein kinase in hypoglycemia sensing in the ventromedial hypothalamus. Diabetes *53*, 1953-1958.

Meier, J. J., Gallwitz, B., Siepmann, N., Holst, J. J., Deacon, C. F., Schmidt, W. E., and Nauck, M. A. (2003). Gastric inhibitory polypeptide (GIP) dose-dependently stimulates glucagon secretion in healthy human subjects at euglycaemia. Diabetologia *46*, 798-801.

Meier, J. J., Kjems, L. L., Veldhuis, J. D., Lefebvre, P., and Butler, P. C. (2006a). Postprandial suppression of glucagon secretion depends on intact pulsatile insulin secretion: further evidence for the intraislet insulin hypothesis. Diabetes *55*, 1051-1056.

Meier, J. J., Nauck, M. A., Pott, A., Heinze, K., Goetze, O., Bulut, K., Schmidt, W. E., Gallwitz, B., and Holst, J. J. (2006b). Glucagon-like peptide 2 stimulates glucagon secretion, enhances lipid absorption, and inhibits gastric acid secretion in humans. Gastroenterology *130*, 44-54.

Mitrakou, A., Kelley, D., Mokan, M., Veneman, T., Pangburn, T., Reilly, J., and Gerich, J. (1992). Role of reduced suppression of glucose production and diminished early insulin release in impaired glucose tolerance. N Engl J Med *326*, 22-29.

Moens, K., Heimberg, H., Flamez, D., Huypens, P., Quartier, E., Ling, Z., Pipeleers, D., Gremlich, S., Thorens, B., and Schuit, F. (1996). Expression and functional activity of glucagon, glucagon-like peptide I, and glucose-dependent insulinotropic peptide receptors in rat pancreatic islet cells. Diabetes *45*, 257-261.

Olsen, H. L., Theander, S., Bokvist, K., Buschard, K., Wollheim, C. B., and Gromada, J. (2005). Glucose stimulates glucagon release in single rat alpha-cells by mechanisms that mirror the stimulus-secretion coupling in beta-cells. Endocrinology *146*, 4861-4870.

Orci, L., Baetens, D., Rufener, C., Amherdt, M., Ravazzola, M., Studer, P., Malaisse-Lagae, F., and Unger, R. H. (1976). Hypertrophy and hyperplasia of somatostatin-containing D-cells in diabetes. Proc Natl Acad Sci U S A *73*, 1338-1342.

Orskov, C., Holst, J. J., and Nielsen, O. V. (1988). Effect of truncated glucagon-like peptide-1 [proglucagon-(78-107) amide] on endocrine secretion from pig pancreas, antrum, and nonantral stomach. Endocrinology *123*, 2009-2013.

Patel, Y. C., Amherdt, M., and Orci, L. (1982). Quantitative electron microscopic autoradiography of insulin, glucagon, and somatostatin binding sites on islets. Science *217*, 1155-1156.

Pederson, R. A., and Brown, J. C. (1978). Interaction of gastric inhibitory polypeptide, glucose, and arginine on insulin and glucagon secretion from the perfused rat pancreas. Endocrinology *103*, 610-615.

Rahier, J., Goebbels, R. M., and Henquin, J. C. (1983). Cellular composition of the human diabetic pancreas. Diabetologia *24*, 366-371.

Raju, B., and Cryer, P. E. (2005). Loss of the decrement in intraislet insulin plausibly explains loss of the glucagon response to hypoglycemia in insulin-deficient diabetes: documentation of the intraislet insulin hypothesis in humans. Diabetes *54*, 757-764.

Raskin, P., and Unger, R. H. (1978). Hyperglucagonemia and its suppression. Importance in the metabolic control of diabetes. N Engl J Med *299*, 433-436.

Ravier, M. A., and Rutter, G. A. (2005). Glucose or insulin, but not zinc ions, inhibit glucagon secretion from mouse pancreatic alpha-cells. Diabetes *54*, 1789-1797.

Rorsman, P., Berggren, P. O., Bokvist, K., Ericson, H., Mohler, H., Ostenson, C. G., and Smith, P. A. (1989). Glucose-inhibition of glucagon secretion involves activation of GABAA-receptor chloride channels. Nature *341*, 233-236.

Salehi, A., Vieira, E., and Gylfe, E. (2006). Paradoxical stimulation of glucagon secretion by high glucose concentrations. Diabetes *55*, 2318-2323.

Scheen, A. J., Castillo, M. J., and Lefebvre, P. J. (1996). Assessment of residual insulin secretion in diabetic patients using the intravenous glucagon stimulatory test: methodological aspects and clinical applications. Diabetes Metab *22*, 397-406.

Schuit, F. C., Derde, M. P., and Pipeleers, D. G. (1989). Sensitivity of rat pancreatic A and B cells to somatostatin. Diabetologia *32*, 207-212.

Schuit, F. C., and Pipeleers, D. G. (1986). Differences in adrenergic recognition by pancreatic A and B cells. Science *232*, 875-877.

Sherwin, R. S., Fisher, M., Hendler, R., and Felig, P. (1976). Hyperglucagonemia and blood glucose regulation in normal, obese and diabetic subjects. N Engl J Med *294*, 455-461.

Sorenson, R. L., Garry, D. G., and Brelje, T. C. (1991). Structural and functional considerations of GABA in islets of Langerhans. Beta-cells and nerves. Diabetes *40*, 1365-1374.

Stagner, J. I., and Samols, E. (1986). Retrograde perfusion as a model for testing the relative effects of glucose versus insulin on the A cell. J Clin Invest *77*, 1034-1037.

Stagner, J. I., Samols, E., and Marks, V. (1989). The anterograde and retrograde infusion of glucagon antibodies suggests that A cells are vascularly perfused before D cells within the rat islet. Diabetologia *32*, 203-206.

Starke, A., Imamura, T., and Unger, R. H. (1987). Relationship of glucagon suppression by insulin and somatostatin to the ambient glucose concentration. J Clin Invest *79*, 20-24.

Tornehave, D., Kristensen, P., Romer, J., Knudsen, L. B., and Heller, R. S. (2008). Expression of the GLP-1 receptor in mouse, rat, and human pancreas. J Histochem Cytochem *56*, 841-851.

Unger, R. H. (1978). Role of glucagon in the pathogenesis of diabetes: the status of the controversy. Metabolism *27*, 1691-1709.

Unger, R. H., and Orci, L. (1977). The role of glucagon in the endogenous hyperglycemia of diabetes mellitus. Annu Rev Med *28*, 119-130.

Vieira, E., Liu, Y. J., and Gylfe, E. (2004). Involvement of alpha1 and beta-adrenoceptors in adrenaline stimulation of the glucagon-secreting mouse alpha-cell. Naunyn Schmiedebergs Arch Pharmacol *369*, 179-183.

Vieira, E., Salehi, A., and Gylfe, E. (2007). Glucose inhibits glucagon secretion by a direct effect on mouse pancreatic alpha cells. Diabetologia *50*, 370-379.

Wakelam, M. J., Murphy, G. J., Hruby, V. J., and Houslay, M. D. (1986). Activation of two signal-transduction systems in hepatocytes by glucagon. Nature *323*, 68-71.

Weinstein, L. S., Yu, S., Warner, D. R., and Liu, J. (2001). Endocrine manifestations of stimulatory G protein alpha-subunit mutations and the role of genomic imprinting. Endocr Rev *22*, 675-705.

Weir, G. C., Knowlton, S. D., Atkins, R. F., McKennan, K. X., and Martin, D. B. (1976). Glucagon secretion from the perfused pancreas of streptozotocin-treated rats. Diabetes *25*, 275-282.

Wendt, A., Birnir, B., Buschard, K., Gromada, J., Salehi, A., Sewing, S., Rorsman, P., and Braun, M. (2004). Glucose inhibition of glucagon secretion from rat alpha-cells is mediated by GABA released from neighboring beta-cells. Diabetes *53*, 1038-1045.

Xu, E., Kumar, M., Zhang, Y., Ju, W., Obata, T., Zhang, N., Liu, S., Wendt, A., Deng, S., Ebina, Y., *et al.* (2006). Intra-islet insulin suppresses glucagon release via GABA-GABAA receptor system. Cell Metab *3*, 47-58.

Yamada, H., Otsuka, M., Hayashi, M., Nakatsuka, S., Hamaguchi, K., Yamamoto, A., and Moriyama, Y. (2001). Ca2+-dependent exocytosis of L-glutamate by alphaTC6, clonal mouse pancreatic alpha-cells. Diabetes *50*, 1012-1020.

Yoon, K. H., Ko, S. H., Cho, J. H., Lee, J. M., Ahn, Y. B., Song, K. H., Yoo, S. J., Kang, M. I., Cha, B. Y., Lee, K. W., *et al.* (2003). Selective beta-cell loss and alpha-cell expansion in patients with type 2 diabetes mellitus in Korea. J Clin Endocrinol Metab *88*, 2300-2308.

Yoshimoto, Y., Fukuyama, Y., Horio, Y., Inanobe, A., Gotoh, M., and Kurachi, Y. (1999). Somatostatin induces hyperpolarization in pancreatic islet alpha cells by activating a G protein-gated K+ channel. FEBS Lett *444*, 265-269.

Zhou, H., Tran, P. O., Yang, S., Zhang, T., LeRoy, E., Oseid, E., and Robertson, R. P. (2004). Regulation of alpha-cell function by the beta-cell during hypoglycemia in Wistar rats: the "switch-off" hypothesis. Diabetes *53*, 1482-1487.

Zhou, H., Zhang, T., Harmon, J. S., Bryan, J., and Robertson, R. P. (2007). Zinc, not insulin, regulates the rat alpha-cell response to hypoglycemia in vivo. Diabetes *56*, 1107-1112.

Part 4

Section D

9

Insulin Therapy and Hypoglycemia - Present and Future

Simona Cernea[1], Ron Nagar[2], Gabriel Bitton[2] and Itamar Raz[3]
[1]*Diabetes, Nutrition and Metabolic Diseases Outpatient Unit, Emergency County Clinical Hospital, Târgu Mureş,*
[2]*InsuLine Medical Ltd., Petach-Tikva,*
[3]*Diabetes Center, Hadassah-Hebrew University Medical School, Jerusalem,*
[1]*Romania*
[2,3]*Israel*

1. Introduction

Over the last few decades the prevalence of diabetes has dramatically grown in most regions of the world. In 2010, 285 million people had diabetes and it is estimated that the number will increase to 438 million in 2030 (1). About 5-10% of them have type 1 diabetes.

Both types of diabetes are characterized by a progressive decline of pancreatic beta cell function and mass. In type 1 diabetes, the chronic autoimmune process causes the selective destruction of insulin-producing beta cells by the auto-reactive T cells in genetically predisposed individuals. There is a continuous loss of functional C-peptide responses and at the time of clinical presentation the beta cell mass is reduced by 70–90 %, as suggested by anatomic studies (2, 3). This results in an inability to secrete sufficient amounts of insulin and loss of metabolic control. As a consequence, exogenous insulin replacement in the form of multiple subcutaneous injections or continuous subcutaneous insulin infusions (CSII) is essential for patients with type 1 diabetes. It prevents death from acute metabolic complications and assures normal growth and development, maintenance of normoglycemia and prevention of end-organ complications.

Type 2 diabetes results from an entirely different pathophysiological process. It is characterized by an increased resistance to insulin action in the peripheral tissues with decreased glucose uptake and enhanced hepatic glucose output associated with impaired insulin-secretory capacity caused by a progressive decline of beta cell function over time. Studies indicate a substantial loss of beta cell mass (of about 25-60 %) by the time of diagnosis, mainly secondary to increased apoptosis and impaired augmentation of cell mass through neogenesis (4, 5). The clinical onset is due to the reduction of beta cell mass per se and to a concomitant dysfunction of residual beta cells (6, 7). The beta cell failure, which seems to occur much earlier during the natural history of the disease than previously thought, results in significant insulin deficiency and by then, insulin administration is required in order to achieve glycemic control (8, 9).

2. Intensive insulin regimens: Evidence for benefit

It is well established that in patients with both types of diabetes obtaining a good metabolic control is of paramount importance because the risk of developing chronic micro- and macrovascular complications is dependent on the degree of glycemic control (10). Current guidelines from professional organizations recommend achieving glycated hemoglobin (HbA1c) levels lower than 7% (and closer to normal values in selected individuals, if this could be achieved without significant increase in hypoglycemic events or other side effects) (11). Several landmark studies emphasize the importance of more physiologic insulin profiles in reaching these goals.

The Diabetes Control and Complications Trial (DCCT) proved that tighter glycemic control after onset obtained with intensive insulin regimens can prevent / delay microvascular complications in patients with type 1 diabetes compared with conventional insulin regimens (12). The follow-up of the DCCT, the Epidemiology of Diabetes Interventions and Complications (EDIC) study provided evidence for the sustained benefit in subjects with prior intensive treatment, even if during the follow-up period the glycemic control was similar to that of subjects previously receiving conventional therapy (13-16). These studies demonstrated that the risk of developing long-term complications is determined both by the degree and the total duration of glycemic exposure. In addition, the DCCT established the relationship between glucose control and residual beta cell function as subjects with stimulated C-peptide concentrations > 0.2 pmol/ml had better outcomes (17, 18). The maintenance of endogenous beta cell function was associated with diminished disease progression, improved long term metabolic control and reduced chronic complications. These studies highlighted the role of insulin therapy over long-term.

In patients with type 2 diabetes similar benefits of intensive insulin regimens have been shown. In the Kumamoto study, which included a smaller patient population, intensive glycemic control obtained by multiple insulin injection therapy delayed the onset and progression of the early stages of diabetic microvascular complications (19, 20). Likewise, the United Kingdom Prospective Diabetes Study (UKPDS) emphasized the role of glycemic control in reducing the incidence of chronic complications in patients with type 2 diabetes, although in this study the intensive treatments were not limited to insulin regimens (21-23). Similar to EDIC, the follow-up of the UKPDS cohort showed the persistence of microvascular benefits in patients formerly treated with intensive regimens (24). A more recent study in subjects with newly diagnosed type 2 diabetes demonstrated that transient intensive insulin therapy (with continuous subcutaneous insulin infusion or multiple daily insulin injections) resulted in favorable outcomes on glycemic control and beta cell function compared to oral hypoglycemic agents (25). Trials in patients with type 2 diabetes of longer duration have also supported the benefits (even if more modest) on the onset / progression of chronic complications (26-28).

3. The importance of controlling postprandial hyperglycemia and hypoglycemic events

To date, the therapeutic interventions have mainly been focused on lowering HbA1c with emphasis on fasting blood glucose levels. However, in order to obtain optimal glycemic control with HbA1c levels < 7%, controlling both fasting and post-meal glycemia is necessary (29, 30).

It is well established that poorly controlled diabetes is associated with development of chronic micro- and macrovascular complications. Experimental studies demonstrated the atherogenic role of postprandial glycemic peaks and the link between the post-meal or post-challenge hyperglycemia (2hPG) and cardiovascular morbidity and mortality. Two meta-analyses have shown an exponential relationship between incidence of cardiovascular events and fasting glucose or 2hPG (31, 32). The relationship was stronger and highly significant for 2hPG and there seemed to be no threshold for 2hPG. Several population-based studies have basically confirmed this finding indicating an increased relative risk (in the range of 1.18 to 3.3) of cardiovascular or coronary heart disease mortality in patients with increased 2hPG (33). It has been reported that in individuals with type 2 diabetes, especially women, postprandial plasma glucose is a stronger predictor of cardiovascular events than fasting glucose levels (34). Another study indicated that both fasting and post-meal glycemia were predictive for cardiovascular events after adjusting for other risk factors in type 2 diabetic subjects (35).

A growing body of evidence shows that there is a relationship between postprandial hyperglycemia and markers of cardiovascular disease such as oxidative stress, carotid IMT and endothelial dysfunction. Oxidative stress has been implicated as a cause of both macro- and microvascular complications of diabetes. The proposed mechanism is that hyperglycemia, insulin resistance and free fatty acids feed into oxidative stress, activation of RAGE and PKC, which leads to vascular inflammation, thrombosis and vasoconstriction (36). Furthermore, increased risk of retinopathy, certain cancers and cognitive dysfunction in elderly was shown to be associated with postprandial hyperglycemia in type 2 diabetic patients (37-39).

The Kumamoto study demonstrated that postprandial glycemia was strongly associated with onset of retinopathy and nephropathy (as were fasting blood glucose and HbA1c) and that control of both fasting glucose levels < 110 mg/dl and post-meal glucose levels < 180 mg/dl prevented the onset and progression of diabetic microvascular complications (19, 20). On the other hand, the cost of strict glycemic control and intensive therapy is an increased risk of hypoglycemia, which per-se is a limiting factor in achieving long-term near-normal glucose control in patients with diabetes (40). Depending on its degree, hypoglycemia can affect physical and cognitive functions and can induce negative psychological and social consequences (41). Studies have consistently indicated a higher rate of hypoglycemia in patients with type 1 diabetes treated to lower HbA1c targets (40, 42). In the DCCT, the frequency of severe hypoglycemia was three times higher in subjects treated with intensive insulin therapy compared with those on conventional therapy, while in the Stockholm Diabetes Intervention Study - severe hypoglycemia occurred 2.5 times more frequently in the intensively treated group (43, 44). Insulin-treated subjects with type 2 diabetes experience severe hypoglycemia less frequently than patients with type 1 diabetes. This fact is explainable in part by the maintenance of some beta cell function (which allows a decrease of insulin secretion when blood glucose falls) and by insulin resistance (41). However, data from UKPDS provide evidence that the risk of hypoglycemia increases with longer duration of insulin treatment. Another study reported similar frequencies of severe hypoglycemia in patients with type 2 and type 1 diabetes after matching for duration of insulin therapy (45, 46). It is plausible that in real life patients on intensive insulin regimens experience higher rates of hypoglycemia, but since there is relatively limited data on the actual frequency of asymptomatic and mild hypoglycemia, episodes of mild hypoglycemia may be underestimated and/or underreported (41).

Hypoglycemia, even mild (especially if it occurs recurrently), can be associated with negative effects, such as impaired autonomic counter-regulation, compromised behavioral defenses against subsequent decreasing glucose concentrations and hypoglycemia unawareness, which causes a vicious cycle of recurrent hypoglycemia (41, 47). Severe hypoglycemia may exert even more serious side effects, such as seizures, unconsciousness (which may be particularly debilitating in the elderly), coma and even death (48). In older patients with type 2 diabetes and a history of severe hypoglycemia, an increased risk of dementia has been reported, particularly for patients who have a history of multiple episodes (49). In the UKPDS, recurrent hypoglycemia was associated with decreased quality of life in patients treated with insulin (50). Moreover, the unpleasant symptoms and negative consequences of hypoglycemia may result in fear and anxiety, lower treatment satisfaction, which in turn may negatively impact the diabetes management and adherence to therapy, precluding a full attainment of the benefits offered by improved glycemic control (48).

Evidence exist that hypoglycemic episodes, especially severe ones, are associated with adverse cardiovascular events (such as prolongation of the QT interval, cardiac arrhythmias, sudden cardiac arrest, and acute myocardial infarction), which are triggered by the stimulation of the sympathetic nervous system and the catecholamine surge (51, 52). Hypoglycemia also has proinflammatory consequences that may augment the risk of plaque inflammation and rupture, causing subsequent cardiovascular events (51). Hypoglycemia, mainly the recurrent and severe episodes, and the presumed ensuing cardiovascular toxicity may increase the susceptibility to poor cardiovascular outcomes, especially in subjects with significant atherosclerosis and functional / structural heart abnormalities. The cause of excess mortality during intensive therapy seen in the ACCORD study is not entirely clear, but it is thought that the most plausible cause is iatrogenic hypoglycemia (51).

Thus, it is equally important to avoid both hyperglycemic surges and hypoglycemic events while striving to obtain a tight metabolic control.

4. Restoring physiological insulin secretory profiles

In the normal, physiologic conditions there is a low basal insulin output that suppresses endogenous hepatic glucose production (overnight and between meals) as well as incremental responses of insulin secretion following food ingestion.

After a meal, blood glucose concentrations start rising within 15 minutes, reach a peak at about 30-45 minutes and within 1-2 hours return to basal levels and remain stable until the next food ingestion (53, 54). The maximal amplitude of glucose excursion depends on the amount and type of carbohydrates ingested (53). These dynamics are mirrored by the prandial insulin secretion profile: there is an initial (first) phase, which peaks in 2-3 minutes and lasts about 10 minutes, then there is a second phase of insulin release that becomes apparent after 10 minutes and continues as long as the glucose concentrations remain elevated and is concordant with the amount of carbohydrates absorbed (54-56). Once the blood glucose levels decrease, insulin secretion returns to baseline values, in order to prevent hypoglycemia in the post-absorptive phase (56).

It is believed that insulin regimens that best mimic the physiological pattern of insulin production are most likely to reach near-normal glycemic control by regulating both fasting and postprandial blood glucose levels (56, 57). These regimens require a sharp increase of insulin levels after meals and flat, nearly constant plasma insulin concentrations in the postabsorbtive / interprandial periods. They are known as basal-bolus therapy because they attempt to replicate the normal insulin secretion by combining basal and meal-time insulin replacements (58).

The "gold-standard" of insulin replacement is CSII by means of a pump, which delivers short-acting insulin in a continuous manner at determined rates and assures a peakless insulin profile between meals and insulin surges at meal-time (56, 58). The short-acting insulin analogues are better suited for CSII because of their faster absorption from subcutaneous tissue (59). The basal insulin rates can be adjusted on an hourly basis according to blood glucose oscillations to meet the 24-hour requirements of each individual and should provide about half of the total daily dose. The prandial doses are calculated by the patients and delivered according to blood glucose monitoring results, target glucose levels, carbohydrate content of the meal, physical activity, insulin sensitivity and other factors (58). Several studies have shown that CSII offers more flexibility and provides better glycemic control with improved HbA1c levels and fewer hypoglycemic events due to lower variability and better reproducibility of insulin absorption (probably resulting from the fact that the subcutaneous insulin depot is smaller) (60, 61). However, the cost of such therapy is too high to be widely available and it also requires significant patient involvement, education and motivation.

Alternatively the basal/bolus replacement can be supplied in the form of multiple daily injections. Traditionally, the regimens consisted of two injections of NPH (in the morning and at bedtime) plus 2-3 injections of regular insulin with meals. The problem with the intermediate-acting insulin preparations like NPH is that their pharmacokinetic profile does not provide a physiologic basal replacement: they have a peak at about 4-6 hours post subcutaneous injection and the action wanes rapidly at about 5-6 hours after the peak (56, 58). This profile increases the risk of nocturnal hypoglycemia (even with a bedtime snack intake), because at the time of their highest concentration (which usually occurs between midnight and 2-3 a.m.) the insulin sensitivity is higher and patients would require less basal insulin (56). Nocturnal hypoglycemia is a serious concern because it causes morning hyperglycemia through the release of counter-regulatory hormones (glucagon, epinephrine, growth hormone, cortisol) and prolonged insulin resistance and influences different physical and psychological functions during the following day. In addition, undetected nocturnal hypoglycemic episodes contribute to hypoglycemia counter-regulatory failure and unawareness, which in turn predisposes to severe hypoglycemia and profoundly impacts on patients' quality of life (62). On the other hand, the time-action profile of the intermediate-acting insulin poses another problem: during the morning hours (after 4 a.m.) the requirement for basal insulin is greater due to increased release of counter-regulatory hormones and by then the insulin action is waning, which results in morning hyperglycemia. An attempt to correct this by increasing the bedtime insulin dose may result in higher risk of nocturnal hypoglycemia.

A different approach of multiple daily injections which attempts to alleviate these problems uses short-acting insulin analogues at meal-time with one or two injections of long-acting insulin analogues (glargine or detemir) and it is the preferred regimen in recent years (58). The long-acting analogues afford less glycemic fluctuations, less variability, reduced risk of hypoglycemic events and a significantly prolonged duration of action (17-24 hours) due to a steady absorption into the circulation and more stable serum concentrations (63, 64). Studies have indicated fewer overall, nocturnal and severe hypoglycemic episodes in both types of diabetes (especially in type 1), while providing similar or slightly improved metabolic control compared with NPH insulin (65-67).

5. The limitations of current prandial insulin treatment for type 1 and type 2 diabetes

Multiple daily insulin injections are the mainstay of insulin delivery for many patients with type 1 diabetes and patients with type 2 diabetes that cannot be controlled with other regimens, especially those with longer duration of the disease and severe insulin deficiency. Despite the evidence and increased awareness of the necessity to achieve strict glycemic control, current insulin therapy has some limitations that preclude reaching the goal of maintaining near-normal glycemia in the long-term, even in compliant patients. The major challenges are related to avoiding postprandial hyperglycemia and late hypoglycemia, which are mainly caused by the mismatch between the time-action profile of the administered insulin and postprandial glucose excursions.

The "conventional" prandial insulin therapy with regular human insulin has its shortcomings in terms of the pharmacokinetic properties which limit their clinical efficacy: the onset of action is slow, the peak is reached in about 2-3 hours and the total duration of action lasts 5-8 hours (68). This is caused by the fact that the dissociation rate of human insulin from hexamers into monomers in the subcutaneous tissues is slow and the absorption into the bloodstream is gradual. Thus, the maximal insulin concentrations do not occur at the time when glucose levels are the highest, and so the short-acting insulin has to be administered 30-45 minutes before meals in order to minimize postprandial hyperglycemia. This is quite inconvenient for patients (and poses a risk of pre-meal hypoglycemia if the food intake is inadvertently delayed) and even so, the time-action profile is not optimal. Glycemic excursions are not properly covered and 4-5 hours post-injection, after the food absorption is completed, there is still some insulin absorption from subcutaneous depot (58). This results in relative hyperinsulinemia, which increases the risk of late postprandial hypoglycemia and would require a snack intake to prevent it. Moreover, the regular human insulin preparations have important intra- and inter-individual variations that result in unpredictable effects and makes it even more difficult to avoid hyper- and hypoglycemia (69).

In order to overcome the problems of non-physiologic pharmacokinetics, the regular human insulins have been largely substituted with the newer insulin analogues that were developed by means of protein engineering and recombinant DNA technology to enable better glycemic control by faster action (70). The insulin analogues have been obtained by substitution or minimal alterations in the amino acid sequence in regions of the molecule not essential for binding to the insulin receptor but pivotal for dimer formation in order to diminish the tendency of self-association between insulin molecules and allow a faster absorption from injection site (70). There are three rapid-acting insulin analogues available at the moment: insulin lispro (based on amino-acid substitution of proline at position B28 and lysine at position B29), insulin aspart (with aspartic acid substituted for proline at position B28) and insulin glulisine (that has an asparagine to lysine substitution at position B3, and a lysine to glutamine acid substitution at position B29) (71). Despite the differences in structure, the three analogues have similar pharmacokinetic and pharmacodynamic properties (70). Their onset of action is more rapid, which permits an administration within 10-15 minutes before meals, the peak is greater and occurs at about 1-2 hours and the total duration of action is shorter (4-5 hours) compared to regular human insulin (Table 1) (58, 68). This allows an improved replacement of mealtime insulin needs with regards to postprandial plasma glucose control and more flexibility than regular insulin. In addition, the insulin analogues have a smaller intra- and inter-individual variability compared to regular insulin which could provide a somewhat improved glycemic control and potentially reduced risk of hypoglycemia (69).

Insulin	Onset of action	Peak action	Total duration of action
Short-acting			
Regular	30-45 min	2-3 h	5-8 h
Rapid-acting			
Lispro Aspart Glulisine	5-15 min	1-2 h	4 h

Table 1. The pharmacodynamic profiles of currently available prandial insulin formulations (68)

However, even with the insulin analogues the synchronization between insulin action and glucose absorption from a meal is still less than ideal, as they do not replicate normal physiology, and many patients still have suboptimal glucose control. Several meta-analyses have suggested that insulin analogues offer rather modest or inconsistent clinical advantages over conventional insulin in terms of lowering HbA1c and reducing hypoglycemia, in children and adults with type 1 diabetes (72-76). Data on the influence on hypoglycemia is particularly inconsistent. Some studies have shown that in fact the overall frequency of hypoglycemic episodes were similar with analogue insulin and regular insulin use in adults with type 1 diabetes and were modestly decreased in children (72-77). Moreover, some reports indicated that the frequency of severe and nocturnal hypoglycemia seemed to be reduced with analogues in adults, but not in prepubertal children, while others found no difference in the frequency of severe or nocturnal hypoglycemia and no evidence for reduction in patient awareness for hypoglycemia with insulin analogues (72-78). It should be noted that hypoglycemia occurrence is not fully attributable to the pharmacokinetic profile of the insulin preparations, but may also result from a mismatch between insulin dose and the carbohydrate content of the meal, delayed food intake or other factors (79).

On the other hand, postprandial hyperglycemia still occurs with the new insulin analogues (80, 81). Hyperglycemic postprandial glucose excursions were found to reach levels over 300 mg/dl in about 50% and over 180 mg/dl in almost 90% of children with type 1 diabetes with good overall metabolic control (82). The findings were confirmed by other studies that indicated postprandial glucose levels higher than 300 mg/dl in subjects with type 1 diabetes receiving multiple insulin injection therapy (83). Targeting postprandial hyperglycemia is important in order to improve HbA1c levels and this has also been recently highlighted by the International Diabetes Federation guidelines (84, 85).

In everyday life the control of postprandial hyperglycemia poses even more challenges due to variations in dietary intake and physical exercise or insulin dosage and timing changes (patients may modify the timing of insulin administration in the sense of dosing immediately before or even after meals in order to fit their lifestyle / daily activity requirements) (86). In addition, lack of predictable insulin response may occur with insulin analogues because their absorption can be affected by various factors such as: mechanics of injection, the injection site, and metabolic factors, similar to regular human insulin (87).

Two meta-analyses indicated that regular human insulin and rapid-acting analogues have comparable frequencies and types of adverse events (other than hypoglycemia), i.e. local site reactions, ketoacidosis and the discontinuation rates during the clinical studies were similar for the two types of insulin preparations (75, 77).

6. Current ultrafast insulin formulations

Thus, the limitations of current insulin formulations and the need for proper postprandial glycemic control have led to research of novel, ultrafast insulin formulations /delivery systems that could eventually better match post-prandial glucose excursions (by speeding the onset of insulin absorption and action coupled with a faster offset of action) and that would offer improved flexibility in terms of injection time relative to a meal (Table 2). By a closer approximation of the normal insulin release, several outcomes could be obtained, i.e. improvement of HbA1c through a better control of postprandial blood glucose, reduced incidence of late-phase hypoglycemia, lower intra-subject variability, and less weight gain.
Recently, stainless steel microneedle syringe devices have been under investigation for intradermal delivery of insulin and their potential to improve postprandial glycemia has been evaluated. The microneedles (34-gauge; an external diameter of approximately 260 μm, 1.25-1.75-mm long) penetrate the stratum corneum and epidermis to reach the dense beds of capillaries and lymphatic vessels of the dermis (88). The dermis layer can facilitate a faster insulin absorption compared to injection into the subcutaneous layer by an increased lymphatic absorption and reach blood circulation.

Insulin	Onset (early T50%)	Peak (T GIRmax)	Offset (late T50%)
Intradermal[90]	28-35 min	105-110 min	271-287 min
rHUPH20+insulin[93]	43-44 min	72-114 min	119-275 min
VIAject[95]	31-35 min	111-136 min	270-297 min
InsuPatch[101]	NA	95 min	NA
Technosphere[105,106]	NA	42-79 min	NA
Oral-lyn[119-121]	23-35 min	40-50 min	56-101 min

Table 2. The pharmacodynamic profiles of ultrafast insulin formulations / delivery systems under development

In animal models the intradermal delivery of insulin by microneedles provided a unique pharmacokinetic profile more closely resembling the intravenous rather than the subcutaneous administration (89). The profile is characterized by an extremely rapid uptake and systemic distribution from the injection site: the time to maximum concentration was significantly reduced (with 64%) for insulin lispro administered intradermaly vs. subcutaneously. In addition, the maximum circulating peak concentrations were elevated several fold (349% for insulin lispro) compared to subcutaneous delivery. Moreover, both regular and analogue insulins, despite their differences in molecular weight, when delivered by microneedles showed a more rapid onset of action than subcutaneous delivery of insulin analogue (lispro) (89).

A clinical study in healthy volunteers that evaluated the pharmacokinetics and pharmacodynamics of intradermal administration of insulin lispro compared to subcutaneous injections under euglycemic clamp conditions, has basically confirmed these findings (90). Delivery via microneedles resulted in faster insulin uptake with decreased time to maximal insulin concentration (by approximately 24 minutes), higher relative bioavailability at early post-injection times and a more physiologic metabolic effect, with faster onset of action (shorter times to maximal and early half-maximal glucose infusion rates) and more rapid offset of action (shorter time to late half-maximal glucose infusion rates) (90). Another clinical study was conducted in patients with type 1 diabetes in order to determine if the more rapid absorption of insulin resulting from microneedle administration translates into a significant reduction in postprandial glucose levels under standardized meal conditions (91). The results indicated that postprandial glucose levels were improved when regular human insulin was delivered intradermaly vs. subcutaneously, but were similar for analogue insulin. In clinical studies the intradermal delivery was generally well tolerated (although some transient, localized wheal formation and redness were noticed at injection sites), but the potential effects of high level or repetitive exposure of protein drugs such as insulin on the lymphatics and immune system need full investigation (90, 91).

Another area of research focuses on the combination of available insulin products with a human recombinant hyaluronidase, which facilitates the local dispersion and absorption of co-administered molecules (92, 93). The human recombinant hyaluronidase is a highly purified neutral pH-active enzyme that depolymerizes hyaluronan in the hypodermis under physiologic conditions. Thus, it decreases the resistance to fluid flow and further contributes to the drug dispersion for better exposure to a larger capillary network (92). Following this, concomitant injection with proteins / drugs such as insulin, is expected to lead to an enhanced absorption and improved bioavailability. Recombinant human hyaluronidase (rHuPH20) is a genetically engineered soluble hyaluronidase approved by the Food and Drug Administration as an adjuvant to enhance permeation of other injected drugs (94). Since rHuPH20 is rapidly metabolized locally, without systemic exposure and because hyaluronan has a fast turn-over, the permeation effects are transient (94).

A phase 1 glucose clamp study in healthy volunteers evaluated the insulin time-concentration curve and pharmacodynamic profiles of insulin analogue (lispro) and of regular human insulin combined with rHuPH20 and reported significantly faster systemic absorption, enhanced insulin plasma concentrations and faster metabolic effects compared with either insulin formulation alone (95). A rise in insulin concentration was observed within 3 minutes following the injection and the enhanced pharmacokinetic and glucodynamic effects early after injection were accompanied by reduced late effects. A second study in healthy subjects also reported a lower intra-subject variability with rHuPH20 coadministration (94). A phase 2 standardized meal-test study in patients with type 1 diabetes examined whether the accelerated insulin absorption has favorable consequences on the control of postprandial glycemic excursions (94). As in the phase 1 studies, the coadministration of rHuPH20 with regular insulin or lispro yielded an accelerated insulin concentration profile that was accompanied by a significant reduction in both mean peak and total post-meal glucose concentrations compared to either insulin alone. Post-meal hypoglycemia was reported to be generally mild and the overall hypoglycemic risk comparable for lispro with or without rHuPH20 and reduced for regular insulin with rHuPH20 compared with regular insulin alone (94). Clinical studies reported a good tolerability profile without severe adverse effects, but there is no safety data so far regarding the repeated or long term exposure to recombinant hyaluronidase.

A third novel ultrafast insulin formulation, VIAjectTM, is currently under clinical development. The main concept of the approach is that instead of altering the structure of insulin molecule, the zinc ions are pulled away from human insulin hexamers and simultaneously charges on the surface of the insulin molecule are masked by the addition of ethylene diamine tetraacetic acid and citric acid (96). This results in destabilization and dissociation of the insulin hexamer and prevents re-association to the hexameric state after subcutaneous injection.

A glucose clamp study in healthy volunteers evaluated the pharmacodynamic, pharmacokinetic and the dose-response properties of the VIAject in comparison with regular human insulin and insulin lispro (96). The results indicated a more rapid increase and decline in serum insulin concentrations after VIAject injection compared to regular human insulin and insulin lispro, but the difference between the later and VIAject failed to reach statistical significance (96). The three dose of ultrafast insulin used in the study showed a linear dose-response relationship. The time-action profile induced by VIAject was faster than either subcutaneously injected human insulin or lispro, with a more rapid onset of action and maximal metabolic activity, while the activity in the first 2 hours after injection was higher. A second glucose clamp study in patients with type 1 diabetes confirmed the faster absorption kinetics and the more rapid onset of insulin action compared to regular human insulin and showed that upon repeated administration, the within-subject variability is lower than that of human insulin (97). Moreover, a more recent meal-test study conducted in patients with type 2 diabetes indicated that treatment with VIAject determined a significant decrease of postprandial oxidative stress and improved endothelial function compared with regular insulin or insulin lispro, while all insulin formulations resulted in comparable improvements in central arterial elasticity (98).

Another innovative approach developed in order to accelerate insulin absorption into the bloodstream is using a technology (InsuPatch™) that heats the tissue locally around the injection site (99). Changes in temperature at injection site are partially responsible for variability in insulin absorption (87). Increased skin temperature results in vasodilatation and improved local perfusion, which enables accelerated and enhanced insulin absorption (100). The InsuPatch™ device is an add-on to the insulin pump and is comprised of a heating pad attached to an insulin infusion set and a controller that monitors the temperature of the pad (99). The heating pad warms in a controlled manner the tissue surrounding the injection site for 30 minutes after insulin delivery, without heating the insulin itself.

A study using a meal tolerance test in subjects with type 1 diabetes treated by CSII tested the effect of InsuPatch™ on rapid-acting insulin absorption and post-challenge glucose excursions. The study found a significant effect of the heating device on the pharmacokinetic parameters: the maximum insulin concentrations increased (by 38%), as well as the total insulin absorption during the first 30, 60 and 90 minutes, (by 57%, 45% and 27%, respectively) as measured by area under the curve (AUC). The time to maximal concentration and time to half maximal concentration significantly decreased, indicating an accelerated insulin absorption. The changes were accompanied by significant reductions in post-challenge glucose levels (both 90 minutes post-meal glucose excursion and AUC 0-120 minutes of glucose concentrations were lowered" before by 39%) (99). The InsuPatchTM was also tested in youth with type 1 diabetes using a euglycemic clamp procedure. The use of the InsuPatchTM was found to decrease time to peak action by more than 40 minutes, whereas the bioavailability and peak responses remained unchanged (101, 102). Such improvements in time-action responses may provide a better control of post-meal glucose excursions (101). Another study that evaluated the effect of the InsuPatchTM heating device on postprandial blood glucose levels after different standardized meals in patients with type 1 diabetes on CSII has confirmed that local heating of the skin around the infusion site significantly increases early post-delivery insulin levels (AUC 0-60 minutes for insulin concentrations above baseline) as well as significantly reduces post-prandial blood glucose (blood glucose at 90 minutes and AUC 0-120 minutes of blood glucose levels) without causing more hypoglycemia (103). Current efforts are being employed in order to optimize the effect of the device on the pharmacokinetic and pharmacodynamic parameters by improving the heating process. The InsuPatch™ device was well tolerated and no serious adverse effects were reported with its use to date (99).

A different strategy that attempts to overcome the barriers and limitations of subcutaneous insulin administration is engaging a diverse route of delivery (i.e. pulmonary). After the discontinuation of the first inhaled insulin product (Exubera), the development of most of the pulmonary administration systems has ceased. One of them though, Technosphere™ insulin, is still being developed and it appears to overcome some of the barriers that contributed to the withdrawal of Exubera (104, 105). Technosphere™ insulin is an ordered lattice array containing recombinant human insulin, formulated as a crystalline dry powder. The Technosphere™ carrier is created with microcrystallized plates of fumaryl diketopiperazine that undergo self-assembly into microparticles with a very large surface area and a high internal porosity which are then lyophilized into a dry powder (104). Insulin is absorbed onto the surface of the particles and is delivered by a high-impedance, low-flow, breath-powered inhaler with a powder de-agglomeration mechanism that allows for a high percentage of the administered insulin to be absorbed. At the neutral pH environment of the lungs, the microparticles dissolve rapidly and insulin is absorbed across the pulmonary epithelium into the systemic circulation, while the carrier is cleared unmetabolized (104, 106).

The pharmacokinetic clamp studies performed in healthy volunteers and patients with type 2 diabetes revealed a very rapid systemic insulin uptake (time to maximal insulin concentration around 15 minutes) with a subsequent fast onset of action (time to maximal metabolic effect of about 40-80 minutes) and a short duration of action (106-109). These characteristics had basically been confirmed by a meal-test study in patients with type 2 diabetes, which demonstrated a more rapid absorption and higher peak insulin levels as well as markedly improved postprandial glycemic control with the inhaled insulin compared with subcutaneous regular human insulin (110). A linear systemic insulin uptake profile was noted in studies employing healthy volunteers inhaling three doses of insulin (106-108). In addition, the within-subject variability of insulin exposure following inhalation of Technosphere™ insulin was lower compared to regular insulin (109). The relative bioavailability was reported to be 26-50% in the first 3 hours after administration (111). Given that other inhaled insulin preparations have been associated with reduced absorption in patients with chronic obstructive pulmonary disease, a study assessing the pharmacokinetic profile and safety of Technosphere™ insulin in nondiabetic patients with chronic obstructive pulmonary disease has shown that insulin absorption was not significantly altered in this group (112). Similarly, the absorption of inhaled insulin appeared not to be altered in a clinically significant manner in smokers (105).

The clinical efficacy of Technosphere™ insulin was assessed in studies of 11 or 12 week-duration in patients with type 2 diabetes (either insulin-naive or treated with basal insulin glargine), which demonstrated significant reductions in postprandial glucose excursions as well as clinically meaningful improvement of glycemic control as evaluated by HbA1c (113, 114). Moreover, a study of longer duration (52 weeks) in subjects with type 2 diabetes compared the inhaled insulin plus insulin glargine with twice daily biaspart insulin and indicated that changes in HbA1c determined by the treatment with inhaled insulin were similar and non-inferior to that with biaspart insulin (115). In addition, the weight gain and the incidence of both mild-to-moderate and severe hypoglycemic events were lower with inhaled insulin therapy.

Considering the issues associated with Exubera in the past, patient satisfaction and acceptance has been evaluated with the new inhaled insulin product. Overall, significant improvements in attitudes toward insulin therapy, treatment satisfaction, and treatment preference were reported with Technosphere™ insulin (105, 116). The therapeutical approach using the new inhaled insulin was implemented without a negative impact on health-related quality of life (116).

To date, Technosphere™ insulin has demonstrated a favorable safety and tolerability profile in clinical studies that collected data in healthy volunteers and patients with diabetes (105). The most frequent treatment-emergent adverse events associated with inhaled insulin in clinical studies were cough and hypoglycemia. Weight gain is commonly associated with insulin therapy. However, data so far indicated that with Technosphere™ insulin the weight gain was actually less compared with subcutaneous prandial insulins (105). While there are no reports of lung cancer or other serious side effects associated with Technosphere™ insulin to date, longer-term safety follow-up and evaluation should be done in subjects treated with this inhaled insulin formulation, especially in smokers and in subjects with respiratory disorders.

Finally, another alternative approach of insulin delivery is through the oral (buccal) route, which offers some advantages: good accessibility, high level of vascularization, relatively large surface for absorption (100–200 cm^2), avoidance of presystemic metabolism in the liver, robustness, direct contact of the drug with the mucosa, weak variations of pH (117, 118). Oral-lyn is a liquid formulation of human regular insulin with very small amounts of generally regarded as safe (GRAS) ingredients, which is delivered to the buccal mucosa with a metered-dose, slightly modified asthma-like spray and used for prandial insulin therapy (117). The device spray the uniform-sized insulin droplets with high speed (100 mph) into the mouth, which then penetrate the superficial layers of the mucosa and get absorbed into the bloodstream.

The pharmacokinetic and pharmacodynamic properties of Oral-lyn have been evaluated in a number of glucose clamp studies, which have demonstrated a significantly more rapid absorption (about 25 minutes) to higher levels than subcutaneous injection of regular human insulin and a rapid return to baseline values (90 minutes after application) (118-121). The profile was paralleled by the glucose infusion rates that reached maximal levels significantly earlier (at about 45 minutes) and then returned back to baseline concentrations after approximately 120 minutes. Increasing doses of Oral-lyn determined a linear dose-response relationship with respect to maximal insulin concentrations, while time to maximal insulin levels was similar across doses (118-121). Additional meal-test studies indicated that the 30- and 60-min glucose levels were significantly lower with oral insulin spray treatment (122, 123). The metabolic effects of Oral-lyn were evaluated in subjects with type 2 diabetes suboptimally controlled with oral hypoglycemic agents and showed that oral insulin spray significantly decreased the 2-hour postprandial glucose increments in comparison with the oral agents alone and that the difference was more pronounced at the end of the 4-h period, due to the rapid onset and wane of action of oral insulin spray (124). In all of the studies Oral-lyn was generally well tolerated, although some individuals experienced transient (1–2 min), mild and self-limited dizziness during dosing with both the oral insulin and placebo spray (122-124). No other significant side effects (including severe hypoglycemia) were noted in studies involving subjects with type 2 diabetes (122).

It should be mentioned that although some of the ultrafast insulin formulations / insulin delivery systems are in early phases of development and/or have not specifically reported for hypoglycemic events, based on their pharmacokinetic properties it can be reasonably expected that they may benefit patients with diabetes by reducing post-meal hyperglycemia with decreasing (or at least without increasing) the risk of hypoglycemic events.

7. Conclusions

The main goal of insulin therapy is to obtain a near-normal glycemic control by mimicking the time-action profile of physiologic insulin secretion as close as possible and with minimal side effects. Management of both types of diabetes is continually evolving as new therapies, including new insulins / insulin delivery systems are still emerging. In real life, with all progress of the recent years, all the above mentioned objectives are difficult to be reached and successful implementation of intensive diabetes management poses true challenges.

Ideally, an insulin-replacement therapeutic approach would keep in check both the fasting and the postprandial glucose concentrations while attaining target HbA1c values, without high glycemic variations and without causing hypoglycemia. Current rapid-acting insulin analogues have a faster pharmacokinetics and action compared with regular human insulin following subcutaneous administration (Table 1). This allows improved control of the post-meal early hyperglycemic surge and late relative hyperinsulinemia, the cause of postprandial hypoglycemia. However, recent meta-analyses showed that in fact the use of insulin analogues had only a modest impact on overall glycemic control and on the rates of side effects, mainly hypoglycemia, compared to conventional insulins (72-76). This is because although improved, the time-action profile still does not exactly replicate normal insulin secretion and therefore there is a mismatch with the blood glucose concentrations curve. Both postprandial hyperglycemia and hypoglycemia have important health consequences as well as on quality of life and failure to address them both may compromise the success of treatment in the short- and long-term.

The extent to which these goals can be met depends on many factors, including the type of diabetes, the stage in the progression of the disease and the pharmacokinetic profile of insulin formulation. If some of these factors are unmodifiable, others are, and efforts are being employed to develop new, improved ultrafast insulin products / delivery systems. They provide even more rapid pharmacokinetic and pharmacodynamic properties compared with current prandial insulin products, which may offer some advantages. The short interval between insulin administration and the appearance of the maximal serum

insulin levels, and the rapid onset of action may have a beneficial effect on the control of post-meal glycemic excursions. Because their action wanes off more rapidly, the risk of postprandial hypoglycemia is decreased. Both requirements seem to be fulfilled by the ultrafast insulins, but their long-term safety and tolerability still remain a concern. Provided that larger clinical studies will confirm their positive safety and tolerability profile, these new technologies will become very attractive candidates for prandial insulin delivery.
However, it should always be kept in mind that the insulin regimens need to be customized to each individual's needs, in order to maximize compliance and optimize glycemic control, while reducing to a minimum the potential unwanted side effects like hypoglycemia and weight gain. Patients with diabetes need substantial psychosocial support, ongoing education and guidance from a diabetes team, in order to set and achieve appropriate, individualized management goals.

8. References

[1] International Diabetes Federation. IDF Diabetes Atlas, 4th edn. Brussels, Belgium: International Diabetes Federation, 2009.
[2] Steele C, Hagopian WA, Gitelman S, Masharani U, Cavaghan M, Rother KI, Donaldson D, Harlan DM, Bluestone J, Herold KC. Insulin secretion in type 1 diabetes. Diabetes 2004; 53: 426–433.
[3] Gepts W. Pathologic anatomy of the pancreas in juvenile diabetes mellitus. Diabetes 1965; 14: 619–633.
[4] Butler AE, Janson J, Bonner-Weir S, Ritzel R, Rizza RA, Butler PC. Beta-cell deficit and increased beta-cell apoptosis in humans with type 2 diabetes. Diabetes 2003; 52(1): 102-110.
[5] Bonner-Weir S. Islet growth and development in the adult. J Mol Endocrinol 2000; 24(3): 297-302.
[6] Donath MY, Halban PA. Decreased beta-cell mass in diabetes: significance, mechanisms and therapeutic implications. Diabetologia 2004; 47(3): 581-589.
[7] Ahrén B. Type 2 diabetes, insulin secretion and beta-cell mass. Curr Mol Med 2005; 5(3): 275-286.
[8] DeFronzo RA. Current issues in the treatment of type 2 diabetes. Overview of newer agents: where treatment is going. Am J Med 2010; 123(3 Suppl): S38-48.
[9] Rolla A. The pathophysiological basis for intensive insulin replacement. Int J Obes Relat Metab Disord 2004, 28 (Suppl. 2): S3-7.
[10] Bretzel R.G. Intensive insulin regimens: Evidence or benefit. Int J Obes Relat Metab Disord 2004, 28 (Suppl. 2): S8-13.
[11] American Diabetes Association. Standards of medical care in diabetes--2011. Diabetes Care 2011; 34 Suppl 1: S11-61.
[12] DCCT: The effect of intensive treatment of diabetes on the development and progression of long-term complications in insulin-dependent diabetes mellitus. The Diabetes Control and Complications Trial Research Group. N Engl J Med 1993; 329: 977–986.
[13] The Diabetes Control and Complications Trial/ Epidemiology of Diabetes Interventions and Complications Research Group. Effect of intensive therapy on

the microvascular complications of type 1 diabetes mellitus. JAMA 2002; 287: 2563-2569.
[14] The Diabetes Control and Complications Trial/ Epidemiology of Diabetes Interventions and Complications Research Group. Sustained effect of intensive treatment of type 1 diabetes mellitus on development and progression of diabetic nephropathy: The Epidemiology of Diabetes Interventions and Complications (EDIC) study. JAMA 2003; 290: 2159-2167.
[15] The Diabetes Control and Complications Trial/ Epidemiology of Diabetes Interventions and Complications Research Group. Retinopathy and nephropathy in patients with type 1 diabetes four years after a trial of intensive therapy. N Engl J Med 2000; 342: 381-389.
[16] Martin CL, Albers J, Herman WH, Cleary P, Waberski B, Greene DA, Stevens MJ, Feldman EL, DCCT/EDIC Research Group. Neuropathy among the diabetes control and complications trial cohort 8 years after trial completion. Diabetes Care 2006; 29: 340–344.
[17] The Diabetes Control and Complications Trial Research Group. Effect of intensive therapy on residual β-cell function in patients with type 1 diabetes in the diabetes control and complications trial. A randomized, controlled trial. Ann Intern Med 1998; 128: 517–523.
[18] Steffes MW, Sibley S, Jackson M, Thomas W. Beta-cell function and the development of diabetes-related complications in the diabetes control and complications trial. Diabetes Care 2003; 26: 832–836.
[19] Shichiri M, Kishikawa H, Ohkubo Y, Wake N. Long-term results of the Kumamoto Study on optimal diabetes control in type 2 diabetic patients. Diabetes Care 2000; 23 Suppl 2: B21-9.
[20] Ohkubo Y, Kishikawa H, Araki E, Miyata T, Isami S, Motoyoshi S, Kojima Y, Furuyoshi N, Shichiri M. Intensive insulin therapy prevents the progression of diabetic microvascular complications in Japanese patients with non-insulin-dependent diabetes mellitus: a randomized prospective 6-year study. Diabetes Res Clin Pract 1995; 28(2): 103-117.
[21] UKPDS: Effect of intensive blood-glucose control with metformin on complications in overweight patients with type 2 diabetes (UKPDS 34). UK Prospective Diabetes Study (UKPDS) Group. Lancet 1998; 352: 854–865.
[22] UKPDS: Intensive blood-glucose control with sulphonylureas or insulin compared with conventional treatment and risk of complications in patients with type 2 diabetes (UKPDS 33). UK Prospective Diabetes Study (UKPDS) Group. Lancet 1998; 352: 837–853.
[23] Stratton IM, Adler AI, Neil HA, Matthews DR, Manley SE, Cull CA, Hadden D, Turner RC, Holman RR. Association of glycaemia with macrovascular and microvascular complications of type 2 diabetes (UKPDS 35): prospective observational study. BMJ 2000; 321: 405- 412.
[24] Holman RR, Paul SK, Bethel MA, Matthews DR, Neil HA: 10-Year Follow-up of intensive glucose control in type 2 diabetes. N Engl J Med 2008; 359: 1577- 1589.
[25] Weng J, Li Y, Xu W, Shi L, Zhang Q, Zhu D, Hu Y, Zhou Z, Yan X, Tian H, Ran X, Luo Z, Xian J, Yan L, Li F, Zeng L, Chen Y, Yang L, Yan S, Liu J, Li M, Fu Z, Cheng H. Effect of intensive insulin therapy on beta-cell function and glycaemic control in

patients with newly diagnosed type 2 diabetes: a multicentre randomised parallel-group trial. Lancet 2008; 371(9626): 1753-1760.

[26] Duckworth W, Abraira C, Moritz T, Reda D, Emanuele N, Reaven PD, Zieve FJ, Marks J, Davis SN, Hayward R, Warren SR, Goldman S, McCarren M, Vitek ME, Henderson WG, Huang GD, VADT Investigators. Glucose control and vascular complications in veterans with type 2 diabetes. N Engl J Med 2009; 360: 129–139.

[27] ADVANCE Collaborative Group, Patel A, MacMahon S, Chalmers J, Neal B, Billot L, Woodward M, Marre M, Cooper M, Glasziou P, Grobbee D, Hamet P, Harrap S, Heller S, Liu L, Mancia G, Mogensen CE, Pan C, Poulter N, Rodgers A, Williams B, Bompoint S, de Galan BE, Joshi R, Travert F. Intensive blood glucose control and vascular outcomes in patients with type 2 diabetes. N Engl J Med 2008; 358:2560–2572.

[28] Ismail-Beigi F, Craven T, Banerji MA, Basile J, Calles J, Cohen RM, Cuddihy R, Cushman WC, Genuth S, Grimm RH Jr, Hamilton BP, Hoogwerf B, Karl D, Katz L, Krikorian A, O'Connor P, Pop-Busui R, Schubart U, Simmons D, Taylor H, Thomas A, Weiss D, Hramiak I, ACCORD trial group. Effect of intensive treatment of hyperglycaemia on microvascular outcomes in type 2 diabetes: an analysis of the ACCORD randomised trial. Lancet 2010; 376: 419–430.

[29] Sorkin JD, Muller DC, Fleg JL, Andres R. The relation of fasting and 2-h postchallenge plasma glucose concentrations to mortality: data from the Baltimore Longitudinal Study of Aging with a critical review of the literature. Diabetes Care 2005; 28(11): 2626-2632.

[30] Woerle HJ, Neumann C, Zschau S, Tenner S, Irsigler A, Schirra J, Gerich JE, Göke B. Impact of fasting and postprandial glycemia on overall glycemic control in type 2 diabetes Importance of postprandial glycemia to achieve target HbA1c levels. Diabetes Res Clin Pract 2007; 77(2): 280-285.

[31] Coutinho M, Gerstein HC, Wang Y, Yusuf S. The relationship between glucose and incident cardiovascular events: a metaregression analysis of published data from 20 studies of 95,783 individuals followed for 12.4 years. Diabetes Care 1999; 22 (2): 233-240.

[32] Levitan EB, Song Y, Ford ES, Liu S. Is nondiabetic hyperglycemia a risk factor for cardiovascular disease? A meta-analysis of prospective studies. Arch Intern Med 2004; 164(19): 2147-2155.

[33] Charpentier G, Riveline JP, dardari D, Varroud-Vial M. Should postprandial hyperglycemia in prediabetic and type 2 diabetic patients be treated? Drugs 2006; 66 (3): 273-286.

[34] Cavalot F, Petrelli A, Traversa M, Bonomo K, Fiora E, Conti M, Anfossi G, Costa G, Trovati M. Postprandial blood glucose is a stronger predictor of cardiovascular events than fasting blood glucose in type 2 diabetes mellitus, particularly in women: lessons from the San Luigi Gonzaga Diabetes Study. J Clin Endocrinol Metab 2006; 91(3): 813-819.

[35] Bonora E, Muggeo M. Postprandial blood glucose as a risk factor for cardiovascular disease in Type II diabetes: the epidemiological evidence. Diabetologia 2001; 44 (12): 2107-2114.

[36] Gerich JE. Clinical significance, pathogenesis, and management of postprandial hyperglycemia. Arch Intern Med 2003; 163(11): 1306-1316.

[37] Shiraiwa T, Kaneto H, Miyatsuka T, Kato K, Yamamoto K, Kawashima A, Kanda T, Suzuki M, Imano E, Matsuhisa M, Hori M, Yamasaki Y. Post-prandial hyperglycemia is an important predictor of the incidence of diabetic microangiopathy in Japanese type 2 diabetic patients. Biochem Biophys Res Commun 2005; 336(1): 339-345.

[38] Abbatecola AM, Rizzo MR, Barbieri M, Grella R, Arciello A, Laieta MT, Acampora R, Passariello N, Cacciapuoti F, Paolisso G. Postprandial plasma glucose excursions and cognitive functioning in aged type 2 diabetics. Neurology 2006; 67(2): 235-240.

[39] Gapstur SM, Gann PH, Lowe W, Liu K, Colangelo L, Dyer A. Abnormal glucose metabolism and pancreatic cancer mortality. JAMA 2000; 283(19): 2552-2558.

[40] Cryer PE. The barrier of hypoglycemia in diabetes. Diabetes 2008; 57(12): 3169–3176.

[41] Rossetti P, Porcellati F, Bolli GB, Fanelli CG. Prevention of hypoglycemia while achieving good glycemic control in type 1 diabetes: the role of insulin analogs. Diabetes Care. 2008; 31 Suppl 2: S113-120.

[42] Diabetes Control and Complications Trial Research Group. Adverse events and their association with treatment regimens in the Diabetes Control and Complications trial. Diabetes Care 1995; 18: 1415–1427.

[43] Diabetes Control and Complications Trial Research Group: The effect of intensive treatment of diabetes on the development and progression of long-term complications in insulin-dependent diabetes mellitus. N Engl J Med 1993; 329: 977–986.

[44] Reichard P, Berglund B, Britz A, Cars I, Nilsson BY, Rosenqvist U. Intensified conventional insulin treatment retards the microvascular complications of insulin-dependent diabetes mellitus (IDDM): the Stockholm Diabetes Intervention Study (SDIS) after 5 years. J Intern Med 1991; 230(2): 101-108.

[45] UKPDS Research Group: Effort of intensive blood glucose control with insulin and sulfonylureas on insulin compared with conventional treatment and risk of complications in patients with type 2 diabetes (UKPDS 33). Lancet 1998; 352: 837–853.

[46] Hepburn DA, MacLeod KM, Pell ACH, Scougal IJ, Frier BM: Frequency and symptoms of hypoglycemia experienced by patients with type 2 diabetes treated with insulin. Diabet Med 1993; 10: 231–237.

[47] Cryer PE. The barrier of hypoglycemia in diabetes. Diabetes. 2008; 57(12): 3169-76.

[48] Barnett AH. Avoiding hypoglycaemia while achieving good glycaemic control in type 2 diabetes through optimal use of oral agent therapy. Curr Med Res Opin 2010; 26(6): 1333-1342.

[49] Whitmer RA, Karter AJ, Yaffe K, Quesenberry CP Jr, Selby JV. Hypoglycemic episodes and risk of dementia in older patients with type 2 diabetes mellitus. JAMA 2009; 301(15): 1565-1572.

[50] United Kingdom Prospective Diabetes Study Group. Quality of life in type 2 diabetic patients is affected by complications but not by intensive policies to improve blood glucose or blood pressure control (UKPDS 37). Diabetes Care 1999; 22:1125-1136.

[51] O'Keefe JH, Abuannadi M, Lavie CJ, Bell DS. Strategies for optimizing glycemic control and cardiovascular prognosis in patients with type 2 diabetes mellitus. Mayo Clin Proc 2011; 86(2): 128-138.

[52] Yakubovich N, Gerstein HC. Serious cardiovascular outcomes in diabetes: the role of hypoglycemia. Circulation. 2011; 123(3): 342-348.

[53] Brand-Miller JC, Stockmann K, Atkinson F, Petocz P, Denyer G. Glycemic index, postprandial glycemia, and the shape of the curve in healthy subjects: analysis of a database of more than 1,000 foods. Am J Clin Nutr 2009; 89(1): 97-105.

[54] Chapelot D, Marmonier C, Valensi P. Predicting more accurately the overall glucose response to a lunch meal by using the postprandial glucose peak. Metabolism 2007; 56(1): 37-43.

[55] Freeman JS. Insulin analog therapy: improving the match with physiologic insulin secretion. J Am Osteopath Assoc 2009; 109(1): 26-36.

[56] Bolli GB. Physiological insulin replacement in type 1 diabetes mellitus. Exp Clin Endocrinol Diabetes 2001; 109 Suppl 2: S317-332.

[57] Robertson C. Physiologic insulin replacement in type 2 diabetes: optimizing postprandial glucose control. Diabetes Educ 2006; 32: 423-432.

[58] Rosenstock J. Insulin therapy: optimizing control in type 1 and type 2 diabetes. Clin Cornerstone 2001; 4(2): 50-64.

[59] Bode BW. Use of rapid-acting insulin analogues in the treatment of patients with type 1 and type 2 diabetes mellitus: insulin pump therapy versus multiple daily injections. Clin Ther 2007; 29 Suppl D: S135-144.

[60] Weissberg-Benchell J, Antisdel-Lomaglio J, Seshadri R. Insulin pump therapy. A meta-analysis. Diabetes Care 2003; 26: 1079-1087.

[61] Pickup J, Mattock M, Kerry S. Glycaemic control with continuous subcutaneous insulin infusion compared with intensive insulin injections in patients with type 1 diabetes: meta-analysis of randomised controlled trial. Br Med J 2002; 324: 1-6.

[62] Jauch-Chara K, Schultes B. Sleep and the response to hypoglycaemia. Best Pract Res Clin Endocrinol Metab 2010; 24(5): 801-815.

[63] Valla V. Therapeutics of diabetes mellitus: focus on insulin analogues and insulin pumps. Exp Diabetes Res. 2010; 2010: 178372.

[64] Heise T, Pieber TR. Towards peakless, reproducible and long-acting insulins. An assessment of the basal analogues based on isoglycaemic clamp studies. Diabetes Obes Metab 2007; 9(5): 648-659.

[65] Monami M, Marchionni N, Mannucci E. Long-acting insulin analogues vs. NPH human insulin in type 1 diabetes. A meta-analysis. Diabetes Obes Metab 2009; 11(4): 372-378.

[66] Horvath K, Jeitler K, Berghold A, Ebrahim SH, Gratzer TW, Plank J, Kaiser T, Pieber TR, Siebenhofer A. Long-acting insulin analogues versus NPH insulin (human isophane insulin) for type 2 diabetes mellitus. Cochrane Database Syst Rev 2007; (2): CD005613.

[67] Monami M, Marchionni N, Mannucci E. Long-acting insulin analogues versus NPH human insulin in type 2 diabetes: a meta-analysis. Diabetes Res Clin Pract 2008; 81(2): 184-189.

[68] Bergental RM. Effective insulin therapy In: DeFronzo RA, Ferrannini E, Keen H, Zimmet P eds. 2004. International Textbook of Diabetes Mellitus, 3rd edition; John Wiley & Sons, Ldt., vol. 1: 995-1015.

[69] Guerci B, Sauvanet JP. Subcutaneous insulin: pharmacokinetic variability and glycemic variability. Diabetes Metab 2005; 31(4 Pt 2): 4S7-4S24.

[70] Rossetti P, Porcellati F, Fanelli CG, Perriello G, Torlone E, Bolli GB. Superiority of insulin analogues versus human insulin in the treatment of diabetes mellitus. Arch Physiol Biochem 2008; 114(1): 3-10.
[71] Evans M, Schumm-Draeger PM, Vora J, King AB. A review of modern insulin analogue pharmacokinetic and pharmacodynamic profiles in type 2 diabetes: improvements and limitations. Diabetes Obes Metab. 2011 published online as doi: 10.1111/j.1463-1326.2011.01395.x.
[72] Siebenhofer A, Plank J, Berghold A, Jeitler K, Horvath K, Narath M, Gfrerer R, Pieber TR. Short acting insulin analogues versus regular human insulin in patients with diabetes mellitus. Cochrane Database Syst Rev 2006; (2): CD003287.
[73] Brunelle BL, Llewelyn J, Anderson JH Jr, et al. Meta-analysis of the effect of insulin lispro on severe hypoglycemia in patients with type 1 diabetes. Diabetes Care 1998; 21:1726–1731.
[74] Siebenhofer A, Plank J, Berghold A, et al. Meta-analysis of short-acting insulin analogues in adult patients with type 1 diabetes: continuous subcutaneous insulin infusion versus injection therapy. Diabetologia 2004; 47: 1895–1905.
[75] Plank J, Siebenhofer A, Berghold A, et al. Systematic review and meta-analysis of short-acting insulin analogues in patients with diabetes mellitus. Arch Intern Med 2005; 165: 1337–1344.
[76] Singh SR, Ahmad F, Lal A, et al. Efficacy and safety of insulin analogues for the management of diabetes mellitus: a meta-analysis. CMAJ 2009; 180: 385–397.
[77] Siebenhofer A, Jeitler K, Berghold A, et al. Severe hypoglycaemia and glycaemic control in type 1 diabetes: meta-analysis of multiple daily insulin injections compared with continuous subcutaneous insulin infusion. Diabet Med 2009; 26:311–312.
[78] Heinemann L. Hypoglycemia and insulin analogues: is there a reduction in the incidence? J Diabetes Complications 1999; 13(2): 105-114.
[79] Kildegaard J, Christensen TF, Hejlesen OK. Sources of glycemic variability - what type of technology is needed? J Diabetes Sci Technol 2009; 3(4): 986-991.
[80] Chapman TM, Noble S, Goa KL. Insulin aspart: a review of its use in the management of type 1 and 2 diabetes mellitus. Drugs 2002; 62(13):1945-1981.
[81] Wilde MI, McTavish D. Insulin lispro: a review of its pharmacological properties and therapeutic use in the management of diabetes mellitus. Drugs 1997; 54(4): 597-614.
[82] Boland E, Monsod T, Delucia M, Brandt CA, Fernando S, Tamborlane WV. Limitations of conventional methods of self-monitoring of blood glucose: lessons learned from 3 days of continuous glucose sensing in pediatric patients with type 1 diabetes. Diabetes Care 2001; 24(11): 1858-1862.
[83] Heptulla RA, Allen HF, Gross TM, Reiter EO. Continuous glucose monitoring in children with type 1 diabetes: before and after insulin pump therapy. Pediatr Diabetes 2004; 5(1): 10-15.
[84] Monnier L, Colette C, Owens DR. Integrating glycaemic variability in the glycaemic disorders of type 2 diabetes: a move towards a unified glucose tetrad concept. Diabetes Metab Res Rev 2009; 25(5): 393-402.
[85] Gallwitz B. Implications of postprandial glucose and weight control in people with type 2 diabetes: understanding and implementing the International Diabetes Federation guidelines. Diabetes Care 2009; 32 Suppl 2: S322-325.

[86] Ramchandani N, Cantey-Kiser JM, Alter CA, Brink SJ, Yeager SD, Tamborlane WV, Chipkin SR. Self-reported factors that affect glycemic control in college students with type 1 diabetes. Diabetes Educ 2000; 26(4): 656-666.

[87] Heinemann L. Variability of insulin absorption and insulin action. Diabetes Technol Ther 2002; 4: 673-682.

[88] Pettis RJ, Hirsch L, Kapitza C, Nosek L, Hövelmann U, Kurth HJ, Sutter DE, Harvey NG, Heinemann L. Microneedle-based intradermal versus subcutaneous administration of regular human insulin or insulin lispro: pharmacokinetics and postprandial glycemic excursions in patients with type 1 diabetes. Diabetes Technol Ther 2011; 13(4): 443-450.

[89] Harvey AJ, Kaestner SA, Sutter DE, Harvey NG, Mikszta JA, Pettis RJ. Microneedle-based intradermal delivery enables rapid lymphatic uptake and distribution of protein drugs. Pharm Res. 2011; 28(1): 107-116.

[90] Pettis RJ, Ginsberg B, Hirsch L, Sutter D, Keith S, McVey E, Harvey NG, Hompesch M, Nosek L, Kapitza C, Heinemann L. Intradermal microneedle delivery of insulin lispro achieves faster insulin absorption and insulin action than subcutaneous injection. Diabetes Technol Ther 2011; 13(4): 435-442.

[91] Pettis RJ, Hirsch L, Kapitza C, Nosek L, Hövelmann U, Kurth HJ, Sutter DE, Harvey NG, Heinemann L. Microneedle-based intradermal versus subcutaneous administration of regular human insulin or insulin lispro: pharmacokinetics and postprandial glycemic excursions in patients with type 1 diabetes. Diabetes Technol Ther 2011; 13(4): 443-450.

[92] Bookbinder LH, Hofer A, Haller MF, Zepeda ML, Keller GA, Lim JE, Edgington TS, Shepard HM, Patton JS, Frost GI. A recombinant human enzyme for enhanced interstitial transport of therapeutics. J Control Release 2006; 114: 230–241.

[93] Pirrello RD, Ting Chen C, Thomas SH. Initial experiences with subcutaneous recombinant human hyaluronidase. J Palliat Med 2007; 10: 861–864.

[94] Muchmore DB, Vaughn DE. Review of the mechanism of action and clinical efficacy of recombinant human hyaluronidase coadministration with current prandial insulin formulations. J Diabetes Sci Technol 2010; 4(2): 419-428.

[95] Vaughn DE, Yocum RC, Muchmore DB, Sugarman BJ, Vick AM, Bilinsky IP, Frost GI. Accelerated pharmacokinetics and glucodynamics of prandial insulins injected with recombinant human hyaluronidase. Diabetes Technol Ther 2009; 11(6): 345-352.

[96] Steiner S, Hompesch M, Pohl R, Simms P, Flacke F, Mohr T, Pfützner A, Heinemann L. A novel insulin formulation with a more rapid onset of action. Diabetologia 2008; 51(9): 1602-1606.

[97] Hompesch M, McManus L, Pohl R, Simms P, Pfützner A, Bülow E, Flacke F, Heinemann L, Steiner SS. Intra-individual variability of the metabolic effect of a novel rapid-acting insulin (VIAject) in comparison to regular human insulin. J Diabetes Sci Technol 2008; 2(4): 568-571.

[98] Forst T, Pfützner A, Flacke F, Krasner A, Hohberg C, Tarakci E, Pichotta P, Forst S, Steiner S. Postprandial vascular effects of VIAject compared with insulin lispro and regular human insulin in patients with type 2 diabetes. Diabetes Care 2010; 33(1): 116-120.

[99] Raz I, Weiss R, Yegorchikov Y, Bitton G, Nagar R, Pesach B. Effect of a local heating device on insulin and glucose pharmacokinetic profiles in an open-label, randomized, two-period, one-way crossover study in patients with type 1 diabetes using continuous subcutaneous insulin infusion. Clin Ther. 2009; 31(5): 980-987.

[100] Sindelka G, Heinemann L, Berger M, Frenck W, Chantelau E. Effect of insulin concentration, subcutaneous fat thickness and skin temperature on subcutaneous insulin absorption in healthy subjects. Diabetologia 1994; 37(4): 377-380.

[101] Cengiz E, Tamborlane WV, Sherr J, Martin M, Steffen AT, Carria L, Weinzimer SA. Faster is better: investigating the effect of a novel warming device on the pharmacodynamics of rapid acting insulin in youth with type 1 diabetes (T1D) Pediatric Diabetes (2010) 11 (Suppl. 14): S99

[102] Cengiz E, Tamborlane WV, Sherr JL, Martin M, Carria L, Sikes KA, Urban AD, Bitton G, Weinzimer SA. Investigating the Effect of a Novel Warming Device on the Pharmacodynamics and Pharmacokinetics of RapidActing Insulin in Youth with Type 1 Diabetes. Journal of Diabetes Science and Technology 2010; 4(2): A23

[103] Freckmann G, Westhoff A, Pleus S, Jendrike N, Zschornack E, Haug C, Krinelke L. Clinical performance of the insulin infusion set InsuPatch that applies local heat to the infusion site. Diabetologia 2010; 53 (Suppl 1): S386.

[104] Richardson PC, Boss AH. Technosphere insulin technology. Diabetes Technol Ther 2007; 9 Suppl 1: S65-72.

[105] Neumiller JJ, Campbell RK, Wood LD. A review of inhaled technosphere insulin. Ann Pharmacother 2010; 44(7-8): 1231-1239.

[106] Steiner, S., Pfutzner, A., Wilson, B.R., Harzer, O., Heinemann, L., Rave, K. TechnosphereTM / Insulin - Proof of concept study with a new insulin formulation for pulmonary delivery. Exp Clin Endocrinol Diabetes 2002, 110: 17-21.

[107] Pfutzner, A., Mann, A.E., Steiner, S.S. TechnosphereTM/ Insulin - A new approach for effective delivery of human insulin via the pulmonary route. Diabetes Technol Ther 2002, 4: 589-594.

[108] Rave K, Potocka E, Heinemann L, Heise T, Boss AH, Marino M, Costello D, Chen R. Pharmacokinetics and linear exposure of AFRESA compared with the subcutaneous injection of regular human insulin. Diabetes Obes Metab 2009; 11(7): 715-720.

[109] Rave K, Heise T, Heinemann L, Boss AH. Inhaled Technosphere insulin in comparison to subcutaneous regular human insulin: time action profile and variability in subjects with type 2 diabetes. J Diabetes Sci Technol 2008; 2(2): 205-212.

[110] Rave K, Heise T, Pfützner A, Boss AH. Coverage of postprandial blood glucose excursions with inhaled technosphere insulin in comparison to subcutaneously injected regular human insulin in subjects with type 2 diabetes. Diabetes Care 2007; 30(9): 2307-2308

[111] Pfützner A, Forst T. Pulmonary insulin delivery by means of the Technosphere drug carrier mechanism. Expert Opin Drug Deliv 2005; 2(6): 1097-1106.

[112] Potocka E, Amin N, Cassidy J, Schwartz SL, Gray M, Richardson PC, Baughman RA. Insulin pharmacokinetics following dosing with Technosphere insulin in subjects with chronic obstructive pulmonary disease. Curr Med Res Opin 2010; 26(10): 2347-2353.

[113] Rosenstock J, Bergenstal R, Defronzo RA, Hirsch IB, Klonoff D, Boss AH, Kramer D, Petrucci R, Yu W, Levy B; 0008 Study Group. Efficacy and safety of Technosphere inhaled insulin compared with Technosphere powder placebo in insulin-naive type 2 diabetes suboptimally controlled with oral agents. Diabetes Care 2008; 31(11): 2177-2182.

[114] Tack CJ, Christov V, de Galan BE, Derwahl KM, Klausmann G, Pelikánová T, Perusicová J, Boss AH, Amin N, Kramer D, Petrucci R, Yu W; 005 Study Group. Randomized forced titration to different doses of technosphere insulin demonstrates reduction in postprandial glucose excursions and hemoglobin A1c in patients with type 2 diabetes. J Diabetes Sci Technol 2008; 2(1): 47-57.

[115] Rosenstock J, Lorber DL, Gnudi L, Howard CP, Bilheimer DW, Chang PC, Petrucci RE, Boss AH, Richardson PC. Prandial inhaled insulin plus basal insulin glargine versus twice daily biaspart insulin for type 2 diabetes: a multicentre randomised trial. Lancet 2010; 375(9733): 2244-2253.

[116] Peyrot M, Rubin RR. Effect of technosphere inhaled insulin on quality of life and treatment satisfaction. Diabetes Technol Ther 2010; 12(1): 49-55.

[117] Bernstein G. Delivery of insulin to the buccal mucosa utilizing the RapidMist system. Expert Opin Drug Deliv 2008; 5(9): 1047-1055.

[118] Heinemann L, Jacques Y. Oral insulin and buccal insulin: a critical reappraisal. J Diabetes Sci Technol 2009;3(3): 568-584.

[119] Cernea S, Kidron M, Wohlgelernter J, Raz I. Dose-response relationship of an oral insulin spray in six patients with type 1 diabetes: a single-center, randomized, single-blind, 5-way crossover study. Clin Ther 2005; 27(10): 1562-1570.

[120] Cernea S, Kidron M, Wohlgelernter J, Modi P, Raz I. Dose-response relationship of oral insulin spray in healthy subjects. Diabetes Care 2005; 28(6): 1353-1357.

[121] Cernea S, Kidron M, Wohlgelernter J, Modi P, Raz I. Comparison of pharmacokinetic and pharmacodynamic properties of single-dose oral insulin spray and subcutaneous insulin injection in healthy subjects using the euglycemic clamp technique. Clin Ther 2004; 26(12): 2084-2091.

[122] Pozzilli P, Manfrini S, Costanza F et al. Biokinetics of buccal spray insulin in patients with type 1 diabetes. Metabolism 2005; 54: 930–934.

[123] Guevara-Aguirre J, Guevara M, Saavedra J, Mihic M, Modi P. Oral spray insulin in treatment of type 2 diabetes: a comparison of efficacy of the oral spray insulin (Oralin) with subcutaneous (SC) insulin injection, a proof of concept study. Diabetes Metab Res Rev 2004; 20: 472–478.

[124] Guevara-Aguirre J, Guevara M, Saavedra J, Mihic M, Modi P. Beneficial effects of addition of oral spray insulin (Oralin) on insulin secretion and metabolic control in subjects with type 2 diabetes mellitus suboptimally controlled on oral hypoglycemic agents. Diabetes Technol Ther 2004; 6: 1–8.

10

Prevention of Hospital Hypoglycemia by Algorithm Design: A Programming Pathway for Electronic Order Entry

Susan S. Braithwaite[1], Lisa Clark[1], Lydia Dacenko-Grawe[1], Radha Devi[1], Josefina Diaz[2], Mehran Javadi[1] and Harley Salinas[1]

[1]*University of Illinois-Chicago; Saint Francis Hospital, Resurrection Health Care*

[2]*University of Illinois-Chicago; Saint Joseph Hospital, Resurrection Health Care*

United States of America

1. Introduction

Caregivers treating hospitalized patients are confronted with the necessity both to control hyperglycemia and also to avoid iatrogenic hypoglycemia. Despite controversy about optimal glycemic targets, a large body of evidence associates uncontrolled hyperglycemia with adverse outcomes, both in the intensive care unit and also on general hospital wards (American Diabetes Association, 2011; Moghissi et al., 2009). On general wards, glycemic control during use of scheduled subcutaneous insulin is superior to that seen during use of sliding scale regimens (Baldwin et al., 2005; Umpierrez et al., 2007). When scheduled insulin was compared to sliding scale treatment among general surgical patients, glycemic control was improved (mean blood glucose 145 ± 32 mg/dL vs. 172 ± 47 mg/dL, $p < 0.01$), and a composite outcome of complications was reduced from 24.3 to 8.6%with odds ratio 3.39 (95% CI 1.50-7.65), $p = 0.003$ (Umpierrez et al., 2011). Nevertheless, the problem of hypoglycemia is a barrier to successful control of hospital hyperglycemia. Among 1718 adult patients admitted at academic medical centers and having hyperglycemia or receiving insulin therapy, hypoglycemia occurred on 2.8% of all hospital days (Boord et al., 2009). Predisposing factors and adverse outcomes associated with hypoglycemia have been examined in observational studies and in clinical trials studying the effect of glycemic control upon nonglycemic outcomes (Bagshaw et al., 2009; Fischer et al., 1986; Finfer et al., 2009; Kagansky et al., 2003; Krinsley et al., 2007; Maynard et al., 2008; Smith et al., 2005; Stagnaro-Green et al., 1995; Turchin et al., 2009; Van den Berghe et al., 2006; Varghese et al., 2007; Vriesendorp et al., 2006; Wexler et al., 2007). Mortality of patients having myocardial infarction is higher at the lowest as well as the highest ranges glucose, such that the relationship between mortality and glucose is described by a J-shaped curve (Kosiborod et al., 2008). Outcomes of hospitalized patients that have been linked to hypoglycemia include increased ICU mortality or hospital mortality rates, adverse events such as seizures, and increased length of stay. In the intensive care unit and on general wards, associated factors identified among patients having hypoglycemia include use of bicarbonate-based substitution fluid during continuous venovenous hemofiltration, need for inotropic support, greater severity of illness, co-administration of octreotide with insulin, comorbidities including chronic kidney disease, sepsis, advanced age, history of diabetes or severe diabetes, and history of prior episodes of hypoglycemia. Of special importance, because of the implication for prevention, is the frequency with which the literature on hospital hypoglycemia describes interruption of normal feedings attributable to hospital routine, or episodes of reduced enteral intake without adjustment of insulin therapy, as a factors predisposing to hypoglycemia.

Mechanisms of potential harm from hypoglycemia are partially understood, but the causal relationships between hypoglycemia or iatrogenic hypoglycemia and outcomes is unclear. Concerning the association of hypoglycemia with adverse outcomes, it remains a tenable explanation at least in part that severity of illness may predispose both to adverse outcomes and to hypoglycemia (Kosiborod et al., 2009; van den Berghe et al., 2006). Proof of permanent injury ascribed to a hypoglycemic episode in the hospital setting sometimes is available, but the case ascertainment rate is low. Although proof of direct harm from identifiable hypoglycemic events within large studies may be not discerned by statistical analysis, yet the harm is uniquely damaging to the individual suffering the hypoglycemic event, so that the reporting of isolated cases remains important (Bhatia et al., 2006; Scalea et al., 2007). Life-changing morbidity or mortality may result from a severe hypoglycemic reaction. It is also suspected that some harms may result from hypoglycemia that are not directly traceable to immediate consequences of a specific hypoglycemic event. Since hospital patients will not be randomized to hypoglycemia or non-hypoglycemia, our understanding of the causes and clinical impact of hypoglycemia will be observational, resulting from analyses of hypoglycemia as a secondary outcome, within trials of therapeutic strategies or interventions aiming at targets other than hypoglycemia, or resulting from analysis of hypoglycemia within cohort studies. For the present, the association of hypoglycemia with adverse outcomes justifies development of strategies for prevention of hypoglycemia in the hospital.

The goal of this chapter is to describe attributes of a programming pathway for computerized order entry that may incorporate the best elements of paper protocols for subcutaneous insulin and that may help prevent hospital hypoglycemia. In designing treatment for the hyperglycemic patient, it is necessary to anticipate events that create risk for hypoglycemia and to meet those events with appropriate revisions of nutritional therapy and scheduled insulin. When insulin orders are in place but patient risk for hypoglycemia is predicted to increase, the components of insulin therapy that might be withheld or reduced may differ, depending upon co-morbidities, anticipated disruption of carbohydrate exposure, alteration of other medical therapies, and classification of diabetes. By juxtaposing elements of care within a checklist of orders, paper protocols present reminders to the prescriber about strategies for hypoglycemia prevention. We believe the main opportunity for improvement within computerized order entry systems is the need to present several different packages of orders at the user interface that match differing patterns of carbohydrate exposure. For each pattern of carbohydrate exposure, the package must include default and acceptable alternative orders that encompass monitoring of blood glucose, scheduled and correction-dose insulin orders, and menus of additional directions associated with the insulin orders.

2. Algorithms for glycemic management in the hospital

Any algorithm must identify a target blood glucose or a target range and define a safe and effective method for attainment and homeostatic maintenance of target range control. Provisions must be in place regardless of algorithm design to make anticipatory adjustments to prevent hypoglycemia in case of sudden change of any of the usual determinants of insulin requirement, such as carbohydrate exposure or concomitant medications. After making brief reference to an algorithmic method for protection against hypoglycemia during intravenous insulin infusion, the literature on electronic order entry of glycemic management plans is briefly referenced, and idealized examples of programmable branching pathways for patients who are eating and not eating will be presented.

2.1 Intravenous insulin infusion

Computerization of intravenous insulin algorithms may be successfully accomplished either through a free standing electronic decision support system or as part of a hospital computer system (Dortch et al, 2008; Hermayer et al. 2007; Junega et al, 2007). The method of computerized order entry that we will use is under construction and will not be presented here, except to say that the algorithms are related to those previously published (Bellam and Braithwaite, 2010; Devi at al, in press 2011). The choice of intravenous insulin protocol depends upon the population treated. The protocols will be designed according to a mathematical rule having population-specific parameters. The protocols are related to column-based tabular protocols in which each column of the table is associated with an assumed maintenance rate of insulin infusion that is thought to be the rate necessary to maintain target range control. Each row of the table represents a range of blood glucose values. The assumed maintenance rate (column assignment) is determined with knowledge of the previous assumed maintenance rate (column assignment) together with the rate of change of blood glucose, at the previous insulin infusion rate. The next insulin infusion rate, at each nursing interaction, depends upon the blood glucose (the row) and the reassigned maintenance rate (column re-assignment, if any). The conservative protocol differs from the standard critical care protocol for intravenous insulin infusion not in the target range blood glucose values, but in the column change rules that result in changing from a lower to a higher maintenance rate (column), or from a higher to a lower assumed maintenance rate (column). That is to say, by analogy with a paper protocol, the column change rules based on rate-of-change of glucose are more conservative under the conservative protocol. We believe that two design features of the intravenous insulin infusion protocols will be shown to be protective against hypoglycemia, namely (1) the column change rules based on rate of change of blood glucose and (2) the near-sigmoidal relationship, at given maintenance rate (within-column), between the insulin infusion rate and the blood glucose.
The protocols for diabetic ketoacidosis and hyperglycemic hyperosmolar state each differ from each other and from the critical care protocols for intravenous insulin infusion by having different column change rules and additionally different target ranges for blood glucose. The target range for blood glucose in treatment of diabetic ketoacidosis or hyperglycemia hyperosmolar coma is higher than for other patients likely to be treated with intravenous insulin infusion. An initially fixed-dose weight-based method for assigning insulin infusion rate during the initial hours of treatment is advocated in the consensus statement of the American Diabetes Association for use during the first several hours of treatment of DKA (Kitabchi et al., 2009). In contrast, a dynamic rule to assign the insulin

infusion rate during treatment of hyperglycemic crisis is employed at our institutions (Devi et al., 2011). The deactivation time for intravenous insulin infusion may be as long as 90 minutes (Mudaliar et al., 2008). A rationale for a dynamic insulin infusion rate in the early hours of treatment for hyperglycemic emergency is that under conventional management late hypoglycemia sometimes complicates the treatment course.

2.2 Algorithms for subcutaneous insulin

Many protocols for hospital care were developed in the era of handwritten order entry. Order sets were developed that served as a checklist to prevent omissions of elements of care. For example, a reminder to have a standing "prn" order for intravenous dextrose under selected conditions or to order an A1C may be part of the order set. Order sets help integrate the components of care with each other. Timing of testing, insulin, and meals may be coordinated by justaposition of related orders on a paper order set. A lynchpin of successful order writing is the coordination of the patterns of glucose monitoring and insulin administration with carbohydrate exposure (Bellam and Braithwaite, 2010; Braithwaite et al., 2007; Campbell et al., 2004; Thompson et al., 2005). If an order set is well designed, by checking boxes and entering numbers the prescriber creates orders that are familiar to and readily interpreted by pharmacy and nursing staff. Lengthy narrative is reduced. Standardization of order entry protects patient safety. A well designed order set facilitates individualization of patient care. Guidelines may be appended to or embedded within order sets, together with references to supportive medical literature (Donaldson et al. 2006; Hermayer et al, 2009; Lee et al. 2008; Maynard et al., 2009; Schnipper et al., 2010; Trujillo et al., 2008; Wexler et al., 2010). Protocols executed through order sets were thought to reduce medical errors, improve safety, and increase adherence to those guidelines that were supported by medical evidence.

As electronic order entry began to gain widespread use, a body of descriptive studies developed concerning the use of structured order sets for electronic order entry for subcutaneous insulin therapy in the hospital. Hermeyer and colleagues described a comprehensive program, including a web-based calculator for the intravenous insulin protocol (Hermeyer et al., 2009). Maynard and colleagues, in a published study of computerized order entry with paper guidelines used on the side, defined time periods 1, 2 and 3 (TP1, TP2, and TP3) during rolling out of the program. Paper statements of guidelines adjunctive to computerized order entry were developed (Lee et al., 2008). The relative risk (RR) of an uncontrolled patient-stay was reduced from baseline to 0.91 (CI 0.85-0.96) in TP2, and to 0.84 (CI 0.77-0.89) in TP3, with more marked effects in the secondary analysis limited to patients with at least 8 point-of-care glucose values (Maynard et al., 2009). The percent of patient-days with hypoglycemia was 3.8%, 2.9%, and 2.6% in the 3 time periods, representing a RR for hypoglycemic day in TP3:TP1 of 0.68 (CI 0.59-0.78). Similar reductions were seen in risk for hypoglycemic patient-stays.

Evidence from cluster randomized studies supports the use of structured order sets to improve glycemic outcomes. Schnipper and colleagues in several stages developed a computerized version of their order entry system for glycemic control (Schnipper et al., 2009; Schnipper et al., 2010; Trujillo et al., 2008). In a cluster randomized design of 179 patients at a single site, two of the four medical services were chosen randomly to receive the intervention using a computerized order set built into the proprietary computer at Brigham and Women's Hospital. The mean percent of glucose readings between 60-180 was

75% in the intervention group and 71% in the usual care group [adjusted RR 1.36 (1.02-1.80)]. With the intervention, there were a lower patient-day weighted mean glucose (148 vs 158, p = 0.04); less use of sliding scale (25% vs 58%, p = 0.01); and no difference in hypoglycemia < 40 mg/dL (0.5% vs 0.3%, p = 0.58). Wexler and colleagues at a single site randomized medical teams to availability of an electronic insulin order template versus usual insulin ordering. Intervention group patients (n=65) had mean glucose of 195 +/- 66 mg/dl. Control group patients (n=63) had mean glucose of 224 +/- 57 mg/dl (P=0.004). In the intervention group, there was no increase in hypoglycemia (Wexler et al., 2010).

With electronic order entry, there is a risk that some of the integration between the components of care might be lost that had been achievable with paper order sets. Under some electronic systems, juxtaposition of related orders is lost. Users might have to navigate between screens to complete a package of orders relating to diabetes encompassing such necessities as a nutrition plan, point-of-care tests, insulin doses, and a treatment plan for hypoglycemia. A plan for continuous enteral tube feedings might be entered on one screen, followed by insulin orders on another screen, and finally orders for point-of-care glucose monitoring and call parameters on a third screen. Orders that are preselected as the likeliest choice, based on absolute rate of utilization, could be programmed as defaults but might be misapplied to subgroups through user failure to deselect and replace the order for the patient at hand. As an example, if the choice "ACHS" appears at the top of a list of possible orders for glucose monitoring as the default (ante cibum and hora somni, before meals and at bedtime), then an order for ACHS timing could be accepted by default, rather than timing more appropriate to the carbohydrate exposure actually planned for a patient who might receive continuous enteral tube feedings.

3. Programming pathway for glycemic management in the hospital

In the United States, in coming years hospitals will strive to comply with "meaningful use" regulations for electronic health records, described in the Health Information Technology for Economic and Clinical Health Act (Blumenthal & Tavenner, 2010). Electronic order entry will gradually replace handwriting of orders. Some systems will sharply restrict the use of free-text entries, creating necessity for a system that will link orders to preprogrammed comments that may be selected by the user. A template similar to that of electronic order entry might be used to facilitate communication among caregivers at the time of patient transfers and discharge. The remainder of this chapter will describe the design of an idealized proposal for a programming pathway for electronic order entry for glycemic management of hospitalized patients.

Within the figures showing the programming pathway, orders that are members of a category or subcategory have the same level of indentation. Pre-assignment of a default choice within-category sometimes is justified either based on frequency of use or medical indications. The user may select or deselect an order by clicking on a button associated with an order at the user interface. In some cases, selection by a provider of one order results in de-selection of another order within the same subcategory or category. In other cases, choices within-category or within sub-category are not mutually exclusive; selection of one order does not result in de-selection of another order (Figure 1). It is envisioned that the user will move through a sequence of those screens within the programming pathway that are determined by having made an early commitment to one branch of the algorithm. When the provider is satisfied that no modifications are required, the provider enters an electronic signature.

SYMBOLS FOR PROGRAMMING

● default choice,
within-category or within a subcategory populated by mutually exclusive choices.

○ alternative, among mutually exclusive choices,
within-category or within a subcategory populated by mutually exclusive choices.

■ default option for selection, not exclusive of other choices,
within-category or within a subcategory populated by options for selection.
SIDE MENU's associated with the order are displayed routinely
unless the order is de-selected, in which case the SIDE MENU vanishes.

□ option for selection,
within-category or within a subcategory populated by options for selection,
none exclusive of other choices.
DROP DOWN MENU's associated with the order are not displayed
until the order is selected.

Fig. 1. Instructions to programmer. Symbols signify the function of buttons at the user interface and define the structure of the program.

3.1 Programming pathway as checklist

Just as structured paper order sets for subcutaneous insulin therapy may protect the patient from omissions of needed elements of care by presenting a checklist, similarly a checklist of reminders for glycemic management may appear within a branching programming pathway. For example, the main trunk of the branching pathway may call for elements of care that are considered to be potentially universally appropriate, such as a standing "prn" order for concentrated intravenous dextrose for treatment of hypoglycemia, a nutrition consult, or an A1C (Figure 2). The programming pathway that we will present goes on to branch into 8 different treatment plans, each having preventive measures related to hypoglycemia that are specific to the components of the treatment plan, embedded as checklist options for selection, such as “reduce” orders for basal insulin for type 2 diabetes or “hold” parameters for prandial insulin (Figure 3).

3.2 Individualization facilitated under the programming pathway

It is necessary to specify precautions against hypoglycemia, but manual entry can be burdensome. Under the branches of the pathway, measures for hypoglycemia prevention could take different forms depending upon the carbohydrate exposure of the patient, including but not limited to the scheduling the monitoring of blood glucose, assignment of call parameters at alert levels of glucose, pattern of insulin administration, or use of the classification of hyperglycemia or diabetes to determine “hold” parameters for specific components of insulin therapy. We believe the ordering of these protective additional directions is more likely to occur when a complete menu of options is presented to the prescriber than when reliance is placed upon provider initiative and recall. To a large extent, manual entry of such safety provisions can be replaced by checking boxes and entering numbers. The programming pathway accommodates the spectrum of reasonable provider treatment preferences. By offering a menu of treatment alternatives and additional directions to the insulin orders, the programming pathway facilitates individualization of care for each patient.

GLYCEMIC MANAGEMENT ORDER SETS
(Opening Screen)

INSTRUCTIONS TO PRESCRIBER:
Orders for diet, maintenance fluids, enteral feedings, and TPN should be placed before proceeding with glycemic management orders.
No orders in this pathway can be finalized if the ***Hypoglycemia*** orders shown immediately below are deselected.

Hypoglycemia

■ Activate hospital hypoglycemia protocol

■ 25 mL of 50 % dextrose in water IV
prn glucose < 80 mg/dL per nursing hypoglycemia protocol
if patient is NPO, intubated or unable to take oral fluids/food
(route IV, order entered in association with POC blood glucose test order)

Requests for Consultations

☐ Nutrition consultation

☐ Endocrine consultation

Diagnostic Tests

☐ A1C

(Continued)

Fig. 2. Opening screen.

3.3 Intravenous insulin algorithm selection under the pathway

The programming pathway specifies options for four different intravenous insulin infusion protocols. A full discussion of these pathways is beyond the scope of the present discussion. For critical care patients requiring an intravenous insulin infusion, to help the user decide whether to order the conservative critical care intravenous insulin infusion protocol or the standard one, the user may find a link to a drop-down guideline for indications for the conservative IV insulin protocol. This states that the conservative IV insulin protocol will be appropriate for patients with renal failure, malnutrition, hepatic failure, sepsis, severe congestive heart failure, adrenal insufficiency, and other conditions that the caregiver judges to create high-risk for hypoglycemia. The conservative protocol also is the protocol to which the prescriber might default, in case a patient already has demonstrated hypoglycemia while on the standard protocol but still requires intravenous insulin infusion therapy (Figure 3).

An American Diabetes Association consensus statement provides a summary of diagnostic criteria for diabetic ketoacidosis or hyperosmolar hyperglycemic state (Kitabchi et al., 2009). The criteria for each can be summarized in a link to a drop-down guideline for diagnosis, accessed from the opening menu (Figure 3). Classification as diabetic ketoacidosis (DKA) is suggested by plasma glucose > 250 mg/dL, arterial pH < 7.3, bicarbonate < 15, anion gap > 12 meq/L, and moderate ketonuria or ketonemia. Classification as hyperglycemic hyperosmolar state (HHS) is suggested by plasma glucose > 600 mg/dl, serum osmolality > 320 mosm/L, arterial pH > 7.3, bicarbonate > 15 meq/L, and minimal ketonuria and ketonemia.

3.4 Subcutaneous insulin algorithm selection under the pathway

For patients who will receive subcutaneous insulin, once the pattern of carbohydrate exposure is determined, then the prescriber can select the appropriate branch of the pathway (Figure 3). Selection of a single branch from the list will launch an appropriate submenu, dependent upon carbohydrate exposure, for the schedule of blood glucose monitoring and the selection and timing of components of insulin administration. One branch of the programming pathway presently under construction will provide for a diabetes hospital patient self-management program. Models for patient self-management in the hospital have been described (Braithwaite et al., 2007; Bailon et al., 2009). The focus of this chapter is on orders for subcutaneous insulin therapy for patients who are not candidates for hospital self-management.

GLYCEMIC MANAGEMENT ORDER SETS
(Opening Screen, Continued)

Choose One Branch of the Pathway for Orders Associated with Insulin Therapy

- ○ GLYCEMIC MANAGEMENT AND SUBCUTANEOUS INSULIN FOR PATIENTS WHO ARE EATING
- ○ GLYCEMIC MANAGEMENT AND SUBCUTANEOUS INSULIN FOR PATIENTS WHO ARE NOT EATING, INCLUDING PATIENTS RECEIVING CONTINUOUS ENTERAL FEEDINGS, CONTINUOUS DEXTROSE-CONTAINING MAINTENANCE FLUIDS, OR NO CARBOHYDRATE EXPOSURE
- ○ GLYCEMIC MANAGEMENT AND SUBCUTANEOUS INSULIN FOR PATIENTS WITH OVERNIGHT ENTERAL FEEDINGS AND DAYTIME MEALS
- ○ CRITICAL CARE INTRAVENOUS INSULIN INFUSION, NON-DKA, NONPREGNANT ADULT
- ○ CONSERVATIVE CRITICAL CARE INTRAVENOUS INSULIN INFUSION, NON-DKA, NONPREGNANT ADULT
  (link to drop-down guideline for indications for conservative IV insulin protocol appears here)
- ○ INTRAVENOUS INSULIN INFUSION PROTOCOL FOR HYPERGLYCEMIC CRISES, NONPREGNANT ADULT, DIABETIC KETOACIDOSIS
  (link to drop-down guideline for diagnosis appears here)
- ○ INTRAVENOUS INSULIN INFUSION PROTOCOL FOR HYPERGLYCEMIC CRISES, NONPREGNANT ADULT, HYPEROSMOLAR HYPERGLYCEMIC STATE
  (link to drop-down guideline for diagnosis appears here)
- ○ DIABETES HOSPITAL PATIENT SELF MANAGEMENT

(Go to First Screen within Selected Branch of the Pathway)

Fig. 3. Selection of branch of the pathway.

3.5 Subcutaneous insulin dose titration after pathway initiation

A method for establishing starting doses of insulin is described in sections that will follow. An associated guideline might state that rewriting of the doses of scheduled insulin should be considered daily. Here, a guideline for revision of scheduled insulin is presented that is appropriate to each subcutaneous pathway.

- review comorbidities and medications affecting insulin requirement and carbohydrate exposure or omission.
- review the medication administration record for confirmation of insulin dosing over the preceding 24 hr.
- add the total amount of scheduled and correction dose insulin delivered in the previous 24 hr to determine total daily dose of insulin actually delivered.
- *if all blood glucose readings were > 180 mg/dL, add 10%* to the total daily dose actually delivered in the previous 24 hr to determine the new total daily dose of scheduled insulin.
- *if any blood glucose was < 80 mg/dL, subtract 20%* from the total daily dose actually delivered in the previous 24 hr to determine the new total daily dose of scheduled insulin.

The new dose of scheduled insulin is reapportioned between the components of scheduled therapy. Once the treatment pattern has been entered, changing of dose or correction dose scale can be accomplished outside of the programming pathway. If there are no further specifications, any standing "additional directions" concerning scheduled insulin may be carried forward.

Therapeutic inertia in changing established insulin regimens is a recognized problem in the care of hospitalized patients. In a study of 52 hospitalized patients treated with 50% dextrose for an episode of hypoglycemia, it was found that subsequent to withholding of insulin at the time of the hypoglycemia, 31% of the patients received no other change in treatment (Garg et al., 2004). The guideline above would give caregivers direction on trouble-shooting of the causes of hypoglycemia and making appropriate revisions of treatment.

3.6 Integration of the components of care under the pathway during placement of orders for subcutaneous insulin

A decision support system helps the prescriber to recognize the components of care under the pattern of treatment that is ordered and the relationship between these components. During widespread adoption of computerization of order entry, a distinct computer order is required separately for feedings, intravenous dextrose, glucose monitoring, each component of insulin therapy, treatment of hypoglycemia, and call parameters. The relationship of these elements of care to each other and their timing must be coordinated. The integration of the components of care, achieved by many paper protocols and order sets, must be preserved. The prescriber must be able to accomplish the goals of glycemic control and hypoglycemia prevention without navigation through multiple screens of an electronic order entry system. Whether patients are eating or not, interruption of carbohydrate exposure is a well verified risk factor for hospital hypoglycemia. The risk arises from hospital routine that interrupts feedings or patient factors that result in poor oral intake (Fischer et al., 1986). Restrictions on free-text entries will necessitate preprogramming of additional directions. In each branch of the pathway that will be shown, in case of reduction of carbohydrate exposure, the insulin orders may be accompanied by standardized statements concerning hypoglycemia

prevention. Examples include additional directions to "hold" prandial insulin in case of meal omission, "hold" prandial insulin on the mornings of dialysis, or "reduce" insulin in case of poor oral intake.
The order entry system should associate the pattern of blood glucose monitoring, the components of insulin administration together with additional directions, the "call" parameters, and the orders for "prn" oral or intravenous carbohydrate. If an order entry system is well designed, the user will encounter a comprehensive electronic menu for prescribing a glycemic management plan, having internally coordinated components, accessible through a single branch of the pathway of order entry. Under each of the first three branches of the pathway, nursing instructions include an assessment of patient needs, including early attention to patient education and eventual discharge planning.

3.6.1 Subcutaneous Insulin for patients who are eating

Basal-prandial-correction therapy is a prescribing pattern for insulin, described in previous reviews, that is especially well suited to insulin treatment of the hospitalized patient who is eating (Hirsch, 2005; Clement et al., 2004). The orders for monitoring and insulin are written in association with a meal plan, usually a consistent carbohydrate diet. Other specifications to the diet are preserved that may be required for care of comorbidities. The nursing orders for monitoring of blood glucose provide options for testing postprandially but recommend restriction of scheduled postprandial testing to conditions in which retrospective review of the results might be used to revise scheduled therapy for special populations or conditions, such as pregnancy or cystic fibrosis (Figure 4). Most patients require either testing with meals; with meals and at bedtime; or with meals, at bedtime, and midsleep.
Prandial insulin coverage is the treatment given to cover meals, and basal insulin is the treatment necessary to prevent unchecked gluconeogenesis and ketogenesis, required whether or not nutrition is provided. The long-acting insulin analogs glargine and detemir are designed to provide basal coverage. Glargine may be given once daily for most patients, and detemir may be given once or twice daily. The rapid-acting insulin analogs lispro, aspart and glulisine are designed to provide prandial coverage and to provide rapid correction of hyperglycemia. Biphasic or premixed insulin therapy provides both basal and prandial insulin coverage. In the hospital, since there is a risk of interruption of meals, it is desirable to use an insulin treatment plan under which the prandial component of treatment can be interrupted without compromise to the basal insulin coverage. For patients eating discrete meals, biphasic insulin therapy in the hospital generally is replaced by treatment separately with basal coverage and prandial coverage. For correction of hyperglycemia, the rapid-acting insulin analogs are given with meals, sometimes for coverage of snacks, and sometimes at bedtime or midsleep.
Some patients having type 2 diabetes who normally require insulin may experience reduction of insulin resistance during fasting and may produce endogenous insulin sufficient that under conditions of reduced oral intake the requirements for exogenous insulin may decline. Others, who normally are insulin independent, may experience stress-related insulin resistance in the hospital sufficient to produce a requirement for exogenous insulin treatment. Dose initiation guidelines for insulin-requiring patients whose dose requirements are not known might be stated conservatively as follows (with reapportionment as indicated for special conditions, as described below):

- daily basal requirement 0.15 units/kg for type 2 diabetes or for stress hyperglycemia, and 0.25 units/kg for type 1 diabetes

- daily prandial requirement 0.15 units/kg for type 2 diabetes or for stress hyperglycemia, and 0.25 units/kg for type 1 diabetes, apportioned between three meals.

The total daily dose of scheduled insulin is apportioned between the scheduled basal and prandial insulin. A guideline concerning the initial percentage distribution of total daily dose of scheduled insulin between the components of therapy may suggest 50% basal and 50% prandial for most patients, but reapportionment for special conditions:

- 50% basal insulin, 50%prandial insulin for many patients
- > 50% basal insulin, < 50%prandial insulin during immediate recovery following heart surgery
- 33% basal insulin , 67%prandial insulin for renal or hepatic failure, malnutrition, or corticosteroid therapy

GLYCEMIC MANAGEMENT AND SUBCUTANEOUS INSULIN FOR PATIENTS WHO ARE EATING

Physician Orders for Nursing Staff

■ Point-of-care blood (POC) blood glucose monitoring with frequency

SIDE MENU

(Prescriber guideline: the post cibum (postprandial, PC) options may be appropriate for pregnant patients, patients having cystic fibrosis, and some other patients in special situations, but are not required for general management of diabetes or hyperglycemia.)

Frequency of Monitoring

● WMEALS, HS (default)	[0800, 1200, 1700 before meals; 2200]
○ WMEALS, HS, 0200	[0800, 1200, 1700 before meals; 2200, 0200]
○ ONCE DAILY	[0800 before breakfast]
○ TWICE DAILY	[0800 before breakfast, 1800]
○ WMEALS	[0800, 1200, 1700 before meals]
○ 2HR PC	
○ 0800 & 2HR PC	
○ WMEALS & 2HR PC	[0800, 1200, 1700 before meals, and 2HR PC]
○ WMEALS & 2HR PC	[0800, 1200, 1700 before meals, 2HR PC, & HS; 7x/d)
○ WMEALS & 2HR PC, 0200	[0800, 1200, 1700 before meals, 2HR PC, HS, & 0200; 8x/d]

■ Call house officer for point-of-care glucose

SIDE MENU

Call Parameters, High Glucose

● > 350 mg/dL (default)
○ > _____ mg/dL

■ Call house officer for point-of-care glucose

SIDE MENU

Call Parameters, Low Glucose

● < 70 mg/dL (default)
○ < _____ mg/dL

■ Assess patient needs in relation to discharge

□ Teach patient survival skills (capillary glucose monitoring, insulin injection if used, hypoglycemia)

(Go to Next Screen within Pathway)

Fig. 4. Nursing orders for patients who are eating. WMEALS = with meals. WMEALS, HS = with meals and at bedtime. Times of meals may differ according to institutional practices.

Under a treatment plan using basal-prandial-correction dose therapy, typically basal insulin is given once daily as long-acting insulin analog. Before development of insulin analogs, NPH insulin had been used to provide basal coverage, and regular insulin to provide prandial coverage and correction of hyperglycemia. In general, during the treatment of type 2 diabetes, in comparison with NPH-based basal insulin regimens there is less hypoglycemia with use of long-acting insulin analog therapy for basal coverage (Rosenstock et al., 2005; Hermansen et al., 2006). However, some patients prefer to be treated with NPH. Morning dosing with NPH insulin may provide both basal and partial prandial insulin coverage. In the ambulatory setting, some patients use NPH insulin to achieve pattern correction; for example, an evening dose of NPH insulin may cover the dawn phenomenon, correcting a pattern of morning hyperglycemia by meeting predawn insulin resistance with increased insulin levels. Under the branch of the pathway for patients who are eating, prescribers are given the alternatives of using a long-acting insulin analog or NPH for basal insulin coverage (Figure 5).

Not uncommonly, in order to correct fasting hyperglycemia, doses of intermediate or long acting insulin may have been increased during normal dietary intake to a dose higher than true basal requirements. If the basal insulin dose is unchanged during NPO status (nihil per os, nothing by mouth), patients having type 2 diabetes may experience hypoglycemia (Olson et al., 2009). It is important that the programming pathway should present options for basal insulin reduction or interruption in case of planned NPO status. On the other hand, if the basal insulin dose is established correctly in type 1 diabetes, the dose during NPO status usually may be preserved (Mucha et al., 2004). Omission of basal insulin during NPO status in type 1 diabetes may result in ketoacidosis. Therefore, the programming pathway provides options for prescribers to reduce basal insulin in type 2 diabetes but to continue basal insulin in type 1 diabetes, in anticipation of NPO status. A prescriber guideline embedded in the order entry screen warns against interruption of basal insulin for type 1 diabetes (Figure 5).

In the treatment of type 2 diabetes, rapid-acting analogs for prandial coverage may produce less hypoglycemia than regular insulin (Anderson et al., 1997; Raymann et al, 2006; Velussi at al. 2002). The provider may see the need to provide differing doses of prandial insulin at different times of day; the programming pathway permits flexibility in the prescribing of prandial doses, allowing either a fixed dose (best ordered usually with a consistent carbohydrate diet) or a variable dose (Figure 6). This programming pathway is designed for use on the assumption that not all nursing staff are trained on recognition of carbohydrate content of meals; therefore, insulin-to-carbohydrate ratios are not prescribed under the branch of the pathway for subcutaneous insulin for patients who are eating. A modification of the pathway might be used by hospitals that routinely train all nurses on advanced carbohydrate counting so that the provider might order and nurses might use an insulin to carbohydrate ratio to assign prandial insulin doses according to what is on the patient's tray. Patients using the skills of advanced carbohydrate counting and already skilled in self management may best be treated under a different branch of the pathway, for diabetes hospital patient self management.

Several additional directions may be selected in conjunction with orders for prandial use of rapid-acting insulin analog that provide protection against hypoglycemia. Most obviously, the direction "HOLD IF NPO" is intended to reduce the risk of administration of prandial insulin at times when meals might be omitted. The order to hold prandial insulin for

GLYCEMIC MANAGEMENT AND SUBCUTANEOUS INSULIN FOR PATIENTS WHO ARE EATING
(Continued)

Scheduled Basal Insulin

☐ Long-acting insulin analog (Long-AA) for basal insulin coverage

DROP DOWN MENU

Long-Acting Analog of Insulin (Long-AA)

● Glargine insulin (route SC, priority routine), dose ______ units
○ Detemir insulin (route SC, priority routine), dose ______ units

Frequency and Time of Medication

● Once daily at 2200 (default for Long-AA)
○ Once daily at 0800
○ Twice daily at 0800 and 2200

Additional Directions

(Prescriber guideline:
true basal insulin requirements should not be withheld for type 1 diabetes)

○ DO NOT WITHHOLD
○ CUT 20% IF NPO
○ CUT 50% IF NPO
○ HOLD IF NPO

☐ NPH for basal insulin coverage, morning dose

DROP DOWN MENU

Morning Dose of NPH

● NPH insulin (route SC, priority routine), ______ units, once daily at 0800

Additional Directions

(Prescriber guideline:
true basal insulin requirements should not be withheld for type 1 diabetes.)

○ DO NOT WITHHOLD
○ CUT 20% IF NPO
○ CUT 50% IF NPO
○ HOLD IF NPO

☐ NPH for basal insulin coverage, evening dose

DROP DOWN MENU

Evening Dose of NPH

○ NPH insulin (route SC, priority routine), ______ units, once daily at 1700
○ NPH insulin (route SC, priority routine), ______ units, once daily at 2200

Additional Directions

(Prescriber guideline:
true basal insulin requirements should not be withheld for type 1 diabetes.)

○ DO NOT WITHHOLD
○ CUT 20% IF NPO
○ CUT 50% IF NPO
○ HOLD IF NPO

(Go to Next Screen within Pathway)

Fig. 5. Basal insulin orders for patients who are eating. The start time and duration for each recurring medication order are to be programmed, but will not shown. SC = subcutaneously; NPO = nihil per os (nothing by mouth). Abbreviations may differ according to institutional policy.

glucose below a given threshold replicates a conservative practice pattern that many users of multiple daily insulin injections employ at home. Acceptable control may be achieved by postprandial administration of rapid-acting insulin analog (Jungmann, 2005). For patients whose oral intake is uncertain, the programming pathway provides the option that the use of prandial insulin might be withheld until 50% of the tray has been taken. For patients with stage V chronic kidney disease having hemodialysis, there may be greater risk for hypoglycemia on hemodialysis days (Kazempour-Ardebili et al., 2009). To permit insulin dose reduction by dose omission of rapid-acting analog at breakfast and lunch on dialysis days, a checkbox is provided specifying that the nurse should withhold the scheduled rapid-acting analog before breakfast and lunch on hemodialysis days (Figure 6).

GLYCEMIC MANAGEMENT AND SUBCUTANEOUS INSULIN FOR PATIENTS WHO ARE EATING
(Continued)

Scheduled Rapid-Acting Analog of Insulin (Rapid-AA)

● Rapid-AA insulin (route SC, priority routine), dose ______ units, every day (default)

SIDE MENU

Frequency and Time of Medication

● WMEALS (default) [0800, 1200, 1700]

Additional Directions

☐ HOLD IF NPO
☐ HOLD IF BG < XXX
☐ HOLD UNTIL 50% OF TRAY IS TAKEN
☐ HOLD SCHEDULED RAPID-AA BEFORE BREAKFAST AND LUNCH ON HEMODIALYSIS DAYS

○ Rapid-AA insulin (route SC, priority routine) every day, dose specified for each meal separately

DROP DOWN MENU

Dose with Frequency and Time of Medication

☐ dose ______ units, every day with breakfast. [0800]
☐ dose ______ units, every day with lunch. [1200]
☐ dose ______ units, every day with supper. [1700]
☐ dose ______ units, every day with HS snack. [2200]

Additional Directions

☐ HOLD IF NPO
☐ HOLD IF BG < XXX
☐ HOLD UNTIL 50% OF TRAY IS TAKEN
☐ HOLD SCHEDULED RAPID-AA BEFORE BREAKFAST AND LUNCH ON HEMODIALYSIS DAYS

(Go to Next Screen within Pathway)

Fig. 6. Prandial insulin (nutritional insulin) for patients who are eating. BG = point-of-care blood glucose.

Frequent dosing with rapid-acting analogs for correction of hyperglycemia creates the risk of "stacking" of effect. When a patient has had hyperglycemia prior to a meal, consideration of another correction dose may arise in the postprandial state. The effect of a previously administered correction dose may not have been fully exerted when the blood glucose is retested. Use of a fixed glucose-dependent correction dose rule, designed to meet specific pre-meal targets, may result in hypoglycemia when applied postprandially, prior to full dissipation of the effects of any earlier correction dose. Therefore, orders for correction doses under the programming pathway are restricted to the following three time plans for administration: with meals; HS (bedtime); 0200. The orders may provide a different scale for each of those three time plans (Figure 6).

GLYCEMIC MANAGEMENT AND SUBCUTANEOUS INSULIN FOR PATIENTS WHO ARE EATING
(Continued)

Bridging Doses of Insulin for Transition from Intravenous Insulin Infusion to Scheduled Subcutaneous Therapy

☐ NPH insulin for transitioning from insulin drip (route SC), dose ______ units

DROP DOWN MENU
(Prescriber guideline: if intravenous insulin infusion will terminate at a time of day when the first daily basal insulin dose is not yet due, a bridging dose of subcutaneous NPH insulin may be used once, to be given at least 2 hr prior to interruption of intravenous insulin infusion.)

Priority
- O Priority stat
- O Priority routine, once at ______

☐ Regular insulin for transitioning from insulin drip (route SC), dose ______ units

DROP DOWN MENU
(Prescriber guideline: if intravenous insulin infusion will terminate at a time of day when the first daily basal insulin dose is not yet due, a bridging dose of subcutaneous regular insulin may be used once, to be given at least 2 hr prior to interruption of intravenous insulin infusion.)

Priority
- O Priority stat
- O Priority routine, once at ______

(Go to Next Screen within Pathway for Correction Dose Insulin, Having Separate Selections "With Meals," "HS," and "0200", Not Shown)

Fig. 7. Bridging doses of insulin for patients who are eating, at the time of transition from intravenous insulin infusion to subcutaneous insulin.

Transitioning guidelines from intravenous insulin infusion to subcutaneous insulin recommend that the provider should order subcutaneous insulin before interruption of insulin infusion (Osburne et al., 2006). Infrequently small amounts of basal and prandial insulin (but not subcutaneous correction doses) may be started more than 2 - 4 hr prior to interruption of intravenous insulin infusion. In order to transition from intravenous insulin to subcutaneous insulin, the 24-hr requirement for scheduled subcutaneous basal insulin that is to be started or added may be about 80% of the 24-hr amount of basal insulin, extrapolated from observation of insulin requirement during the last 6-8 hr of intravenous insulin infusion. To avoid overestimation of basal dose requirement, observation must be made during a timeframe of medical stability during which there have been no meals, such as midnight to 0800; there must be no change of carbohydrate-containing maintenance fluids, enteral feedings, or total parenteral nutritional at the time of transition to subcutaneous insulin therapy; there must have been independence from pressors and continuous veno-venous hemodialysis; and there must be no change of corticosteroid dose. If the time of transition occurs at a time of day that differs from the usual time of administration of long-acting insulin analog, then a bridging dose of regular or intermediate-acting insulin may be given (Figure 7).

3.6.2 Subcutaneous insulin for patients who are not eating

The patient receiving continuous exposure to carbohydrate as intravenous dextrose or enteral feedings, or the patient receiving no carbohydrate, generally should have glucose monitoring at time intervals that are equally spaced (Figure 8). The order "ACHS" for a patient who has been made "NPO" is meaningless. Therefore, the branch of the programming pathway for patients who are not eating starts with the default order for monitoring of point-of-care blood glucose every 6 hr.

During NPO status, the dose of insulin required to cover dextrose-containing maintenance fluids, total parenteral nutrition (TPN), or enteral tube feedings is described as nutritional insulin. Outside of the programming pathway, the provider may include insulin among the TPN additives. long-acting insulin analog sometimes is used for coverage of continuous enteral feedings. Under such a regimen, safety precautions must be in place for dextrose infusion in case of interruption of enteral feedings. A barrier to creating a universal rule is that patient tolerance for intravenous fluids differs according to condition. Safety data about use of basal insulin during enteral feedings, conducted with careful definition of insulin dose, has been generated in the context of a clinical trial, such that close supervision of the patients can be assumed to have occurred (Koryotkoski et al., 2009).

Personal observation of isolated cases of severe hypoglycemia outside of the research context has led to concern that safety of covering enteral feedings with long-acting analog, demonstrated under controlled research conditions, is not generalizable. In actual practice, use of long-acting analog to cover enteral feedings can be complicated by protracted hypoglycemia, a special risk in case of unforeseen interruption of enteral feedings. When NPH and regular insulin are used every 6 hours, each insulin dose is smaller than under a once-daily glargine program, and the frequency of insulin administration provides deliberate stacking of effect. The use of more frequent and smaller doses of intermediate acting insulin achieves control superior to that of sliding scale insulin; such therapy is intended to reduce the risk of prolonged exposure to high doses of long-acting insulin in case of sudden interruption of enteral feedings, and to reduce the importance of reliance upon the antidote of intravenous dextrose, in case of feeding interruptions.

A "sliding scale" regimen of NPH insulin every 4 hr or every 6 hr has been examined, compared to sliding scale aspart insulin alone for treatment of patients receiving enteral feedings (Cook, A. et al., 2009). Amber Cook and colleagues use a standardized rule for altering the NPH dose based on response of blood glucose. In our programming pathway, and on the antecedent paper order sets, in contrast to the closely related regimen of Amber Cook at al., we specify an option for use of mixtures of NPH and regular insulin every 6 hours. The prescribing style is intended to achieve flat-line coverage of insulin effect. The method described in our guideline is to administer equal doses of insulin every 6 hours, apportioned as 2/3 NPH and 1/3 regular insulin, with instructions to withhold the regular insulin in case of glucose below a given threshold.

GLYCEMIC MANAGEMENT AND SUBCUTANEOUS INSULIN FOR PATIENTS WHO ARE NOT EATING, INCLUDING PATIENTS RECEIVING CONTINUOUS ENTERAL FEEDINGS, CONTINUOUS DEXTROSE-CONTAINING MAINTENANCE FLUIDS, OR NO CARBOHYDRATE EXPOSURE

Physician Orders for Nursing Staff

(Orders to "call," assess," and "teach" to be programmed, but not shown here)

■ POC (point-of-care) blood glucose monitoring Q6HRS [0600, 1200, 1800, 2400]

Scheduled Intermediate-Acting Insulin

● NPH insulin (route SC, priority routine), dose ______ units
(Prescriber guideline: Prescribe equal total doses of scheduled insulin every 6 hr, apportioned as 2/3 NPH, 1/3 regular insulin.)

SIDE MENU
(Start time for order and duration of order to be programmed, but not shown here)

Frequency and Time of Medication

● Q6HRS (default for NPH insulin)
○ Q12HRS

Additional Directions

☐ HOLD IF TUBE FEEDS STOP
☐ HOLD X6 HR BEFORE TUBE FEEDS WILL STOP
☐ HOLD IF INFUSION RATE OF DEXTROSE-CONTAINING MAINTENANCE FLUIDS IS REDUCED
☐ CALL M.D. IF UNPLANNED INTERRUPTION OF TUBE FEEDS OCCURS TO CONSIDER DEXTROSE-CONTAINING FLUID ORDER

Scheduled Regular Insulin

● Regular insulin (route SC, priority routine), dose _____ units
(Prescriber guideline: Prescribe equal total doses of scheduled insulin every 6 hr, apportioned as 2/3 NPH, 1/3 regular insulin.)

SIDE MENU
(Start time for order and duration of order to be programmed, but not shown here)

Frequency and Time of Medication

● Q6HRS (default for regular insulin)
○ Q12HRS

Additional Directions

☐ HOLD IF TUBE FEEDS STOP
☐ HOLD X6 HR BEFORE TUBE FEEDS WILL STOP
☐ HOLD IF INFUSION RATE OF DEXTROSE-CONTAINING MAINTENANCE FLUIDS IS REDUCED
☐ HOLD IF BG < XXX
☐ CALL M.D. IF UNPLANNED INTERRUPTION OF TUBE FEEDS OCCURS TO CONSIDER DEXTROSE-CONTAINING FLUID ORDER

(Go to Next Screen within Pathway)

Fig. 8. Nursing orders and scheduled insulin orders for patients who are not eating, including patients receiving continuous dextrose-containing maintenance fluids, continuous enteral feedings, or no carbohydrate exposure.

The algorithm we use does not provide a protocolized rule for changing the NPH dose based on glycemic response, but rather alters insulin delivery below a given glucose threshold by protocolized omission of scheduled regular insulin. The prescriber within the programming pathway is invited to provide the additional direction for scheduled regular insulin "HOLD FOR BG < XXX" (where BG = point-of-care blood glucose).

Transitioning guidelines from intravenous insulin infusion to subcutaneous insulin for the prescriber include the following, with recognition that the guidelines may not be appropriate for every case, and that individualization is required:

- Order subcutaneous insulin before interruption of insulin infusion. Infrequently small amounts of scheduled NPH and regular insulin (but not sliding scale) may be started more than 2 - 4 hr prior to interruption of intravenous insulin infusion.
- Prescribe equal total doses of scheduled insulin every 6 hr, apportioned as 2/3 NPH, 1/3 regular insulin.
- In order to transition from intravenous insulin to subcutaneous insulin, the 24-hr requirement for scheduled NPH and regular insulin that is to be started or added may be about 80% of the 24-hr amount of intravenous insulin, extrapolated from observation of insulin requirement during the last 6-8 hr of intravenous insulin infusion. To avoid overestimation of dose requirement, observation must be made during a timeframe of medical stability; there must be no change of carbohydrate-containing maintenance fluids, enteral feedings, or total parenteral nutrition at the time of transition to subcutaneous insulin therapy; there must have been independence from pressors and CVVHD; and there must be no change of corticosteroid dose.

A set of dose initiation guidelines is given for insulin-requiring patients whose dose requirements are not known. The total daily dose of insulin for coverage of enteral feedings or continuous intravenous dextrose exposure may be calculated conservatively as follows:

- 24 hr basal requirement is 0.15 units/kg for type 2 diabetes or for stress hyperglycemia, and 0.25 units/kg for type 1 diabetes.
- nutritional requirement is 1 unit per 10 gm of carbohydrate per 24 hr, as determined by review of maintenance fluid or enteral tube feeding composition and delivery rate.
- for type 2 diabetes or stress hyperglycemia, during continuous carbohydrate exposure, the total daily dose of insulin is the sum of the 24 hr basal and nutritional components of therapy.
- the total daily dose of insulin is apportioned between NPH and regular insulin as above.

On a periodic basis, the caregiver then may alter the scheduled NPH and insulin by revising the scheduled insulin orders, using a guideline as shown above for re-establishing total daily dose (see section 3.5), and reapportioning the dose between NPH and regular insulin.

To prevent inadvertent interruption of basal insulin for type 1 diabetes patients who are not eating, a special provision is available, in the branch of the programming pathway for patients who are not eating, to maintain basal dose requirements of long-acting insulin analog treatment when interruption of carbohydrate exposure necessitates interruption of nutritional insulin (Figure 9).

3.6.3 Subcutaneous insulin for patients with overnight enteral feedings and daytime meals

For patients whose oral intake is temporarily poor but likely to improve, overnight enteral tube feedings may be used during transition from negligible oral intake to a full meal plan. Premixed 70% human insulin isophane suspension/30% human insulin (70/30 NPH / regular insulin) may be used as premedication to cover overnight enteral feedings (Figure

10). The need for correction dose insulin is likely to occur during and at the end of each feeding. As the patient's intake of oral feedings improves, correction dose insulin during the day may be required. For patients having type 1 diabetes, additionally daily use of long acting insulin analog should be ordered, in an amount restricted to the basal dose, together with the regimen of premixed insulin that is being used for nutritional coverage and regular insulin for correction dose coverage. Once dietary intake is adequate, overnight enteral feedings and the accompanying premedication with 70/30 isophane NPH/regular insulin no longer are required. Once the patient is eating, a new basal-prandial-correction insulin regimen may be required.

3.6.4 Diabetes hospital patient self management

In the ambulatory setting, skilled use of a flexible insulin program may reduce the frequency of hypoglyemia (Samann et al., 2006). Patients competent at diabetes self-management, for example patients using multiple daily injections or insulin pump therapy, under defined conditions can be treated in the hospital with continuation of their usual program of self-management (Braithwaite et al., 2007; Bailon et al., 2009). A full description of such a program is beyond the scope of this chapter. A hallmark feature is the utilization of the skills of advanced carbohydrate counting to permit matching of mealtime insulin bolus doses to carbohydrate intake, and the use of a rule for establishment of correction doses for treatment of hyperglycemia.

GLYCEMIC MANAGEMENT AND SUBCUTANEOUS INSULIN FOR PATIENTS WHO ARE NOT EATING
INCLUDING PATIENTS RECEIVING CONTINUOUS ENTERAL FEEDINGS,
CONTINUOUS DEXTROSE-CONTAINING MAINTENANCE FLUIDS, OR NO CARBOHYDRATE EXPOSURE
(Continued)

Scheduled Long-Acting Analog of Insulin (Long-AA)
(Prescriber guideline: this order for type 1 diabetes is restricted to basal dose requirements;
the order may be used for the basal dose requirement, together with
an NPH and regular insulin regimen for nutritional coverage and/or correction dose insulin coverage.)

○ Glargine insulin (route SC, priority routine), dose ______ units
○ Detemir insulin (route SC, priority routine), dose ______ units

DROP DOWN MENU
(Start time for order and duration of order to be programmed, but not shown here)

Frequency and Time of Medication
● Once daily at 2200 (default for glargine)
○ Once daily at 0800
○ Twice daily at 1000 and 2200

Additional Directions
(Prescriber guideline:
true basal insulin requirements should not be withheld for type 1 diabetes.)
● DO NOT WITHHOLD

(Go to Next Screen within Pathway, Correction Dose Insulin As Needed Every 6 hr, Not Shown)

Fig. 9. Basal insulin orders for type 1 diabetes patients who are not eating.

GLYCEMIC MANAGEMENT AND SUBCUTANEOUS INSULIN
FOR PATIENTS WITH OVERNIGHT ENTERAL FEEDINGS AND DAYTIME MEALS

Physician Orders for Nursing Staff
(Orders to "call," assess," and "teach" to be programmed, but not shown here)

■ POC (point-of-care) blood glucose monitoring with frequency

SIDE MENU
Frequency of Monitoring
● WMEALS, HS, 0200 [0800, 1200, 1700 before meals; 2200, 0200]
○ WMEALS, HS [0800, 1200, 1700 before meals; 2200]

Scheduled Premixed 70% Human Insulin Isophane Suspension and 30% Human Insulin
(Prescriber guideline: this order provides coverage for overnight enteral feedings; cancel this order when overnight enteral feedings are discontinued.)

■ Premixed 70% human insulin isophane suspension and 30% human insulin (route "SC", priority "premedication"), dose ______ units.

SIDE MENU
(Start time for order and duration of order to be programmed, but not shown here)
Frequency and Time of Medication
● Once q PM as premedication to enteral feeding (default)
○ Once daily at 1800 as premedication to enteral feeding
○ Once daily at 2000 as premedication to enteral feeding
○ Once daily at 2200 as premedication to enteral feeding
Additional Directions
■ HOLD IF NO TUBE FEEDS (tube feedings, enteral feedings)
□ CALL M.D. IF UNPLANNED INTERRUPTION OF TUBE FEEDS OCCURS TO CONSIDER DEXTROSE-CONTAINING FLUID ORDER

Scheduled Long-Acting Analog of Insulin (Long-AA, Abbreviated Display of Order)
(Prescriber guideline: this order for type 1 diabetes is restricted to basal dose requirements; the order may be used for the basal dose requirement together with an NPH and regular insulin regimen for nutritional coverage and/or correction dose coverage)

○ Glargine insulin (route SC, priority routine), dose ______ units
○ Detemir insulin (route SC, priority routine), dose ______ units

DROP DOWN MENU
(Frequency and time of medication, start time for order,duration of order, and additional directions to be programmed, but not shown here)

(Go to Next Screen within Pathway, Correction Dose Insulin ACHS and 0200, Not Shown)

Fig. 10. Insulin orders for patients having overnight enteral tube feedings and daytime meals.

4. Conclusion

A programming pathway for computerized order entry is described that will present templates to the prescriber for well-established strategies for control of hyperglycemia and prevention of hospital hypoglycemia. There is not yet an embodiment of the plan within an existing electronic health record, nor is the content specifically yet endorsed by the healthcare system of the authors, but rather the plan is proposed in general terms as a springboard for development and for modification to meet local needs. A user of the electronic order entry system may opt out of the programming pathway. The pathway is intended to both standardize order entry and also to facilitate individualization of care by the provider and for the patient. An opening screen offers default orders that will be universally desirable for glycemic management and then asks the user to choose a branch of the programming pathway based on route of insulin (intravenous or subcutaneous) and, for subcutaneous insulin regimens, based upon carbohydrate exposure. Within each branch of the pathway for subcutaneous insulin, it is possible to complete related orders without navigation between screens and without use of free-text, by entering numbers and selecting additional directions from side menus and drop down menus. User guidelines are displayed or available by computer link. By grouping and prioritizing related orders (especially the plans for nutrition, glucose monitoring, and insulin) and by offering appropriate additional directions within a branch of the pathway, the integration of the components of care, achievable on paper order sets by juxtaposition, is preserved under the electronic order entry system by user choice of a branch of the programming pathway.

5. Acknowledgement

The authors would like to acknowledge the work of the Diabetes Council of the Resurrection Health Care System and the input of members of the nursing, nutrition services, pharmacy, resident physician, attending physician, and administrative staff.

6. References

American Diabetes Association. 2011. Standards of medical care in diabetes - 2011. Diabetes Care 34 (Suppl 1):S11-S61.

Anderson, J. H., Jr., R. L. Brunelle, P. Keohane, V. A. Koivistos, M. E. Trautmann, L. Vignati, and R. DiMarchi. 1997. Mealtime treatment with insulin analog improves postprandial hyperglycemia and hypoglycemia in patients with non-insulin-dependent diabetes mellitus. Multicenter Insulin Lispro Study Group. *Arch Intern Med* 157 (11):1249-55.

Bagshaw, S. M., M. Egi, C. George, and R. Bellomo. 2009. Early blood glucose control and mortality in critically ill patients in Australia. *Crit Care Med* 37 (2):463-70.

Bhatia, A., B. Cadman, and I. Mackenzie. 2006. Hypoglycemia and Cardiac Arrest in a Critically Ill Patient on Strict Glycemic Control. *Anesth Analg* 102 (2):549-551.

Baldwin, D., G. Villanueva, R. McNutt, and S. Bhatnagar. 2005. Eliminating Inpatient Sliding-Scale Insulin: A reeducation project with medical house staff. *Diabetes Care* 28 (5):1008-1011.

Bellam, H., and S. S. Braithwaite. 2010. Hospital hypoglycemia: from observation to action. *Insulin Journal* 5 (1):16-36.

Blumenthal, D., and M. Tavenner. 2010. The "Meaningful Use" Regulation for Electronic Health Records. *New England Journal of Medicine* 363 (6):501-504.

Boord, J.A. , R.A. Greevy, SS Braithwaite, et al. 2009. Evaluation of hospital glycemic control at US academic medical centers. Hospital Medicine 4:35–44.

Braithwaite, S. S., B. Robertson, H. P. Mehrotra, L. M. McElveen, and C. L. Thompson. 2007. Managing hyperglycemia in hospitalized patients. *Clin Cornerstone* 8 (2):44-54; discussion 55-7.

Campbell, K B, and S S Braithwaite. 2004. Hospital Management of Hyperglycemia. Clin Diabetes 22 (2):81-88.

Clement S., S.S. Braithwaite, M.F. Magee, et al. 2004. Management of Diabetes and Hyperglycemia in Hospitals. Diabetes Care 27(2):553-591.

Cook, A., D. Burkitt, L. McDonald, and L. Sublett. 2009. Evaluation of Glycemic Control Using NPH Insulin Sliding Scale Versus Insulin Aspart Sliding Scale in Continuously Tube-Fed Patients. *Nutrition in Clinical Practice* 24 (6):718-722.

Bailon, RM, B.J. Partlow, V. Miller-Cage, M.E. Boyle, J.C. Castro, P.B. Bourgeois, C.B. Cook. 2009. Continuous subcutaneous insulin infusion (insulin pump) therapy can be safely used in the hospital in select patients. Endocr Pract. Jan-Feb;15(1):24-9.

Devi, R., G. Selvakumar, L. Clark, C. Downer, and S.S. Braithwaite. 2011. A dose-defining algorithm for attainment and maintenance of glycemic targets during intravenous insulin infusion and fluid therapy of hyperglycemic crisis. *Diabetes Management* 1 (4):397–412

Donaldson, S., G. Villanuueva, L. Rondinelli, and D. Baldwin. 2006. Rush University guidelines and protocols for the management of hyperglycemia in hospitalized patients: elimination of the sliding scale and improvement of glycemic control throughout the hospital. *Diabetes Educ* 32 (6):954-62.

Dortch, M. J., N. T. Mowery, A. Ozdas, L. Dossett, H. Cao, B. Collier, G. Holder, R. A. Miller, and A. K. May. 2008. A Computerized Insulin Infusion Titration Protocol Improves Glucose Control With Less Hypoglycemia Compared to a Manual Titration Protocol in a Trauma Intensive Care Unit. *JPEN J Parenter Enteral Nutr* 32 (1):18-27.

Finfer S., D.R. Chittock, S.Y. Su, et al. 2009. Intensive versus conventional glucose control in critically ill patients. N Engl J Med 360(13):1283-97.

Fischer, K F, J A Lees, and J H Newman. 1986. Hypoglycemia in hospitalized patients. *N Engl J Med* 315:1245-50.

Garg, R., H. Bhutani, A. Jarry, and M. Pendergrass. 2007. Provider response to insulin-induced hypoglycemia in hospitalized patients. *J Hosp Med* 2 (4):258-60.

Hermansen, K., M. Davies, T. Derezinski, G. Martinez Ravn, P. Clauson, and P. Home. 2006. A 26-week, randomized, parallel, treat-to-target trial comparing insulin detemir with NPH insulin as add-on therapy to oral glucose-lowering drugs in insulin-naive people with type 2 diabetes. *Diabetes Care* 29 (6):1269-74.

Hermayer, K.L., D.E. Neal, T.V. Hushion, M.G. Irving, P.C. Arnold, L.Kozlowski, M.R. Stroud, F.B. Kerr, and J.M. Kratz. 2007. Outcomes of a Cardiothoracic Intensive Care Web-Based Online Intravenous Insulin Infusion Calculator Study at a Medical University Hospital. *Diabetes Technology & Therapeutics* 9:523-534.

Hermayer, K.L., P. Cawley, P. Arnold, A. Sutton, J. Crudup, L. Kozlowski, and T.V. Hushion. 2009. Impact of improvement efforts on glycemic control and hypoglycemia at a university medical center. *J. Hosp. Med.* 4 (6):331-339.

Hirsch, I.B. 2005. Insulin analogues. N Engl J Med. 352(2):174-83.

Juneja, R., C. Roudebush, N. Kumar, A. Macy, A. Golas, D. Wall, C. Wolverton, D. Nelson, J. Carroll, and S. Flanders. 2007. Utilization of a computerized intravenous insulin infusion program to control blood glucose in the intensive care unit. *Diabetes Technol Ther* 9:232-240.

Jungmann E. 2005. Intensified insulin therapy of type 2 diabetes mellitus: pre- or postprandial injection of aspart insulin? Dtsch Med Wochenschr 130(20):1254-1257.

Kagansky, N, S Levy, E Rimon, L Cojocaru, A Fridman, Z Ozer, and H Knobler. 2003. Hypoglycemia as a predictor of mortality in hospitalized elderly patients. *Arch Intern Med* 163:1825-1829.

Kitabchi, A. E., G. E. Umpierrez, J. M. Miles, and J. N. Fisher. 2009. Hyperglycemic crises in adult patients with diabetes. Diabetes Care 32 (7):1335-43.

Kazempour-Ardebili, S., V. L. Lecamwasam, T. Dassanyake, A. H. Frankel, F. W. K. Tam, A. Dornhorst, G. Frost, and J. J. O. Turner. 2009. Assessing Glycemic Control in Maintenance Hemodialysis Patients With Type 2 Diabetes. *Diabetes Care* 32 (7):1137.

Korytkowski, M. T., R. J. Salata, G. L. Koerbel, F. Selzer, E. Karslioglu, A. M. Idriss, K. K.W. Lee, A. J. Moser, and F. G.S. Toledo. 2009. Insulin Therapy and Glycemic Control in Hospitalized Patients With Diabetes During Enteral Nutrition Therapy: A randomized controlled clinical trial. *Diabetes Care* 32 (4):594-596.

Kosiborod, M, S.E. Inzucchi, H.M. Krumholz, L. Xiao, P.G. Jones, S. Fiske, F.A. Masoudi, S.P. Marso, J.S. Spertus. 2008. Glucometrics in patients hospitalized with acute myocardial infarction: defining the optimal outcomes-based measure of risk. Circulation 117(8):1018-27.

Kosiborod, M., S.E. Inzucchi, A. Goyal, H.M. Krumholz, F.A. Masoudi, L. Xiao, and J.A. Spertus. 2009. Relationship between spontaneous and iatrogenic hypoglycemia and mortality in patients hospitalized with acute myocardial infarction. *JAMA* 301 (15):1556-64.

Krinsley, J. S., and A. Grover. 2007. Severe hypoglycemia in critically ill patients: risk factors and outcomes. *Crit Care Med* 35 (10):2262-7.

Lee, J., B. Clay, Z. Zelazny, and G. Maynard. 2008. Indication-based ordering: a new paradigm for glycemic control in hospitalized inpatients. *J Diabetes Sci Technol* 2 (3):349-56.

Maynard, G. A., M. P. Huynh, and M. Renvall. 2008. Iatrogenic Inpatient Hypoglycemia: Risk Factors, Treatment, and Prevention: Analysis of Current Practice at an Academic Medical Center With Implications for Improvement Efforts. *Diabetes Spectr* 21 (4):241-247.

Maynard, G., J. Lee, G. Phillips, E. Fink, and M. Renvall. 2009. Improved inpatient use of basal insulin, reduced hypoglycemia, and improved glycemic control: effect of structured subcutaneous insulin orders and an insulin management algorithm. *J Hosp Med* 4 (1):3-15.

Moghissi E.S., M.T. Korytkowski, M. DiNardo, et al. 2009. American Association of Clinical Endocrinologists and American Diabetes Association Consensus Statement on Inpatient Glycemic Control. Endocrine Practice 15(4):1-17.

Mucha, G. T., S. Merkel, W. Thomas, and J. P. Bantle. 2004. Fasting and Insulin Glargine in Individuals With Type 1 Diabetes. *Diabetes Care* 27 (5):1209-1210.

Mudaliar, S., P. Mohideen, R. Deutsch, T. P. Ciaraldi, D. Armstrong, B. Kim, X. Sha, and R. R. Henry. 2002. Intravenous Glargine and Regular Insulin Have Similar Effects on Endogenous Glucose Output and Peripheral Activation/Deactivation Kinetic Profiles. *Diabetes Care* 25 (9):1597-1602.

Olson, R. P., M. A. Bethel, and L. Lien. 2009. Preoperative hypoglycemia in a patient receiving insulin detemir. *Anesth Analg* 108 (6):1836-8.

Osburne, R. C., C. B. Cook, L. Stockton, M. Baird, V. Harmon, A. Keddo, T. Pounds, L. Lowey, J. Reid, K. A. McGowan, and P. C. Davidson. 2006. Improving Hyperglycemia Management in the Intensive Care Unit: Preliminary Report of a Nurse-Driven Quality Improvement Project Using a Redesigned Insulin Infusion Algorithm. *The Diabetes Educator* 32 (3):394-403.

Rayman, G., V. Profozic, M. Middle. 2006. Insulin glulisine imparts effective glycaemic control in patients with Type 2 diabetes. Diabetes Res Clin Pract. 76(2):304-312.

Rosenstock, J., G. Dailey, M. Massi-Benedetti, A. Fritsche, Z. Lin, and A. Salzman. 2005. Reduced hypoglycemia risk with insulin glargine: a meta-analysis comparing insulin glargine with human NPH insulin in type 2 diabetes. *Diabetes Care* 28 (4):950-5.

Scalea, T. M., G. V. Bochicchio, K. M. Bochicchio, S. B. Johnson, M. Joshi, and A. Pyle. 2007. Tight glycemic control in critically injured trauma patients. *Ann Surg* 246 (4):605-10; discussion 610-2.

Schnipper, J. L., C. D. Ndumele, C. L. Liang, and M. L. Pendergrass. 2009. Effects of a subcutaneous insulin protocol, clinical education, and computerized order set on the quality of inpatient management of hyperglycemia: results of a clinical trial. *J Hosp Med* 4 (1):16-27.

Schnipper, J. L., C. L. Liang, C. D. Ndumele, and M. L. Pendergrass. 2010. Effects of a computerized order set on the inpatient management of hyperglycemia: a cluster-randomized controlled trial. *Endocr Pract* 16 (2):209-18.

Smith, W. D., A. G. Winterstein, T. Johns, E.Rosenberg, and B. C. Sauer. 2005. Causes of hyperglycemia and hypoglycemia in adult inpatients. *Am J Health Syst Pharm* 62 (7):714-719.

Stagnaro-Green, A, M K Barton, P L Linekin, E Corkery, K deBeer, and S H Roman. 1995. Mortalilty in hospitalized patients with hypoglycemia and severe hyperglycemia. *Mount Sinai Journal of Medicine* 62 (6):422-426.

Thompson, C. L., K. C. Dunn, M. C. Menon, L. E. Kearns, and S. S. Braithwaite. 2005. Hyperglycemia in the Hospital. *Diabetes Spectr* 18 (1):20-27.

Turchin, A., M. E. Matheny, M. Shubina, J. V. Scanlon, B. Greenwood, and M. L. Pendergrass. 2009. Hypoglycemia and clinical outcomes in patients with diabetes hospitalized in the general ward. *Diabetes Care* 32 (7):1153-7.

Trujillo, J. M., E. E. Barsky, B. C. Greenwood, S. A. Wahlstrom, S. Shaykevich, M. L. Pendergrass, and J. L. Schnipper. 2008. Improving glycemic control in medical inpatients: a pilot study. *J Hosp Med* 3 (1):55-63.

Umpierrez, G. E., J. P. Kelly, J. E. Navarrete, M. M. C. Casals, and A. E. Kitabchi. 1997. Hyperglycemic Crises in Urban Blacks. *Archives of Internal Medicine* 157 (6):669-675.

Umpierrez, G. E., D. Smiley, A. Zisman, L. M. Prieto, A. Palacio, M. Ceron, A. Puig, and R. Mejia. 2007. Randomized Study of Basal-Bolus Insulin Therapy in the Inpatient Management of Patients With Type 2 Diabetes (RABBIT 2 Trial). *Diabetes Care* 30 (9):2181-2186.

Umpierrez, G. E., D. Smiley, S. Jacobs, L. Peng, A. Temponi, P. Mulligan, D. Umpierrez, C. Newton, D. Olson, and M. Rizzo. 2011. Randomized Study of Basal Bolus Insulin Therapy in the Inpatient Management of Patients With Type 2 Diabetes Undergoing General Surgery (RABBIT 2 Surgery). *Diabetes Care* 34 (2):256-261.

Van den Berghe, G., A. Wilmer, I. Milants, P. J. Wouters, B. Bouckaert, F. Bruyninckx, R.Bouillon, and M. Schetz. 2006. Intensive Insulin Therapy in Mixed Medical/Surgical Intensive Care Units: Benefit Versus Harm. *Diabetes* 55 (11):3151-3159.

Varghese, P., V. Gleason, R. Sorokin, C. Senholzi, S. Jabbour, and J. E. Gottlieb. 2007. Hypoglycemia in hospitalized patients treated with antihyperglycemic agents. *J Hosp Med* 2 (4):234-40.

Velussi, M. 2002. Lispro insulin treatment in comparison with regular human insulin in type 2 diabetic patients living in nursing homes. *Diabetes Nutr Metab* 15 (2):96-100.

Vriesendorp, T., S. van Santen, H. De Vries, E. de Jonge, F. Rosendaal, M. Schultz, and J. Hoekstra. 2006. Predisposing factors for hypoglycemia in the intensive care unit. *Crit Care Med* 34 (1):96-101.

Wexler, D. J., J. B. Meigs, E. Cagliero, D. M. Nathan, and R. W. Grant. 2007. Prevalence of Hyper- and Hypoglycemia Among Inpatients With Diabetes: A national survey of 44 U.S. hospitals. *Diabetes Care* 30 (2):367-369.

Wexler, Deborah J., Peter Shrader, Sean M. Burns, and Enrico Cagliero. 2010. Effectiveness of a Computerized Insulin Order Template in General Medical Inpatients With Type 2 Diabetes. *Diabetes Care* 33 (10):2181-2183.

11

Hypoglycemia Prevention in Closed-Loop Artificial Pancreas for Patients with Type 1 Diabetes

Amjad Abu-Rmileh[1] and Winston Garcia-Gabin[2]

[1]*Research Group on Statistics, Applied Economics and Health (GRECS), University of Girona*

[2]*Automatic Control Laboratory, KTH Royal Institute of Technology*

[1]*Spain*

[2]*Sweden*

1. Introduction

The current chapter addresses the problem of hypoglycemia in type 1 diabetes from biomedical and control engineering points of view. It gives a general introduction to the artificial pancreas system, and the risk of hypoglycemia in closed-loop insulin treatment. Then, it provides a review on the state of the art in hypoglycemia control, and the recent approaches in dealing with hypoglycemia in closed-loop artificial pancreas systems. Next, different control techniques that can be used to minimize the risk of hypoglycemia and improve the control outputs are presented.

Since the Diabetes Control and Complications Trial (DCCT), tight glycemic control has been established as the control objective in the treatment of patients with type 1 diabetes mellitus (T1DM) (DCCT Research Group (1993)), except if some contraindication exists. However, there still lacks a universal, efficient and safe system able to normalize the glucose levels of patients. The intensive insulin therapy required to achieve the tight glycemic control, based on the injection of basal and bolus insulin to reproduce its physiological secretion, has as counteraction an increase in the risk of significant and severe hypoglycemia with all their consequences. Therefore, hypoglycemia is considered as one of the major limiting factors in achieving tight glycemic control in T1DM (Cryer (2008)).

With the inability of conventional therapy to achieve satisfactory glycemic control, and the development in continuous glucose monitoring (CGM) systems and the increasing use of insulin pumps, the idea of developing an artificial pancreas is viewed as the ideal solution for glycemic control in T1DM (Bequette (2005); Hovorka et al. (2006); Kumareswaran et al. (2009)). The artificial pancreas is an automated closed-loop system that maintains blood glucose levels within the desired range and prevents hypoglycemia, while minimizing or eliminating the need for patient intervention. The artificial pancreas replaces the β-cells functions in glucose sensing and insulin delivery. It consists of three main components (Figure 1): a glucose sensor to measure glucose concentration, a pump for insulin delivery, and a closed-loop control algorithm to bridge between the glucose measurements and the dose of insulin to be delivered. As other medical devices, the architecture of closed-loop artificial pancreas should include strict safety measures implemented as safety module or supervision system, to evaluate the performance of the control algorithm and apply fault detection techniques (Doyle III et al. (2007)).

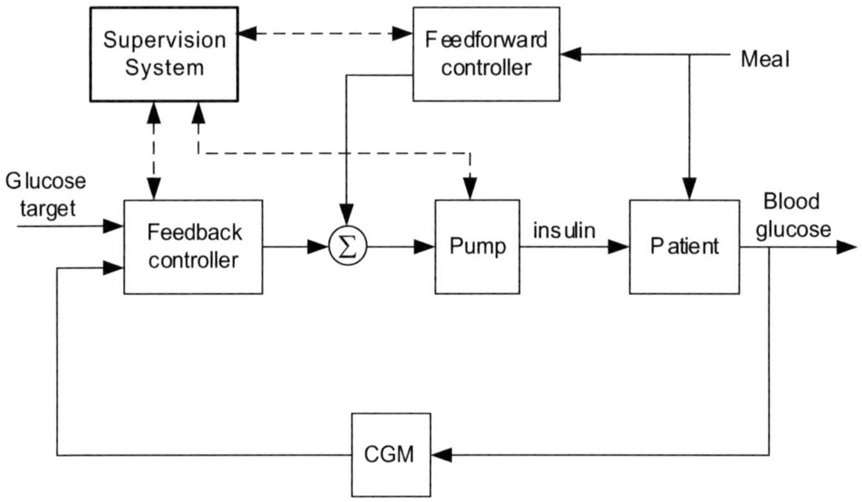

Fig. 1. Artificial pancreas components with patient in the loop. Control algorithm may use feedback or feedforward-feedback control loops

Closed-loop control of blood glucose has been a subject of continuous research for more than 40 years, however, till now no commercially available product does exist. The continuous subcutaneous insulin infusion (CSII) pumps are being widely used, and a number of CGM systems have received regulatory approval (Kumareswaran et al. (2009)). Although the sensors and pumps systems still have some limitations, their use in an open-loop combination resulted in better clinical outcomes over conventional injections therapy (Klonoff (2005); Kumareswaran et al. (2009)). Thus, the primary limitations to develop such an artificial pancreas are the development of reliable closed-loop control algorithms, and the availability of robust and precise glucose sensors. However, recent research in the development of the artificial pancreas suggests that types of the automatic glucose control system are likely to come to market in the near future.

1.1 Patient modeling

The artificial pancreas automatically regulates the blood glucose level based on the glucose measurements, the insulin infusions and in model-based control approaches, on the mathematical insulin-glucose model (diabetic patient model) used to design the controller. Also, these models are essential for testing and validating the artificial pancreas in simulation studies (i.e. *in-silico*) before putting it into clinical use with real patients. Thus, one essential task in the development of artificial pancreas is to obtain a model of T1DM patient, which can help in the development of a closed-loop control system.

Several models with different structures and degrees of complexity are being used to describe the glucoregulatory system - mainly as insulin-glucose and meal-glucose relationships - in T1DM. Most of these are first principle models represented by differential and algebraic equations and based on existing knowledge and hypotheses regarding the underlying physiological system. Among the models that have been frequently used to represent the

diabetic patient in artificial pancreas studies are: the *Meal model* (Dalla Man et al. (2006; 2007)), *Hovorka model* (Hovorka et al. (2004; 2002)), the minimal model (Bergman et al. (1979)), and *Sorensen model* (Sorensen (1985)). Extensive reviews on available models can be found in Chee & Fernando (2007) and Cobelli et al. (2009). Some of these models have been implemented in simulation environments designed to support the development of the closed-loop artificial pancreas (Kovatchev et al. (2009); Wilinska et al. (2010)).
Due to the complex nature of the insulin-glucose system, different empirical models have been proposed to relate insulin input to glucose response (see for example Eren-Oruklu et al. (2009b); Finan et al. (2009)). Empirical models develop a functional relationship between insulin and glucose based on empirical observations (i.e. collected patient data). These models do not describe the physiological model, but they explicitly address inter-patient variability since the data-driven model is specific to individual patient dynamics. Empirical models are more suitable for real-time parameter estimation and updating due to their simple structure in comparison with complex first order models.

1.2 Control problems

The feasibility of closed-loop artificial pancreas systems and their advantage over conventional treatment has been proved in several clinical studies (Atlas et al. (2010); Clarke et al. (2009); Hovorka et al. (2010); Steil et al. (2011; 2006); Weinzimer et al. (2008)), and a wide spectrum of control algorithms has been proposed to close the control loop, including classical and modern control strategies. Many reviews on closed-loop algorithms are available, see for example (Bequette (2005); Chee & Fernando (2007); Doyle III et al. (2007); El-Youssef et al. (2009); Takahashi et al. (2008)).
However, blood glucose control in T1DM is still one of the difficult control problems to be solved in biomedical engineering. In addition to the inherent complexity of glucoregulatory system, which includes the presence of nonlinearities, and time-varying and patient-specific dynamics, there exist other problems, such as noisy measurements, limitations of the models used to develop the control algorithms, as well as the limitations of the subcutaneous route used for glucose sensing and insulin delivery (e.g. technological and physiological delays and subcutaneous tissues dynamics). The aforementioned challenges make it very difficult to find a general and reliable solution to the nonlinear problem of glycemic control. Therefore, the design of a robust closed-loop control algorithm is an essential step for the progress of the artificial pancreas.
For closed-loop artificial pancreas system to be optimal and replicate the normal insulin secretion, the insulin therapy should respect the fact that hypoglycemia is not a naturally occurring episode in T1DM. Also, hypoglycemia is believed to be more dangerous in short term than hyperglycemia. Therefore, in order to achieve tight control while not substituting the problem of hyperglycemia for the life-threatening hypoglycemia, the insulin therapy in T1DM should be optimized so that it reduces the risk of hyperglycemic events in both frequency and magnitude, without provoking significant or severe hypoglycemia as a result of excessive or ill-timed insulin infusion.

2. Hypoglycemia in closed-loop artificial pancreas

Hypoglycemia is the most common complication of insulin therapy in T1DM and continuously limits the efforts to improve glycemic control. Therefore, hypoglycemia prevention should be unavoidably considered among the main objectives in the development of the closed-loop artificial pancreas systems. Severe hypoglycemia episodes are a

well-known cause of death in diabetic patients, and are more commonly seen during the night than during the day. Given that the first generations of the artificial pancreas are not expected to achieve complete regulation of the glucose levels during the 24 hours period, first generations of the artificial pancreas might be focusing on critical aspects like preventing hypoglycemia episodes during night (Hovorka et al. (2010)).
Currently, the vast majority of closed-loop artificial pancreas works focuses on the achievement of tight control during daily life conditions (i.e. 24 hours control), and therefore addresses both hyper- and hypoglycemia in fasting and postprandial conditions. Various strategies are employed in these works to avoid fasting, postprandial and nocturnal hypoglycemia. Mostly, the control algorithms use changes in the target blood glucose to adjust the doses of insulin to prevent hypoglycemia (i.e. higher target glucose level during night and postprandial periods) (Eren-Oruklu et al. (2009a); Marchetti et al. (2008); Weinzimer et al. (2008)). In other works, hypoglycemia prediction algorithms were tested, and short-term suspension of insulin pump was used as safety approach when hypoglycemia is predicted (Lee & Bequette (2009)). Also, variations in insulin sensitivity during the day (due to the 24 hours circadian cycle in insulin sensitivity), have been considered in the design of artificial pancreas control algorithms, and used to adjust the basal insulin requirements during the day (Garcia-Gabin et al. (2009); Steil et al. (2003); Wang et al. (2009)).
Another strategy used to avoid hypoglycemia is the double hormone closed-loop system, which uses glucagon infusion in response to low glucose levels. In T1DM, insulin deficiency is often accompanied by the loss of glucagon secretory response to hypoglycemia. Furthermore, insulin therapy causes even more degradation in the functionality of other counterregulatory hormones (Briscoe & Davis (2006)), and consequently, results in higher possibility for hypoglycemic risk. Different artificial pancreas studies have demonstrated that glucagon infusion significantly reduces the risk of insulin-induced hypoglycemia in T1DM (Castle et al. (2010); El-Khatib et al. (2009; 2010); Ward et al. (2008)).

2.1 Overnight hypoglycemia control

Overnight closed-loop insulin delivery has received great interest because it addresses the critical problem of nocturnal hypoglycemia. Furthermore, prevention of nocturnal hypoglycemia and achieving good control overnight can help in improving the quality of glycemic control during the day (Hovorka et al. (2010)) (e.g. starting the day with acceptable glucose levels). A number of clinical and *in-silico* studies attempts to deal with the hypoglycemia prevention - mainly nocturnal hypoglycemia - as the primary control objective. In (Wilinska et al. (2009)), a manual closed-loop insulin delivery system was employed during night period using model predictive control (MPC) algorithm and CGM measurements (CGM readings were provided to the MPC by medical staff), and aimed at regulating glucose level overnight to avoid nocturnal hypoglycemia. In (Hovorka et al. (2010)), the system was tested in a clinical study with children and adolescents. Earlier version of this MPC algorithm was tested in previous clinical study to evaluate its control and prediction performance during fasting conditions (Shaller et al. (2006)). An automated closed-loop insulin delivery system was tested in a multinational clinical trial (Bruttomesso et al. (2009); Clarke et al. (2009)). The system used a personalized MPC algorithm developed in (Magni et al. (2007)). The system was developed completely *in-silico* and then tested in the clinical trial.
The studies concluded that the MPC algorithm is well suited for glucose control under fasting and overnight conditions in T1DM patients. The studies showed that the artificial pancreas is superior to open-loop control in preventing overnight hypoglycemia where significant

reduction in overnight hypoglycemia episodes was observed with closed-loop control in comparison with standard therapy. Also, during closed-loop period, the blood glucose level was within the target glycemic range for a longer time period, and the frequency of low glucose values was reduced.

2.2 Hypoglycemia alarm systems

Beside control algorithms, several algorithms for hypoglycemia detection and prediction are proposed as alarm systems to avoid hypoglycemia. The progress in CGM systems has made it possible to develop such real-time algorithms to reduce the hypoglycemic risk. These algorithms can be used to detect occurring hypoglycemia or warn about a pending hypoglycemic episode. The algorithms are based mainly on a combination of CGM data and a set of defined threshold of glucose and glucose rate of change. Different estimation and prediction approaches (e.g. linear and statistical prediction, Kalman filter optimal estimation, time series, etc.) have been proposed to develop these algorithms (Buckingham et al. (2009); Cameron et al. (2008); Hughes et al. (2010); Palerm et al. (2005); Sparacino et al. (2007)). Nguyen et al. (2009) used a specialized sensor (*Hypoglycemia monitor*) for nocturnal hypoglycemia detection, based on bayesian neural networks approach. The sensor measures specific physiological parameters continuously trying to detect the hypoglycemic events. In Skladnev et al. (2010), a data fusion approach was used to enhance the hypoglycemia alarm of CGM systems. The CGM information (data and alarms) was fused with autonomic nervous system responses that were detected by the specialized *Hypoglycemia monitor*. The data fusion method was able to improve nocturnal hypoglycemia alarms, and reduced the number of undetected hypoglycemic events.
Hypoglycemia prediction/detection algorithms are usually coupled with specific supporting actions to improve their efficiency in preventing hypoglycemia. Different actions have been proposed, such as gradual insulin attenuation (Hughes et al. (2010)), pump suspension (Buckingham et al. (2009); Lee & Bequette (2009)), glucose infusion (Choleau et al. (2002)), and audible (Buckingham et al. (2009); Weinzimer et al. (2008)) or visual (Hughes et al. (2010)) alarms to alert the patient about actual or impending hypoglycemia. The statistical and linear hypoglycemia predictors with pump suspension algorithm proposed in (Buckingham et al. (2009)) were used in a clinical study, and proved to be effective in preventing hypoglycemia without provoking rebound hyperglycemia after the suspension of the pump.

3. Hypoglycemia prevention by control algorithm improvement

To improve the performance of the closed-loop system, and significantly reduce the risk of hypoglycemia, the control system of the artificial pancreas can be augmented with different control techniques. Such techniques can be introduced either by modifying the controller structure (i.e. internal), or by implementing the additional technique separately (i.e. external component). The increased cost or complexity that could be added to the system by incorporating such techniques can be justified by the improved performance of the system in dealing with life-threatening hypoglycemia. Both external and internal techniques have been tested and proved to provide satisfactory results, and to outperform the stand-alone closed-loop controllers.

3.1 Model predictive control

Several studies have concluded that model predictive control (widely known as MPC) is expected to be the core of closed-loop control algorithm in the near future artificial pancreas.

Therefore, MPC is discussed in some details in this chapter. MPC is a control strategy that has developed considerably over the past few decades. Basically, MPC is based on a model of the system to be controlled. The model is used to predict the future system outputs, based on the past and current values and on the proposed optimal future control actions. These actions are calculated by optimizing a cost function where the future tracking error is considered, as well as the system constraints if any (Maciejowski (2002)). MPC employs a receding horizon strategy; repeated displacement of the time horizon, while only applying the first control signal in the calculated sequence at each time step, with the rest of the sequence being discarded.

MPC has many virtues that make it a competitive candidate for the blood glucose control problem: (1) The prediction nature of MPC allows for anticipatory and careful insulin delivery to avoid large fluctuations in glucose levels. Such feature is important for avoiding overdosing and hypoglycemic risk. (2) The ability of MPC to handle constraints on system inputs and outputs is a major advantage of MPC over other control strategies. These constraints are very critical when dealing with the human body, and allow to satisfy hardware specifications of the insulin pump. (3) The applicability of MPC to systems with time delays can be useful to overcome the physiological and technological delays associated with the subcutaneous route. (4) MPC allows the introduction of feedforward control action to compensate for known sources of disturbance affecting the system, such as meal intake. These advantages of MPC over other control strategies have promoted the use of MPC in the field of insulin delivery. Different MPC schemes are being used in artificial pancreas research, where the applicability of such control strategy has been demonstrated in *in-silico* studies (see for instance (Abu-Rmileh et al., 2010a; Dua et al., 2009; Grosman et al., 2010; Hovorka et al., 2004; Lee & Bequette, 2009; Magni et al., 2007; Parker et al., 1999)), and clinical trials as mentioned earlier.

3.2 Unequal penalization

Closed-loop control schemes can be designed so that unequal penalties are used upon hyperglycemia and hypoglycemia. The reason for such unequal penalties is that in diabetes therapy, the performance requirement of a controller has asymmetric nature, as hypoglycemic events are much less tolerable than hyperglycemia. Since hypoglycemia is believed to be more life-threatening in the short term, the control algorithm should be more aggressive in avoiding hypoglycemic episodes than in correcting hyperglycemic events.

MPC is one control strategy that permits to incorporate this kind of unequal penalization. To achieve such requirements of asymmetrical response, an asymmetric cost function is used in the optimization algorithm in MPC. The asymmetric cost function imposes different weight on hypoglycemia than on hyperglycemia, in contrast to conventional cost functions that impose the same weight on hypoglycemic and hyperglycemic events. As stated before, MPC calculates the insulin control action u_k, by optimizing a quadratic cost function, penalizing predicted output deviations and control signal along some prediction horizons. The asymmetric cost function has the form:

$$\min_{\Delta u} J = \sum_{j=1}^{N_p} \|w^y(\hat{y}(k+j|k) - r(k+j))\|^2 + \sum_{j=1}^{N_u} \|w^{\Delta u}(\Delta u(k+j|k)\|^2 + q\varepsilon^2 \quad (1)$$

Subject to the following constraints:

$$\begin{aligned} u_{min} &\leq u_k \leq u_{max} \\ \Delta u_{min} &\leq \Delta u_k \leq \Delta u_{max} \\ y_{min} - \varepsilon\Phi_{min} &\leq y_k \leq y_{max} + \varepsilon\Phi_{max} \end{aligned} \tag{2}$$

where $\hat{y}(k+j|k)$ is the j-step prediction of the output on data up to instant k, $r(k+j)$ is the target glucose level, Δu is the insulin input increment, N_p and N_u are the prediction and control horizons, and $w^{\Delta u}$, w^{y} are weights on the insulin increments and the error between $y(k)$ and $r(k)$ respectively, ε is a slack variable used for output constraints softening (to avoid infeasibility problems in the optimization), q is the weight on the slack variable ε, $u_{min/max}$, $\Delta u_{min/max}$ and $y_{min/max}$ are the constraints imposed on the input, input increments, and output respectively, and Φ_{min}, Φ_{max} are the relaxation variables.

The cost function in equation (1) is asymmetric in the sense that the lower and upper output constraints are subjected to unequal relaxation bands and therefore, the constraints have different levels of softness. The unequal softness levels could be achieved by introducing the nonnegative relaxation variables Φ_{min}, Φ_{max} which represent the concern for relaxing the corresponding constraint; the larger Φ, the softer the constraint. MPC with asymmetric cost function was tested with different diabetic patient models, and showed an excellent ability to minimize the hypoglycemic events, especially in postprandial period (Abu-Rmileh & Garcia-Gabin (2010a;b); Kirchsteiger & Del Re (2009)). Kirchsteiger & Del Re (2009) give a comparison between symmetric and asymmetric cost function MPC's, where the latter shows superior performance in avoiding hypoglycemia.

In Dua et al. (2009), a multi-programming MPC is used, and provided with different techniques to avoid hypoglycemia. In the multi-programming approach, the optimization problem in MPC is solved by searching for optimal solution within some valid regions (search regions) defined by the constraints and the parameters of the cost function. The main advantage of the multi-parametric MPC is that it provides the same performance as traditional MPC with lower computational load. The controller is provided with asymmetric cost function, and higher priority is given to the satisfaction of constraints imposed on hypoglycemia. Another type of asymmetric performance is presented in Grosman et al. (2010) to minimize the undesirable hypoglycemic and hyperglycemic events. The proposed MPC uses a glycemic zone rather than a fixed glucose level as a target (Zone-MPC). Three different zones are defined (permitted, lower, and upper zones), where the control objective is adjusting the insulin input to maintain glucose level within the permitted zone.

3.3 Gain scheduling

Gain scheduling (GS) is a well-known technique for controlling nonlinear systems by linear controllers. Briefly, GS is one of the simplest forms of adaptive control that employs different control structures in the different operating ranges of the nonlinear system. In glucose control, GS was inspired from the natural pancreas where the level of insulin activity varies between different glycemic ranges; being dominant in the hyperglycemic range, in balance with glucagon action in normoglycemia, and almost inactive in the hypoglycemic range where glucagon is dominant.

From an engineering perspective, a simple nonlinearity test (e.g. steady state insulin-glucose relationship) can be used to show that insulin has a nonlinear effect on blood glucose in different glycemic ranges (see Figure 2). Linear control algorithms are intended to control linear systems, and they usually offer poor results when used to control nonlinear systems in regions far from where the linear model used was obtained. Therefore, nonlinear control or multiple linear controllers should be applied to handle each glycemic range separately and mimic the natural pancreas secretions. The use of multiple linear controllers by gain scheduling approach is discussed here, while nonlinear control is addressed later in this chapter.

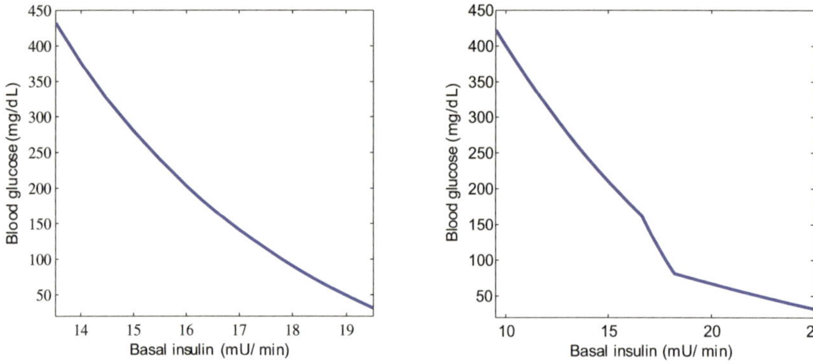

(a) Smooth nonlinearity (*Meal model*) (b) Strong nonlinearity (*Hovorka model*)

Fig. 2. Nonlinear steady-state insulin-glucose behavior in different models of diabetic patients

The idea behind using the GS strategy in artificial pancreas is to use multiple linear controllers to deal with the system nonlinear behavior and maintain the ability of handling each glycemic range separately according to its dynamics. Since most of the closed-loop control strategies use insulin only, the control algorithm should provide the different levels of insulin activity in different glycemic ranges by employing the GS technique. GS scheme requires the assignation of scheduling parameters that can be used to select the suitable linear controller for each range. The GS strategy overcomes the limitations of the linear control approach which is only valid in the neighborhood of a single operating point, and provides a performance similar to nonlinear controllers with lower complexity.
A simplified diagram of the GS control is shown in Figure 3. As it can be seen in the figure, the measured glucose level is used as a scheduling variable, and also delivered to the controllers box as feedback signal. The controllers receive the desired glucose level (glucose target) to calculate the required insulin based on the difference between target glucose and CGM measurements, and the glycemic range defined by the GS selection. A control approach combining linear MPC with GS was tested in (Abu-Rmileh & Garcia-Gabin (2010a;b)), and proved to enhance the performance of the closed-loop controller in avoiding hypoglycemia.

3.4 Meal announcement

Regulation of blood glucose level after a meal is one of the main challenges for the fully developed artificial pancreas. Meals usually lead to a significant glucose flux into the blood stream. If feedback control is used to eliminate the meal effect, the controller reacts only after a rise in glucose has occurred and been detected by the CGM sensor. Elevated glucose level can lead to insulin overdosing, resulting in postprandial hypoglycemia (Steil et al. (2006)).

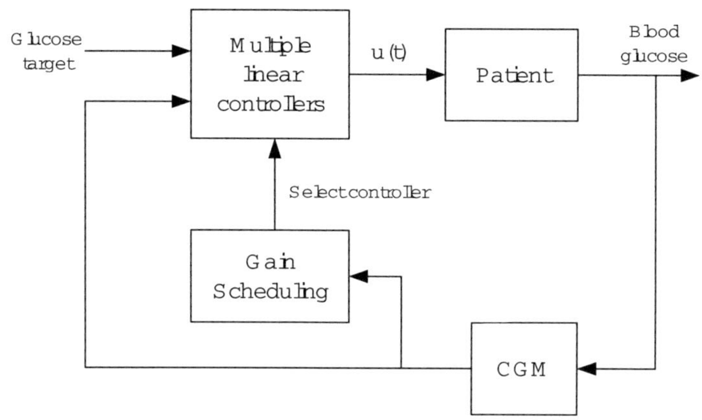

Fig. 3. Gain scheduling control scheme; the CGM output is delivered to the controllers box as a feedback signal, and to GS to select the controller to be used.

To avoid the limitation of purely reactive feedback control action and improve the controller response against meal effect, feedforward control (i.e. meal announcement) can be used. Feedforward is a well-known control technique used to eliminate the disturbance effect when the source of disturbance can be measured. In blood glucose control, the meal intake can be viewed as a known source of disturbance, and feedforward control can be used for meal announcement. In case information is given to the artificial pancreas system about the upcoming meal (size and time), a feedforward scheme may be implemented to deliver additional meal-time insulin bolus (Figure 1).
For the design of the feedforward controller, the effect of meal on blood glucose level should be modeled. The system model (insulin-glucose) in the feedforward element describes or predicts how each change in insulin will affect glucose, while the disturbance model (meal-glucose) is used to describe or predict how each change in meal will affect glucose. Let G_s and G_d be the system and disturbance models respectively, the feedforward control u_{ff} is calculated as:

$$u_{ff} = -\frac{G_d}{G_s} \times Meal \tag{3}$$

Feedforward controllers can range from simple scaling multipliers (static feedforward) to sophisticated differential equations (dynamic feedforward). Dynamic models give a better description of actual system and disturbance behaviors, often achieving improved disturbance rejection performance. However, the dynamic feedforward can be difficult to obtain and implement. In specific control algorithms such as MPC, the feedforward control signal can be calculated by the controller itself rather than using a separate feedforward controller. If the meal effect is included in the prediction model of the MPC, the controller predicts the future glucose levels as a function of insulin-glucose dynamics, CGM measurements, and meal information. Consequently, the meal effect on blood glucose will be considered in calculating the future insulin dose (i.e. predictive feedforward). In this controller configuration, the insulin dose has two parts: feedback insulin delivered in fasting conditions, and feedforward insulin bolus used at meal time to obtain better meal compensation.

The different configurations of feedforward (static, dynamic, and predictive) are being used in the artificial pancreas research, and their feasibility in improving the overall controller performance has been demonstrated in different clinical and simulation studies (Abu-Rmileh & Garcia-Gabin (2010a;b); Abu-Rmileh et al. (2010b); Lee & Bequette (2009); Marchetti et al. (2008); Weinzimer et al. (2008)). Since the feedforward action starts to deliver insulin before the meal effect appears in the CGM feedback loop, lower fluctuations in glucose levels are observed, with higher percentage of time within the acceptable glycemic range. An example of the improved performance achieved with feedforward control is shown in Figure 4. Finally, it should be mentioned that meal announcement must be done carefully, since an excess of insulin or badly-timed bolus may induce undesirable hypoglycemia episodes.

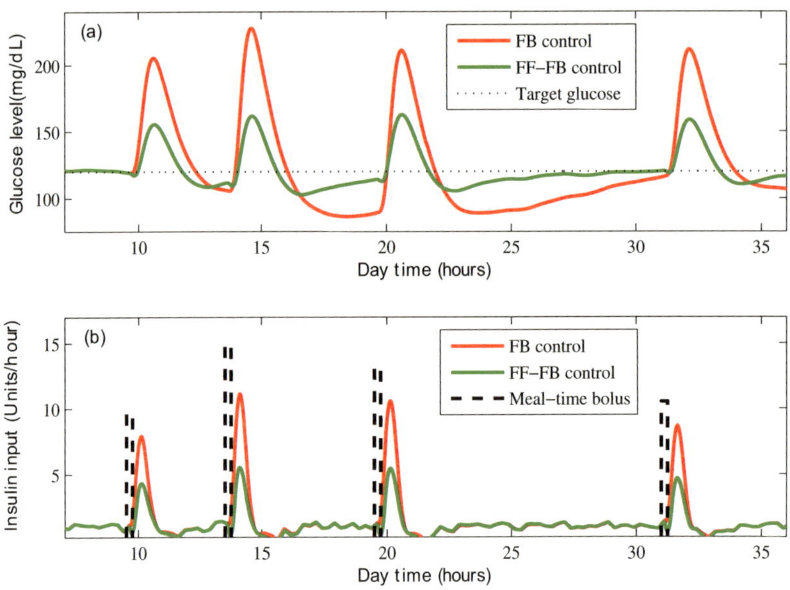

Fig. 4. Feedback (FB) vs. feedforward-feedback (FF-FB) control performance, (a) glucose level (b) insulin input

3.5 Meal detection

Beside feedback and feedforward control, meal detection techniques can be used to deal with meal challenge. Although feedforward-feedback control achieves better results than feedback alone, it is not uncommon that patients forget to announce upcoming meals. Therefore, a system for meal compensation that does not require information from the patient, would be preferable. The CGM measurements along with a set of thresholds on glucose levels and glucose rates of change (i.e. first and second derivative), can be used to build meal detection/compensation algorithms. When a meal is detected, the algorithm can be used to initiate extra meal-time insulin dose, or to activate an alarm for the patient. The meal-time dose can be delivered as insulin bolus or micro boluses, or a gain scheduling scheme can be used to adjust the controller output when a meal is detected. Meal detection and CGM-activated insulin dose remove the need for patient's interventions, and make the closed-loop artificial pancreas fully automatic. Meal detection algorithms also reduce the hypoglycemic risk produced by erroneous insulin bolus or skipped meal, which may occur in the case of feedforward meal announcement.

Three main types of meal detection algorithms currently exist. A voting scheme is used in (Dassau et al. (2008)) to detect meals based on a combination of four different methods for calculating glucose rates of change. Another algorithm is proposed in (Lee & Bequette (2009); Lee et al. (2009)), where the meal detection algorithm is developed by using a finite impulse response filter and a set of threshold values. The algorithm estimates the meal size at the time of detection. Since the main objective of the development of meal detection algorithms is the application to closed-loop artificial pancreas, Lee & Bequette (2009) tested the design algorithm in combination with a MPC closed-loop controller, and demonstrated that meal detection strategy is efficient and outperforms the stand-alone feedback control scheme. Cameron et al. (2009) presented a probabilistic and evolving algorithm to detect the meal and predict its shape, and to estimate the total appearance of glucose from the meal. The algorithm has proved to enhance the meal-compensation ability of the feedback controller.

3.6 Time delay compensation

It is well-known that the time delay in the subcutaneous route is a major challenge in the development of the artificial pancreas (Hovorka (2006)). Both physiological and technological delays exist in glucose sensing and insulin delivery. Such time delays can result in poorly controlled glucose since hypoglycemia can be induced and remains undetected for a significant time period. In an attempt to eliminate or minimize the effect of time delay, closed-loop control structures with time-delay compensation features can be used to improve the control outputs and reduce the hypoglycemic risk produced by physiological and technological delays.

Smith predictor structure is a control scheme that presents good properties in controlling systems with long time delay. The idea behind Smith predictor is to incorporate the system model within the closed-loop control structure (i.e. the system model becomes an explicit part of the controller). Thus, the design of Smith predictor scheme requires a model of the system dynamics and an estimate of the system time delay t_0. In the Smith predictor scheme, there are two parallel paths for the control signal $u(t)$ (see Figure 5); one passing through the real system (the patient), and one passing through the model of the system G_s. The function of the parallel path containing the model is to generate the difference $e_m(t)$ between the actual system output $y(t)$ and a model-based prediction of the control signal effect on the system output $y_m(t)$. The Smith predictor uses the model to predict the delay-free response of the system $y_{\bar{m}}(t)$. Then, it compares this prediction to the target glucose level $r(t)$ to decide what control actions are needed. To avoid drifting and reject external disturbances, the Smith predictor also compares the actual system output with a prediction that takes the time delay into account. The error $e_m(t)$ contributes to the overall error signal $e(t)$ delivered to the feedback controller.

The Smith predictor structure has been recently used in artificial pancreas studies (Abu-Rmileh et al. (2010a;b)). With an initial estimation of the time delay, the Smith predictor shows the ability to minimize the effect of time delays and the associated risk of hypoglycemia, and to enhance the controller performance. As mentioned before, the MPC strategy, which has been extensively studied in artificial pancreas applications, is another competitive control algorithm with inherited ability to deal with system time delays (Hovorka (2006)).

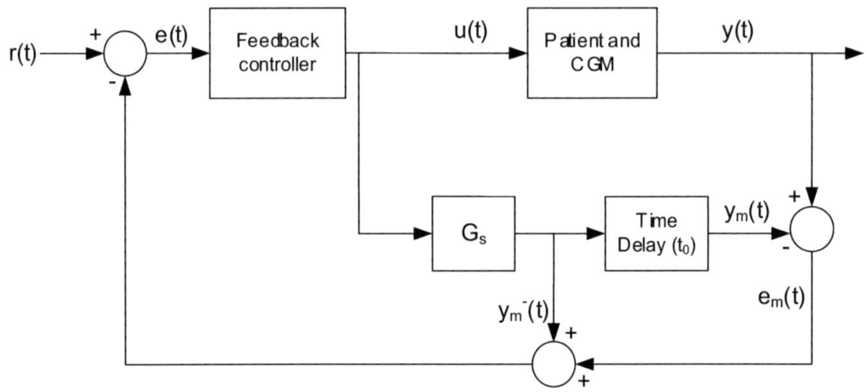

Fig. 5. Smith predictor control structure for time-delay compensation

3.7 Insulin on board and insulin feedback

As discussed previously, the use of subcutaneous route faces a challenging problem represented by the delayed insulin action. The effect of subcutaneous insulin may remain active over an extended time period (3-5 hours) after administration. Insulin on board (IOB) is a term used to describe how much insulin is still active from previous doses. Modern insulin pumps include the IOB option that helps in calculating the next required insulin dose. Therefore, IOB curves (time-action profiles) can be used in the development of artificial pancreas control algorithms to consider the effect of previous insulin, and provide a type of safety measure to avoid the problem of overdosing and the associated hypoglycemia. Ellingsen et al. (2009) developed a MPC scheme with IOB constraints. The IOB was used as dynamic safety constraints with a set of curves, to account for the time profile of delayed insulin action. Lee et al. (2009) used the IOB safety constraints in an integrated control scheme for the artificial pancreas that includes MPC strategy, meal detection algorithm, IOB constraints, and pump suspension option to avoid hypoglycemia.

Another technique used to reduce insulin infusion is the *insulin feedback*, initially introduced by Steil et al. (2004). The algorithm aims at reproducing as close as possible the insulin secretion from the natural pancreas. The idea behind this technique is to consider that a part of previous insulin is still active, and can cause further reduction in glucose level. Based on a pharmacokinetic model (Steil et al. (2006)), the algorithm estimates the plasma insulin level, and reduces the output of a proportional-integration-derivative (PID) controller by using the insulin feedback term, that is proportional to the estimated plasma insulin. Different versions of the algorithm have been used in clinical studies (Steil et al. (2011; 2006); Weinzimer et al. (2008)). In a recent study (Steil et al. (2011)), the insulin feedback has been used to improve the PID controller response in avoiding hypoglycemia after breakfast, and has achieved the desired performance.

3.8 Nonlinear modeling and control

Since the effect of insulin is nonlinear across the different glycemic ranges, the use of nonlinear models able to describe this nonlinear behavior would facilitate the design of more robust nonlinear control strategies, to handle the difference between glycemic ranges and their insulin requirements. Nonlinear models are more flexible in capturing complex behavior than the linear models, and consequently, the nonlinear control strategies are considered to be more suitable for this type of systems than linear control strategies. Therefore, nonlinear control is believed to be more appropriate for the closed-loop artificial pancreas, and will enhance hypoglycemia prevention features of closed-loop systems due to its ability to provide particular insulin profile for each glycemic region. However, the identification of nonlinear models is still a challenging task in the artificial pancreas research. In order to be used in closed-loop control, such nonlinear model should be sufficiently accurate to capture the main system behavior and nonlinearity, while being relatively simple to be identified from the available data such as CGM measurements, and insulin and meal information.

Nonlinear control strategies like nonlinear MPC (NMPC) and sliding mode control (SMC), have shown superior performance over classical linear controllers in the blood glucose control problem. Most of the available MPC strategies are based on a linear model of the system. For systems that are highly nonlinear, the performance of a linear MPC can be poor. This has motivated the design of the NMPC, where a more accurate nonlinear model of the system is used for prediction and optimization. NMPC has been used in a number of artificial pancreas studies (Hovorka et al. (2010; 2004); Schlotthauer et al. (2005); Trajanoski & Wach (1998)).

SMC is a nonlinear robust procedure to synthesize controllers for linear and nonlinear systems. The design of SMC algorithm includes two main steps. 1) Choosing a switching (sliding) surface, along which the system can slide to its desired final value. The sliding surface is designed so that it describes the desired system dynamics. The sliding surface divides the phase plane into regions where the switching function has different signs. 2) By using appropriate control law: make the system reach the switching surface *(reaching phase)*, and keep it on the surface *(sliding phase)*. The structure of the controller is intentionally altered as its state crosses the surface in accordance with a prescribed control law. SMC exhibits good robustness against parameter variations, modeling errors and disturbances.

SMC algorithms have been employed successfully in different *in-silico* studies of artificial pancreas (Abu-Rmileh et al. (2010a;b); Kaveh & Shtessel (2008)). The combination between SMC and Smith predictor used in (Abu-Rmileh et al. (2010a;b)) is simple in its formulation and implementation, yet has some good features such as accuracy and robustness, insensitivity to internal and external disturbances, time-delay compensation and finite time convergence. These features make the proposed control algorithm suitable for the blood glucose problem which incorporates many sources of uncertainty and disturbances, and imposes some specific time requirements to avoid hypoglycemia and extended hyperglycemia. Other nonlinear control and modeling techniques have been used in the artificial pancreas research. Brief descriptions of frequently used approaches are given here, while comprehensive reviews are provided in Bequette (2005); Chee & Fernando (2007); El-Youssef et al. (2009); Takahashi et al. (2008)).

As mentioned before, the glucoregulatory system is nonlinear and difficult to model mathematically. Therefore, empirically-based and model-free control techniques such as fuzzy and neural network systems would be key components in artificial pancreas control systems. Fuzzy systems are based on the idea that input-output relationships are not crisp, but can change gradually from one state to the next, and partial membership rather than crisp membership can be used to adjust the control action. Fuzzy logic control takes the input variables and maps them into fuzzy levels by sets of membership functions. Each input variable has determined value's degree of membership in a fuzzy set. The process of converting crisp input values to fuzzy values is called *fuzzification*. The fuzzy controller makes decisions for what action to take based on a set of rules. The set of rules are built generally based on expert knowledge. The input signal is processed applying the corresponding rules and generating a result for each, then combining the results of these rules. Finally, the fuzzy controller output is obtained via *defuzzification* combining result back into a specific crisp control output value. Different fuzzy control schemes have been implemented in artificial pancreas studies (see for example Atlas et al. (2010); Campos-Delgado et al. (2006); Ibbini (2006); Ibbini & Massadeh (2005)). In Atlas et al. (2010), a personalized fuzzy logic controller has been validated clinically, and proved to minimize hyperglycemic peaks while preventing hypoglycemia.

Neural networks are modeling techniques that result in a nonlinear model based on experimental data. It is a black-box model organized in sequential layers containing neurons. The network output is obtained as a weighted sum of inputs through the hidden layers. The weights are found during a training process by minimizing the error between desired and network output. Neural networks show excellent adaptation and learning ability. Neural networks deal with the blood glucose problem without explicit description of the exact model of the insulin-glucose system. Such approach is very useful in irregular situations (e.g. patients have a disease or abnormal conditions) that limit the usability of normal models (Takahashi et al. (2008)). Neural networks have been used to obtain insulin-glucose models for the design of nonlinear closed-loop controllers (El-Jabali (2005); Schlotthauer et al. (2005); Takahashi et al. (2008); Trajanoski & Wach (1998)). A combination between fuzzy logic and neural network (neuro-fuzzy) control strategy was applied by Dazzi et al. (2001) in clinics, and proved to provide superior glycemic control compared to conventional algorithms, with hypoglycemic events reduced to half.

Adaptive control is another approach used for glucose regulation. The complexity of glucose control mechanism highlights the need for an adaptive control algorithm to compensate for variations in patient dynamics (e.g. time-varying insulin sensitivity, stress and physical exercise) or disturbances by adapting the controller and model parameters to the changing patient conditions (Eren-Oruklu et al. (2009a); Hovorka (2005)). Adaptive control includes several configurations that allow not only outputs of the controller to be changed over time, but also the method by which those outputs are generated; the controller continuously monitors its own adaptation through a defined metric, and is capable of altering its own control scheme to better meet the adaptation criterion. For blood glucose control, different adaptation schemes have been employed (Chee & Fernando (2007)), in systems that use the sensor measurements to track the changes in glucose dynamics and update the controller structure to assign the required insulin regime. In model-based adaptive control, patient model is used to predict future glucose levels based on current and past insulin infusions. The model parameters are continuously updated and used in the control algorithm to calculate the required insulin. Adaptive control strategies have the ability to individualize the control scheme and/or patient model to represent the inter- and intra-patient variability. Adaptive schemes have achieved safe control while avoiding hypoglycemia in spite of all the challenges facing the closed-loop artificial pancreas (Eren-Oruklu et al. (2009a); Shaller et al. (2006)).

4. Conclusions

Closed-loop insulin delivery by the artificial pancreas gives hope to achieve tight glycemic control in T1DM by reducing the risk of hypoglycemia while solving the problem of hyperglycemia. The prevention of life-threatening hypoglycemia is considered as a possible goal for the first generation of the artificial pancreas before reaching the fully developed device that mimics the function of natural pancreas in night, fasting and prandial conditions. The closed-loop system can be subjected to different modifications to implement control techniques that reduce the risk of hypoglycemia. The feasibility of some of these techniques

has been tested and proved to improve the performance of the closed-loop control and reduce the hypoglycemia episodes. Other techniques are still under study.
While partial results obtained in different artificial pancreas studies are promising, several aspects regarding the fully developed artificial pancreas are still open, and further improvements are needed. Obtaining models from patient's input-output data using advanced modeling techniques is recommended for blood glucose control. Nonlinear identification of insulin-glucose models for control is desirable. Development of advanced control techniques is needed due to the nonlinear behavior, unmodeled disturbances, delay and inaccuracy in measurements, together with modeling errors and patient variability.
Another required improvement is the modeling of different meal contents, since most of the available models are restricted to carbohydrates effect. Using multiple variable control (i.e. considering insulin, glucagon, exercise, stress, etc.), and incorporating the effect of insulin sensitivity change during the day in the control algorithm design, would increase the reliability of models in representing the real conditions of the diabetic patient, and consequently, improve the overall performance of the designed artificial pancreas.
Although the nonlinearity in the insulin-glucose system is quite obvious, the available hypoglycemia detection and prediction algorithms do not consider the nonlinear nature of the system through the different glycemic ranges (Chan et al. (2010)). Taking into account the nonlinearity of the system would be a possible way to enhance the performance of the algorithms and increase their effectiveness in preventing hypoglycemia (Chan et al. (2010)). The inclusion of IOB effect in predicting future hypoglycemic episodes could be another technique to improve the feasibility of these algorithms (Buckingham et al. (2009)). Finally, improving the accuracy and reliability of CGM systems is an essential task, since both control algorithms and hypoglycemia alarms depend widely on CGM measurements. Poorly functioning sensor increases the risk of system-induced and undetected hypoglycemia, while accurate sensor improves the control quality and reduces the risk.

5. Acknowledgement

The first author acknowledges the support of the University of Girona through the (BR-UdG) research grant.

6. References

Abu-Rmileh, A. & Garcia-Gabin, W. (2010a). Feedforward-feedback multiple predictive controllers for glucose regulation in type 1 diabetes, *Computer Methods and Programs in Biomedicine* 99(2): 113–123.

Abu-Rmileh, A. & Garcia-Gabin, W. (2010b). A Gain Scheduling Model Predictive Controller for Blood Glucose Control in Type 1 Diabetes, *IEEE Transaction on Biomedical Engineering* 57(10): 2478–2484.

Abu-Rmileh, A., Garcia-Gabin, W. & Zambrano, D. (2010a). Internal model sliding mode control approach for glucose regulation in type 1 diabetes, *Biomedical Signal Processing and Control* 5(2): 94 – 102.

Abu-Rmileh, A., Garcia-Gabin, W. & Zambrano, D. (2010b). A robust sliding mode controller with internal model for closed-loop artificial pancreas, *Medical and Biological Engineering and Computing* 48(12): 1191 – 1201.

Atlas, E., Nimri, R., Miller, S., Gurmberg, E. & Phillip, M. (2010). MD-logic artificial pancreas system: A pilot study in adults with type 1 diabetes mellitus, *Diabetes Care* 33(5): 1072–1076.

Bequette, B. (2005). A critical assessment of algorithms and challenges in the development of a closed-loop artificial pancreas, *Diabetes Technology and Therapeutics* 7(1): 28–46.

Bergman, R., Ider, Y., Bowden, C. & Cobelli, C. (1979). Quantitative estimation of insulin sensitivity, *American Journal of Physiology* 236: E667.

Briscoe, V. & Davis, S. (2006). Hypoglycemia in type 1 and type 2 diabetes: Physiology, pathophysiology, and management, *Clinical Diabetes* 24(3): 115–121.

Bruttomesso, D., Farret, A., Costa, S., Marescotti, M. C., Vettore, M., Avogaro, A., Tiengo, A., Dalla Man, C., Place, J., Facchinetti, A., Guerra, S., Magni, L., De Nicolao, G., Cobelli, C., Renard, E. & Maran, A. (2009). Closed-loop artificial pancreas using subcutaneous glucose sensing and insulin delivery and a model predictive control algorithm: preliminary studies in padova and montpellier., *Journal of Diabetes Science and Technology* 3(5): 1014–1021.

Buckingham, B., Cobry, E., Clinton, P., Gage, V., Caswell, K., Kunselman, E., Cameron, F. & Chase, H. P. (2009). Preventing hypoglycemia using predictive alarm algorithms and insulin pump suspension, *Diabetes Technology and Therapeutics* 11(2): 93–97.

Cameron, F., Niemeyer, G. & Buckingham, B. A. (2009). Probabilistic evolving meal detection and estimation of meal total glucose appearance., *Journal of diabetes science and technology* 3(5): 1022–1030.

Cameron, F., Niemeyer, G., Gundy-Burlet, K. & Buckingham, B. (2008). Statistical hypoglycemia prediction, *Journal of Diabetes Science and Technology* 2(4): 612–621.

Campos-Delgado, D., Hernandez-Ordoñez, M., Femat, R. & Gordillo-Moscoso, A. (2006). Fuzzy-based controller for glucose regulation in type 1 diabetic patients by subcutaneous route, *IEEE Transations on Biomedical Engineering* 53(11): 2201–2210.

Castle, J., Engle, J., El-Youssef, J., Massoud, R., Yuen, K., Kagan, R. & Ward, W. (2010). Novel use of glucagon in a closed-loop system for prevention of hypoglycemia in type 1 diabetes, *Diabetes Care* 33(6): 1282 – 1287.

Chan, A., Heinemann, L., Anderson, S., Breton, M. & Kovatchev, B. (2010). Nonlinear metabolic effect of insulin across the blood glucose range in patients with type 1 diabetes mellitus., *Journal of diabetes science and technology* **4**(4): 873–881.

Chee, F. & Fernando, T. (2007). *Closed-Loop Control of Blood Glucose*, Springer-Verlag, London.

Choleau, C., Dokladal, P., Klein, J. ., Kenneth Ward, W., Wilson, G. S. & Reach, G. (2002). Prevention of hypoglycemia using risk assessment with a continuous glucose monitoring system, *Diabetes* 51(11): 3263–3273.

Clarke, W. L., Anderson, S., Breton, M., Patek, S., Kashmer, L. & Kovatchev, B. (2009). Closed-loop artificial pancreas using subcutaneous glucose sensing and insulin delivery and a model predictive control algorithm: the virginia experience., *Journal of Diabetes Science and Technology* 3(5): 1031–1038.

Cobelli, C., Dalla Man, C., Sparacino, G., Magni, L., De Nicolao, G. & Kovatchev, B. (2009). Diabetes: Models, signals, and control, *IEEE Reviews in Biomedical Engineering* 2: 54 –96.

Cryer, P. (2008). Hypoglycemia: Still the limiting factor in the glycemic management of diabetes, *Endocrine Practice* 14(6): 750–756.

Dalla Man, C., Camilleri, M. & Cobelli, C. (2006). A system model of oral glucose absorption: validation on gold standard data, *IEEE Transactions on Biomedical Engineering* 53(12): 2472–2478.

Dalla Man, C., Rizza, R. & Cobelli, C. (2007). Meal simulation model of the glucose-insulin system, *IEEE Transactions on Biomedical Engineering* 54(10): 1740–1749.

Dassau, E., Bequette, B., Buckingham, B. & Doyle III, F. (2008). Detection of a meal using continuous glucose monitoring: Implications for an artificial β-cell, *Diabetes care* 31(2): 295–300.

Dazzi, D., Taddei, F., Gavarini, A., Uggeri, E., Negro, R. & Pezzarossa, A. (2001). The control of blood glucose in the critical diabetic patient: a neuro-fuzzy method, *Journal of Diabetes and its Complications* 15(2): 80–87.

DCCT Research Group (1993). The effect of intensive treatment of diabetes on the development and progression of long term complications in insulin-dependent diabetes mellitus, *New England Journal of Medicine* 329(14): 977–986.

Doyle III, F., Jovanovic, L. & Seborg, D. (2007). Glucose control strategies for treating type 1 diabetes mellitus, *Journal of Process Control* 17(7): 572–576.

Dua, P., Doyle III, F. & Pistikopoulos, E. (2009). Multi-objective blood glucose control for type 1 diabetes, *Medical and Biological Engineering and Computing* 47(3): 343–52.

El-Jabali, A. (2005). Neural network modeling and control of type 1 diabetes mellitus, *Bioprocess and Biosystems Engineering* 27(2): 75–79.

El-Khatib, F. H., Jiang, J. & Damiano, E. R. (2009). A feasibility study of bihormonal closed-loop blood glucose control using dual subcutaneous infusion of insulin and glucagon in ambulatory diabetic swine., *Journal of Diabetes Science and Technology* 3(4): 789–803.

El-Khatib, F. H., Russell, S. J., Nathan, D. M., Sutherlin, R. G. & Damiano, E. R. (2010). A bihormonal closed-loop artificial pancreas for type 1 diabetes, *Science Translational Medicine* 2(27).

El-Youssef, J., Castle, J. & Ward, W. (2009). A review of closed-loop algorithms for glycemic control in the treatment of type 1 diabetes, *Algorithms* 2(1): 518–532.

Ellingsen, C., Dassau, E., Zisser, H., Grosman, B., Percival, M., Jovanovic, L. & Doyle 3rd., F. (2009). Safety constraints in an artificial pancreatic β cell: an implementation of model predictive control with insulin on board., *Journal of Diabetes Science and Technology* 3(3): 536–544.

Eren-Oruklu, M., Cinar, A., Quinn, L. & Smith, D. (2009a). Adaptive control strategy for regulation of blood glucose levels in patients with type 1 diabetes, *Journal of process control* 19(8): 1333–1346.

Eren-Oruklu, M., Cinar, A., Quinn, L. & Smith, D. (2009b). Estimation of future glucose concentrations with subject-specific recursive linear models, *Diabetes Technology and Therapeutics* 11(4): 243–253.

Finan, D., Palerm, C., Doyle, F., Seborg, D., Zisser, H., Bevier, W. & Jovanovic, L. (2009). Effect of input excitation on the quality of empirical dynamic models for type 1 diabetes, *AICHE Journal* 55(5): 1135–1146.

Garcia-Gabin, W., Zambrano, D., et al. (2009). A sliding mode predictive control approach to closed-loop glucose control for type 1 diabetes, *7th IFAC Symposium on Modelling and Control in Biomedical Systems*, Aalborg, Denmark, pp. 85–90.

Grosman, B., Dassau, E., Zisser, H., Jovanovic, L. & Doyle III, F. (2010). Zone model predictive control: A strategy to minimize hyper- and hypoglycemic events, *Journal of Diabetes Science and Technology* 4(4): 961–975.

Hovorka, R. (2005). Management of diabetes using adaptive control, *International Journal of Adaptive Control and Signal Processing* 19(5): 309–325.

Hovorka, R. (2006). Continuous glucose monitoring and closed-loop systems, *Diabetic Medicine* 23: 1–12.

Hovorka, R., Allen, J. M., Elleri, D., Chassin, L. J., Harris, J., Xing, D., Kollman, C., Hovorka, T., Larsen, A. M. F., Nodale, M., De Palma, A., Wilinska, M. E., Acerini, C. L. & Dunger, D. B. (2010). Manual closed-loop insulin delivery in children and adolescents with type 1 diabetes: a phase 2 randomised crossover trial, *The Lancet* 375(9716): 743–751.

Hovorka, R., Canonico, V., Chassin, L., Haueter, U., Massi-Benedetti, M., Orsini Federici, M., Pieber, T., Schaller, H., Schaupp, L., Vering, T. & Wilinska, M. (2004). Nonlinear model predictive control of glucose concentration in subjects with type 1 diabetes, *Physiological Measurements* 25(4): 905–920.

Hovorka, R., Shojaee-Moradie, F., Carroll, P., Chassin, L., Gowrie, I., Jackson, N., Tudor, R., Umpleby, A. & Jones, R. (2002). Partitioning glucose distribution/transport, disposal, and endogenous production during ivgtt, *American Journal of Physiology - Endocrinology and Metabolism* 282(5): 992–1007.

Hovorka, R., Wilinska, M., Chassin, L. & Dunger, D. (2006). Roadmap to the artificial pancreas, *Diabetes Research and Clinical Practice* 74(2): S178–S182.

Hughes, C., Patek, S., Breton, M. & BP, K. (2010). Hypoglycemia prevention via pump attenuation and red-yellow-green "traffic" lights using continuous glucose monitoring and insulin pump data, *Journal of diabetes science and technology* 4(5): 1146–1155.

Ibbini, M. (2006). A PI-fuzzy logic controller for the regulation of blood glucose level in diabetic patients, *Journal of Medical Engineering and Technology* 30(2): 83 – 92.

Ibbini, M. & Massadeh, M. (2005). A fuzzy logic based closed-loop control system for the blood glucose level regulation in diabetes, *Journal of Medical Engineering and Technology* 29(2): 64 – 69.

Kaveh, P. & Shtessel, Y. (2008). Blood glucose regulation using higher order sliding mode control, *International Journal of Robust and Nonlinear Control* 18: 557 – 569.

Kirchsteiger, H. & Del Re, L. (2009). Reduced hypoglycemia risk in insulin bolus therapy using asymmetric cost functions, *Asian Control Conference*, pp. 751–756.

Klonoff, D. (2005). Continuous glucose monitoring, roadmap for 21st century diabetes therapy, *Diabetes Care* 28(5): 1231–1239.

Kovatchev, B., Breton, M., Dalla Man, C. & Cobelli, C. (2009). In silico preclinical trials: a proof of concept in closed-loop control of type 1 diabetes, *Journal of Diabetes Science and Technology* 3(1): 44–55.

Kumareswaran, K., Evans, M. & Hovorka, R. (2009). Artificial pancreas: an emerging approach to treat type 1 diabetes, *Expert Reviews of Medical Devices* 6(4): 401–410.

Lee, H. & Bequette, B. (2009). A closed-loop artificial pancreas based on model predictive control: Human friendly identification and automatic meal disturbance rejection, *Biomedical Signal Processing and Control* 4(4): 347–354.

Lee, H., Buckingham, B., Wilson, D. & Bequette, B. (2009). A closed-loop artificial pancreas using model predictive control and a sliding meal size estimator., *Journal of Diabetes Science and Technology* 3(5): 1082–1090.

Maciejowski, J. (2002). *Predictive Control with Constraints*, Prentice Hall.

Magni, L., Raimondo, D., Bossi, L., Dalla Man, C., De Nicolao, G., Kovatchev, B. & Cobelli, C. (2007). Model predictive control of type 1 diabetes: an in silico trial, *Journal of Diabetes Science and Technology* 1(6): 804–812.

Marchetti, G., Barolo, M., Jovanovic, L., Zisser, H. & Seborg, D. (2008). A feedforward-feedback glucose control strategy for type 1 diabetes mellitus, *Journal of Process Control* 18(2): 149–162.

Nguyen, H., Ghevondian, N. & Jones, T. (2009). Real-time detection of nocturnal hypoglycemic episodes using a novel non-invasive hypoglycemia monitor, *Proceedings of the 31st Annual International Conference of the IEEE Engineering in Medicine and Biology Society: Engineering the Future of Biomedicine, EMBC 2009*, pp. 3822–3825.

Palerm, C. C., Willis, J. P., Desemone, J. & Bequette, B. W. (2005). Hypoglycemia prediction and detection using optimal estimation, *Diabetes Technology and Therapeutics* 7(1): 3–14.

Parker, R., Doyle lll, F. & Peppas, N. (1999). A model-based algorithm for blood glucose control in type 1 diabetic patients, *IEEE Transactions on Biomedical Engineering* 46(2): 148–157.

Schlotthauer, G., Gamero, L., Torres, M. & Nicolini, G. (2005). Modeling, identification and nonlinear model predictive control of type i diabetic patient, *Medical Engineering and Physics* 28(3): 240 – 250.

Shaller, H. C., Schaupp, L., Bodenlenz, M., Wilinska, E., Chassin, L. J.and Wach, P., Vering, T., Hovorka, R. & Pieber, T. R. (2006). On-line adaptive algorithm with glucose prediction capacity for subcutaneous closed loop control of glucose: evaluation under fasting conditions in patients with type 1 diabetes, *Diabetic Medicine* 23(1): 90–93.

Skladnev, V., Tarnavskii, S., McGregor, T., Ghevondian, N., Gourlay, S. & Jones, T. (2010). Hypoglycemia alarm enhancement using data fusion, *Journal of Diabetes Science and Technology* 4(1): 34–40.

Sorensen, J. (1985). *A physiologic Model of Glucose Metabolism in Man and its Use to Design and Assess Improved Insulin Therapies for Diabetes*, PhD thesis, Department of Chemical Engineering, MIT.

Sparacino, G., Zanderigo, F., Corazza, S., Maran, A., Facchinetti, A. & Cobelli, C. (2007). Glucose concentration can be predicted ahead in time from continuous glucose monitoring sensor time-series, *IEEE Transactions on Biomedical Engineering* 54(5): 931 –937.

Steil, G., Palerm, C., Kurtz, N., Voskanyan, G., Roy, A., Paz, S. & Kandeel, F. (2011). The effect of insulin feedback on closed loop glucose control, *Journal of Clinical Endocrinology & Metabolism*, DOI:10.1210/jc.2010-2578.

Steil, G., Pantaleon, A. & Rebrin, K. (2004). Closed-loop insulin delivery - the path to physiological glucose control, *Advanced Drug Delivery Reviews* 56(2): 125–144.

Steil, G., Rebrin, K., Darwin, C., Hariri, F. & Saad, M. (2006). Feasibility of automating insulin delivery for the treatment of type 1 diabetes, *Diabetes* 55(12): 3344–3350.

Steil, G., Rebrin, K., Janowski, R., Darwin, C. & Saad, M. (2003). Modeling β-cell insulin secretion - implications for closed-loop glucose homeostasis, *Diabetes Technology and Therapeutics* 5(6): 953–964.

Takahashi, D., Xiao, Y. & Hu, F. (2008). A survey of insulin dependent diabetes part II: Control methods, *International Journal of Telemedicine and Applications* .

Trajanoski, Z. & Wach, P. (1998). Neural predictive controller for insulin delivery using the subcutaneous route, *IEEE Transactions on Biomedical Engineering* 45(9): 1122 – 1234.

Wang, Y., Percival, M., Dassau, E., Zisser, H., Jovanovic, L. & Doyle 3rd., F. (2009). A novel adaptive basal therapy based on the value and rate of change of blood glucose, *Journal of diabetes science and technology* 3(5): 1099–1108.

Ward, W., Engle, J., Duman, H., Bergstrom, C., Kim, S. & Federiuk, I. (2008). The benefit of subcutaneous glucagon during closed-loop glycemic control in rats with type 1 diabetes, *IEEE Sensors Journal* 8(1): 89 – 96.

Weinzimer, S., Steil, G., Karena, S., Dziura, J., Kurtiz, N. & Tamborlane, W. (2008). Fully automated closed-loop insulin delivery versus semiautomated hybrid control in pediatric patients with type 1 diabetes using an artificial pancreas, *Diabetes Care* 31(5): 934–939.

Wilinska, M., Budiman, E., Taub, M., Elleri, D., Allen, J., Acerini, C., Dunger, D. & Hovorka, R. (2009). Overnight closed-loop insulin delivery with model predictive control: assessment of hypoglycemia and hyperglycemia risk using simulation studies., *Journal of Diabetes Science and Technology* 3(5): 1109–1120.

Wilinska, M., Chassin, L., Acerini, C., Allen, J., Dunger, D. & Hovorka, R. (2010). Simulation environment to evaluate closed-loop insulin delivery systems in type 1 diabetes, *Journal of Diabetes Science and Technology* 4(1): 132–144.

12

Glucose Homeostasis – Mechanism and Defects

Leszek Szablewski
Medical University of Warsaw
Poland

1. Introduction

Glucose is an essential metabolic substrate of all mammalian cells. D-glucose is the major carbohydrate presented to the cell for energy production and many other anabolic requirements. Glucose and other monosaccharides are transported across the intestinal wall to the hepatic portal vein and then to liver cells and other tissues. There they are converted to fatty acids, amino acids, and glycogen, or are oxidized by the various catabolic pathways of cells.

Most tissues and organs, such as the brain, need glucose constantly, as an important source of energy. The low blood concentrations of glucose can causes seizures, loss of consciousness, and death. On the other hand, long lasting elevation of blood glucose concentrations, can result in blindness, renal failure, vascular disease, and neuropathy. Therefore, blood glucose concentrations need to be maintained within narrow limits. The process of maintaining blood glucose at a steady-state level is called glucose homeostasis. This is accomplished by the finely hormone regulation of peripheral glucose uptake, heaptic glucose production and glucose uptake during carbohydrate ingestion. This maintenance is achieved through a balance of several factors, including the rate of consumption and intestinal absorption of dietary carbohydrate, the rate of utilization of glucose by peripheral tissues and the loss of glucose through the kidney tubule, and the rate of removal or release of glucose by the liver and kidney. To avoid postprandial hyperglycemia (uncontrolled increases in blood glucose levels following meals) and fasting hypoglycemia (decreased in blood glucose levels during periods of fasting), the body can adjust levels by a variety of cellular mechanisms. Important mechanisms are conveyed by hormones, cytokines, and fuel substrates and are sensed through of cellular mechanisms.

Diabetes mellitus is one of the clinical manifestations of long-term metabolic abnormalities involving multiple organs and hormonal pathways that impair the body's ability to maintain glucose homeostasis. As a result of impaired glucose homeostasis is a hyperglycemia. Prolonged elevation of blood glucose concentrations causes a number of complications like blindness, renal failure, cardiac and peripheral vascular disease, neuropathy, foot ulcers, and limb amputation. Vascular complications represent the leading cause of mortality and morbidity in diabetic patients.

Hypoglycemia is abnormally low levels of sugar (glucose) in the blood. Low levels of sugar in the blood interfere with the function of much organ system. A person with hypoglycemia may feel weak, drowsy, confused, hungry, and dizzy. The other signs of low blood sugar are: paleness, headache, irritability, trembling, sweating, rapid heart beat, and a cold. The most common cause of hypoglycemia is a complication of diabetes. Low level of glucose in the blood occurs most often in people who use insulin to lower their blood sugar. Hypoglycemia can occur as a side effect of some oral diabetes medication that increases insulin production. People with diabetes who reduce food intake to lose weight are more likely to have hypoglycemia.

2. Role of glucose in mammalian cells metabolism

2.1 Glucose as a source of cellular energy

Glucose is rapidly metabolized to produce ATP (adenosine triphosphate), a high energy end product. Glucose is oxidized through a large series of reactions that extract the greatest amount of possible energy from it. If glucose metabolism occurs in the presence of oxygen (aerobically), the net production are 36 molecules of ATP from one molecule of glucose, and 2 molecules of ATP, if glucose metabolism occurs in the absence of oxygen (anaerobically). For details see [Szablewski, 2011].

2.1.1 Glycolysis

Glycolysis is the first pathway which begins the complete oxidation of glucose to pyruvate. It takes place in the cytoplasm of the cell. Glycolysis occurs virtually in all tissues. This pathway is unique in the sense that it can proceed in both aerobic and anaerobic conditions. Glycolysis is the pathway which cleaves the six carbon glucose molecule into two molecules of the three carbon compound pyruvate. The end result of glycolysis is two molecules of ATP and two molecules of $NADH+H^+$ (Nicotinamide adenine dinucleotide - reduced form). NAD is used as an electron acceptor. This cofactor is present only in limited amounts and once reduced to $NADH+H^+$, as in this reaction, it must be re-oxidized to NAD to permit continuation of the pathway. This process occurs by the one of the two methods: aerobic metabolism of glucose or anaerobic glycolysis.

2.1.2 Oxidative decarboxylation

During aerobic metabolism of glucose in the mitochondria, pyruvate is oxidized. During this reaction NAD is uses as an electron and proton acceptor, and pyruvate is converted to acetyl coenzyme-A (abbreviated as "acetyl-CoA"). The carboxyl group of pyruvate leaves the molecule as CO_2 and the remaining two carbons become acetyl-CoA. This reaction occurs twice since each glucose (six carbons) produce 2 pyruvates (three carbons each). Consequently, these processes produce 2 $NADH+H^+$, 2 Acetyl-CoA, and 2 CO_2.

2.1.3 Krebs cycle

Further series of reactions, all which occur inside mitochondria (mitochondrial matrix) of eukaryotic cells, is collectively called "Krebs Cycle", also known as the "Citric Acid Cycle" or the "Tricarboxylic Acid Cycle". In this cycle, acetyl-CoA is oxidized ultimately to CO_2. It is to note, that the molecules that are produced in these reactions can be used as building blocks for a large number of important processes, including the synthesis of fatty acids, steroids, cholesterol, amino acids, and the purines and pyrimidines. Fuel for Krebs cycle comes from lipids, carbohydrates, and proteins, which produce the molecule acetyl-CoA. While the Krebs cycle does produce CO_2, this cycle does not produce significant chemical energy in the form of ATP directly. This cycle produces $NADH+H^+$ and $FADH_2$, which feed into the respiratory cycle, also located inside mitochondria (inner mitochondrial membrane). It is electron transport chain that is responsible for production of large quantities of ATP. The electron transport chain converts $NADH+H^+$ and $FADH_2$ into reactants that the Krebs cycle requires to function. If oxygen is not present, the electron transport chain cannot function, which halts the Krebs cycle.

2.1.4 Electron transport chain

Oxidative phosphorylation is a series of reactions that utilize the energy from $NADH+H^+$ and $FADH_2$ electron carriers to produce more ATP. Embedded in the inner membrane of the mitochondria are the series of proteins that use the stored energy from $NADH+H^+$ and $FADH_2$ to pump protons into the membrane space. This results in an electrical and chemical gradient of protons. The enzyme ATP synthase (ATPase) uses the proton gradient to drive the reaction of producing ATP from ADP and inorganic phosphate. The electron transport chain consists of a series of proteins (called cytochromes) that are embedded in the inner mitochondria membrane and an enzyme ATP synthase. There are four complexes, namely, I, II, III, and IV. In complex IV, the electrons are combined with protons and oxygen to form water, the final end-product. The oxygen acts as the final electron acceptor and without oxygen, soothe reaction does not proceed and therefore only anaerobic respiration is possible. The end result of electron transport chain is three molecules of ATP, if a donor of protons and electrons is $NADH+H^+$ and one molecule of H_2O. If a donor of protons and electrons is $FADH_2$, the end result of electron transport chain is two molecules of ATP and one molecule of H_2O.

2.1.5 The metabolism of lactate

The anaerobic glycolysis occurs in the absence of oxygen (anaerobically). During anaerobic glycolysis, earlier obtained pyruvate is reduced to a compound called lactate. This reduction of pyruvate to lactate is coupled to the oxidation of $NADH+H^+$ to NAD. Glycolysis and reduction of pyruvate to lactate are coupled to the net production of two molecules of ATP from one molecule of glucose. Accumulation of lactate also causes a reduction in intracellular pH. Therefore lactate is removed to other tissues and dealt with by one of the two mechanisms: 1) Lactate is converted back to pyruvate. This process is enzymatically catalyzed by lactate dehydrogenase. In this reaction, lactate becomes oxidized (loses two electrons) and is converted to pyruvate. The pyruvate then proceeds to be further oxidized by a second mechanism, the aerobic metabolism of glucose. 2) Conversion of lactate to glucose in the process of gluconeogenesis.

2.2 Gluconeogenesis

Gluconeogenesis is a metabolic pathway that results in the generation of glucose from non-carbohydrate carbon substrate such as lactate, glycerol, and glucogenic amino acids. One common substrate is lactic acid formed in the skeletal muscle in the absence of oxygen. It may also come from erythrocytes, which obtain energy solely from glycolysis. The lactic acid is released to the blood stream and transported into liver. Here it is converted to glucose. The glucose is then returned to the blood for use by muscle as an energy source and to replenish glycogen stores. This cycle is termed the "Cori cycle". The gluconeogenesis of the cycle is net consumer energy, costing the body four moles of ATP more than are produced during glycolysis. Therefore, the cycle cannot be sustained indefinitely. The process of gluconeogenesis uses some of the reactions of glycolysis (in reverse direction) and some reactions unique to this pathway to re-synthesize glucose. This pathway requires an energy input, but has a role of maintaining a circulating glucose concentration in the blood stream even in the absence of dietary supply. Fatty acids cannot be converted into glucose in animals with the exception of odd-chain acids, which yield propionyl-CoA, a precursor of succinyl-CoA. Glycerol, which is a part of all triacylglycerols, can also be used in gluconeogenesis. On the other hand, in humans and other mammals, in which glycerol is derived from glucose, glycerol is sometimes not considered a true gluconeogenic substrate, as it cannot be used to generate new glucose. For details see [Szablewski, 2011].

2.3 Glycogenesis

Glycogenesis is the process of glycogen synthesis in which glucose molecules are added to chains of glycogen to storage in liver and muscle. This process acts during rest periods following the Cori cycle, in the liver, and also activated by insulin in response to high glucose levels. For details see [Szablewski, 2011].

2.4 Glycogenolysis

When the blood sugar levels fall, glycogen stored in the tissue, especially glycogen of muscle and liver may be broken down. This process of breakdown of glycogen is called "Glycogenolysis" (also known as "Glycogenlysis"). Glycogenolysis occurs in the liver and muscle. Hepatocytes can consume glucose-6-phosphate in glycolysis, or remove the phosphate group and release the free glucose into the blood stream for uptake by other cells. Since muscle cells lack enzyme glucose-6-phosphatase, they cannot convert glucose-6-phosphate into glucose and therefore use the glucose-6-phosphate for their own energy demands. For details see [Szablewski, 2011].

2.5 Pentose phosphate pathway

The pentose phosphate pathway (also called "Phosphogluconate pathway" or "Hexose monophosphate shunt") is primarily a cytoplasmic anabolic pathway that converts the six carbons of glucose to five carbons (pentose) sugars and reducing equivalents. The primary functions of this pathways are: 1) To generate reducing equivalents ($NADH+H^+$) for reductive biosynthesis reactions within cells; 2) To provide the cell with ribose-5-phosphate for the synthesis of the nucleotides and nucleic acids; 3) To metabolize dietary pentose sugars derived from the digestion of nucleic acids as well as rearrange the carbon skeleton of dietary carbohydrates into glycolytic/gluconeogenic intermediates. This pathway is an alternative to glycolysis. While it does involve oxidation of glucose, its primary role is anabolic rather than catabolic. It is to note, that 30% of the oxidation of glucose in the liver occurs via the pentose phosphate pathway. For details see [Szablewski, 2011].

2.6 Lipogenesis

Lipogenesis is the process by which simple sugars such as glucose are converted to fatty acids. Lipogenesis starts with acetyl-CoA and builds up by the addition of two carbon units. Fatty acids are subsequently esterified with glycerol to form triglycerides that are packed in very low-density lipoprotein (VLDL) and secreted from the liver. For details see [Szablewski, 2011].

3. Glucose homeostasis

3.1 Definition of glucose homeostasis

Most tissues and organs need glucose constantly, as an important source of energy. The low blood concentrations of glucose can cause seizures, loss of consciousness, and death. On the other hand, long lasting elevation of glucose concentrations, can result in blindness, renal failure, vascular disease etc. therefore, blood glucose concentrations need to be maintained within narrow limits. The process of maintaining blood glucose at a steady-state level is called "glucose homeostasis" [DeFronzo, 1988]. This is accomplished by the finely hormone regulation of peripheral glucose uptake, hepatic glucose production, and glucose uptake during carbohydrates ingestion. For details see [Szablewski, 2011].

3.2 Mechanisms of glucose homeostasis

To avoid postprandial hypoglycemia and fasting hypoglycemia, the body can adjust glucose levels by secreting two hormones, insulin and glucagon that work in opposition to each other. During periods of hyperglycemia, the β-cells of the pancreatic islets of Langerhans secrete more insulin. Insulin is synthesized in β-cells of pancreas in response to an elevation in blood glucose and amino acid after a meal. The major function of insulin is to counter the concerned action of a number of hyperglycemia-generating hormones to maintain low blood glucose levels. It also plays an important role in the regulation of glucose metabolism. This hormone regulates glucose metabolism at many sites reducing hepatic glucose output, via decreased gluconeogenesis and glycogenolysis, facilitates the transport of glucose into striated muscle and adipose tissue, and inhibits glucagon secretion. Insulin is not secreted if the blood concentration is ≤ 3 mmol/L, but is secreted in increasing amounts as glucose concentrations increase beyond this threshold [Gerich, 1993]. When blood glucose levels increase over about 5 mmol/L the β-cells increase their output of insulin. The glucagon producing α-cells of the pancreatic islets of Langerhans remain quiet, and hold on their hormone. It is to note, that postprandially, the secretion of insulin occurs in two phases. An initial rapid release of preformed insulin, followed by increased insulin synthesis and release in response to blood glucose. Long-term release of insulin occurs if glucose concentrations remain high [Aronoff et al., 2004; Cryer, 1992]. On the other hand, during periods of hypoglycemia, the α-cells of the pancreatic islets of Langerhans secrete more glucagon. It is the principal hormone responsible for maintaining plasma glucose at appropriate levels during periods of increased functional demand [Cryer, 2002]. This hormone counteracts hypoglycemia and opposes insulin actions by stimulating hepatic glucose production. It induces a catabolic effect, mainly by activating liver glycogenolysis and gluconeogenesis, which results in the release of glucose to the bloodstream, thereby increasing blood glucose levels. The digestion and absorption of nutrients are associated also with increased secretion of multiple gut hormones that act on distal targets. There are more than 50 gut hormones and peptides synthesized and released from the gastrointestinal tract. These hormones are synthesized by specialized enteroendocrine cells located in the epithelium of the stomach, small bowel, and large bowel. It was demonstrated that ingest food caused a more potent release of insulin than glucose infused intravenously [Perley & Kipnis, 1967]. This effect, termed the "incretin effect" suggests that signals from the gut are important in the hormonal regulation of glucose disappearance. Incretin hormones are peptide hormones secreted from the gut and specific criteria have to be fulfilled for an agent to be called an incretin. They have a number of important biological effects, as for example, release of insulin, inhibition of glucagon, maintenance of β-cells mass, and inhibition of feeding. Several incretin hormones have been characterized, but currently, GLP-1 (Glucagon-Like Peptide-1) and GIP (Glucose-Dependent Insulinotropic Polypeptide) are the only known incretins. Both GLP-1 and GIP are secreted in a nutrient-dependent manner and stimulate glucose-dependent insulin secretion. Gut hormones are secreted at low basal levels in the fasting state. The secretion of gut hormones is regulated, at least in part, by nutrients. Plasma levels of most gut hormones rise quickly within minutes of nutrient uptake and fall rapidly thereafter mainly because they are cleared by the kidney and are enzymatically inactivated [Drucker, 2007].

4. Defects in glucose homeostasis

4.1 Hyperglycemia

Hyperglycemia is the technical term for high blood glucose (sugar). It develops when there is too much sugar in the blood. High blood glucose happens when the body has too little insulin or when the body cannot use insulin properly. Hyperglycemia is a serious health problem for those with diabetes. In people with diabetes, there are two specific types of hyperglycemia that occur. Fasting hyperglycemia is defined as a blood sugar greater than 90 - 130 mg/dL (5 - 7.2 mmol/L) after fasting for at least 8 hours. Postprandial (after-meal hyperglycemia) is defined as a blood sugar usually greater than 180 mg/dL (10 mmol/L). Hyperglycemia in diabetes may be caused by: skipping or forgetting insulin or oral glucose-lowering medicine, eating too many grams of carbohydrates for the amount of insulin administered, eating too much food and having too many calories, infection, illness, increased stress, decreased activity or exercising less than unusual, strenuous physical activity. Early signs and symptoms of hyperglycemia include the following: increased thirst, headaches, difficulty concentrating, blurred vision, frequent urination, fatigue (weak, tired feeling), weight loss, blood sugar more than 180 mg/dL (10 mmol/L), high levels of sugar in the urine. Prolonged hyperglycemia in diabetes may result in: vaginal and skin infections, slow-healing cuts and sores, decreased vision, nerve damage causing painful cold or insensitive feet, stomach and intestinal problems. In people without diabetes postprandial or post-meal sugars rarely go over 140 mg/dL (7.8 mmol/L), but occasionally, after a large meal, a 1 - 2 hour post-meal glucose levels can reach 180 mg/dL (10 mmol/L). Blood glucose levels can vary from day to day. An occasional high level (above 10 mmol/L) is not problem, as long as it returns to normal (below 7 mmol/L; 126 mg/dL) within 12 - 24 hours. Persistently high blood glucose levels (above 15 mmol/L; 270 mg/dL) for more than 12 - 24 hours can result in the symptoms of hyperglycemia. For details see [Szablewski, 2011].

4.1.1 Impaired glucose tolerance and impaired fasting glucose

There are two forms of pre-diabetes: impaired glucose tolerance (IGT) and impaired fasting glucose (IFG). Impaired glucose tolerance is a transition phase between normal glucose tolerance and diabetes, also referred to as prediabetes. In impaired glucose tolerance, the levels of blood glucose are between normal and diabetic. People with IGT do not have diabetes. Each year, only 1 - 5% of people whose test results show IGT actually develop diabetes. Weight loss and exercise may help people with IGT return their glucose levels to normal. Impaired glucose tolerance is a combination of impaired secretion of insulin and reduced insulin sensitivity (insulin resistance). Fasting blood glucose levels are normal or moderately raised. IGT is diagnosed when: 1) plasma glucose, two hours after consuming 75 g glucose, appears to be superior to 7.8 mmol/L (normal level) but remains inferior to 11.1 mmol/L (diabetes level). The level of plasma glucose is measured by means of an Oral Glucose Tolerance Test (OGTT). The procedure typically involves testing glucose levels after an eight hour fasting period, and measuring it again two hours after drinking a sugar solution. Generally, if the test shows blood glucose levels in the 140 and 199 mg/dL range, two hours after the drink, this could signify impaired glucose tolerance. 2) Fasting plasma glucose is less than 7.0 mmol/L (6.1 - 6.9 mmol/L), a level above normal, but below the threshold for diagnosis of diabetes. Impaired glucose tolerance is often affiliated with several other similar related risk factors such as high blood pressure (hypertension), increased LDL-cholesterol, reduced HDL-cholesterol. A person has impaired fasting glucose when fasting plasma glucose is 100 to 125 mg/dL. This level is higher than normal but less than the level indicating a diagnosis of diabetes. Diabetes mellitus is characterized by recurrent or persistent hyperglycemia and is diagnosed by demonstrating any one of the following: fasting plasma glucose level ≥ 7.0 mmol/L (126 mg/dL), plasma glucose ≥ 11.1 mmol/L (200 mg/dL) two hours after a 75 g oral glucose load as in a glucose tolerance test, symptoms of hyperglycemia and casual plasma glucose ≥ 11.1 mmol/dL, glycated hemoglobin (HbA_{1C}) ≥ 6.5%.

4.1.2 Type 1 diabetes mellitus

Type 1 diabetes mellitus (previously known as juvenile or insulin-dependent diabetes) results due to autoimmune progressive destruction of insulin-producing β-cells by CD4+ and CD8+ T cells and macrophages infiltrating the islets [Foulis et al., 1991]. Although, the etiology of type 1 diabetes is believed to have a major genetic component, studies on the risk of developing type 1 suggest that environmental factor may be important etiological determinants. Evidence of an autoimmune etiology is found in about 95% of these cases and is classified as type 1A, and the remaining 5% lacks defined markers of autoimmunity and therefore are classified as type 1B, also termed idiopathic [Todd, 1999]. Type 1 diabetes is observed in approximately 10% of patients with diabetes mellitus [Gilespie, 2006]. Type 1 diabetes is a complex polygenic disorder. It cannot be classified strictly by dominant, recessive, or intermediate inheritance, making identification of diseases susceptibility or resistant gene difficult [Atkinson & Eisenbarth, 2001; Rabinovitch, 2000]. The lifetime of type 1 diabetes risk for a number of the general population is often quoted as 0.4%. Eight-five percent of cases of type 1 diabetes occur in individuals with no family of the disease. Differences in risk also depend on which parent has diabetes. The risk increases to 1 - 2% if the mother has diabetes and intriguingly to 3 - 7% if the father has diabetes [Haller & Atkinson, 2005; Warram et al., 1988]. The sibling risk is 6% [Risch, 1987]. Monozygotic twins have a concordance rate of 30 to 50%, whereas dizygotic twins have a concordance rate of 6 to 10% [Haller & Atkinson, 2005]. Disease susceptibility is highly associated with inheritance of the HLA (Human Leukocyte Antigen) alleles DR3 and DR4 as well as the associated alleles DQ2 and DQ8. More than 9% of patients with type 1 diabetes express either DR3DQ2 or DR4DQ8. Heterozygous genotypes DR3/DR4 are most common in children diagnosed with type 1 diabetes prior to the age of 5 (50%) [Atkinson & Eisenbarth, 2001]. Individuals with the HLA haplotype DRB1*Q302-DQA1*0301, especially when combined with DRB*10201-DQA1*0501 are highly susceptible (10 - 20-fold increase) to type 1 diabetes. On the other hand, HLA class II haplotypes such as DR2DQ6 confer dominant protection [Todd & Wicker, 2001]. Individuals with the haplotype DRB1*0602-DQA1*0102 rarely develop type

1 diabetes [Peakman, 2001]. Candidate genes studies also identified the insulin gene as the second most important genetic susceptibility factor [Bell et al., 1984]. Whole genome screen has indicated that there are at least 15 other loci associated with type 1 diabetes [Concannon et al., 1998; Cox et al., 2001]. To date, no single gene is either necessary or sufficient to predict the development of type 1 diabetes. Although type 1 diabetes is likely a polygenic disorder, epidemiological pattern of type 1 diabetes suggests that environmental factors are involved [Dorman & Bunker, 2000].

4.1.3 Type 2 diabetes mellitus

Type 2 diabetes mellitus, previously called non-insulin-dependent diabetes mellitus, is a complex heterogeneous group of metabolic disorders including hyperglycemia and impaired insulin action and/or insulin secretion. Current theories of type 2 diabetes include a defect in insulin-mediated glucose uptake in muscle, a dysfunction of the pancreatic β-cells, a disruption of secretory function of adipocytes, and an impaired insulin action in liver [Lin & Sun, 2010]. The etiology of human type 2 diabetes is multifactorial with genetic background and environmental factors of the modern world which favor the development of obesity. Several findings indicate that genetics is an important contributing factor. It has been estimated that 30 - 70% of type 2 diabetes risk can be attributed to genetics [Poulsen et al., 1999]. The lifetime risk of type 2 diabetes is about 7% in a general population, about 40% in offspring of one parent with type 2 diabetes, and about 70% if both parents have type 2 diabetes [Majithia & Florez, 2009]. Patterns of inheritance suggest that type 2 diabetes is both polygenic and heterogeneous - i.e. multiple genes are involved and different combinations of genes play a role in different subsets of individuals [Doria et al., 2008]. Genetic research effort have led to the identification of at least 27 type 2 diabetes susceptibility genes [Staiger et al., 2009] and most recent genome-wide association studies have identified 20 common genetic variants associated with type 2 diabetes [Ridderstral & Groop, 2009]. Since skeletal muscle accounts for ~ 75% of whole body insulin-stimulated glucose uptake, defects in this tissue play a major role in glucose homeostasis in patients with type 2 diabetes [Bjornholm & Zierath, 2005]. Insulin resistance in skeletal muscle is among the earliest detectable defects in humans with type 2 diabetes [Mauvais-Jarvis & Kahn, 2000]. Type 2 diabetic patients are characterized by a decreased fat oxidative capacity and high levels of circulating free fatty acid [Blaak et al., 2000]. The latter is known to cause insulin resistance by reducing stimulated glucose uptake most likely via accumulation of lipid inside the muscle cell [Boden, 1999]. A reduced fat oxidative capacity and metabolic inflexibility are important components of skeletal muscle insulin resistance [Phielix & Mensink, 2008].

4.1.4 Gestational diabetes mellitus

Gestational diabetes mellitus is defined as "carbohydrate intolerance with onset or first recognition during pregnancy" [Metzger, 1991]. This definition includes pregnancies in which the following occur: insulin therapy is required, diabetes persists after delivery, and diabetes may have been present, but not recognized, prior to the pregnancy [Avery & Rossi, 1994]. Women at risk of type 2 diabetes are at risk of gestational diabetes mellitus [Cheung, 2009]. Gestational diabetes mellitus is a heterogeneous disorder in which age, obesity, and genetic background contribute to the severity of the disease. Multiparous women have a very high prevalence of gestational diabetes mellitus [Wagaarachchi et al., 2001]. There has been relatively little research in the area of gestational diabetes genetics [Watanabe et al., 2007].There is evidence for clustering of type 2 diabetes and impaired glucose tolerance in families with gestational diabetes mellitus [McLellan et al., 1995] and evidence for higher prevalence of type 2 diabetes in mothers of women with gestational diabetes [Martin et al., 1985]. The pathophysiology of gestational diabetes remains controversial. Gestational diabetes mellitus may reflect a predisposition to type 2 diabetes under the metabolic conditions of pregnancy or it may represent the extreme manifestation of metabolic alterations that normally occur in pregnancy [Butte, 2000]. Women with gestational diabetes have decreased insulin sensitivity in comparison with control groups. Gestational diabetes induces a state of dyslipidemia consistent with insulin resistance. During pregnancy, women with gestational diabetes do have high serum triacylglycerol concentrations but lower LDL-cholesterol concentrations than do healthy pregnant women [Koukkou et al., 1996]. During pregnancy, gestational diabetes is associated with a number of complications for child. Because insulin does not cross the placenta, the fetus is exposed to the maternal hyperglycemia. The fetal pancreas is capable of responding to this hyperglycemia [Scollan-Kolippoulos et al., 2006]. The fetus becomes hyperinsulinemic, which in turn promotes growth and subsequent macrosomia [Perkins et al., 2007]. Fetus born to mother with gestational diabetes has higher risk of developing macrosomia, neonatal hypoglycemia, hyperbilirubinemia, shoulder dystonia with its attendant risk of brachial injury and clavicle fracture, etc [Ecker et al., 1997; Hapo Study Group, 2008; Hod et al., 1991; Langer & Mazze, 1988; Persson & Hanson, 1998]. These complications have been reported with varying frequency [Garner, 1995]. Additionally, there are some data that suggest an increase in fetal malformation and perinatal mortality [Sepe et al., 1985]. Cesarean sections are also more common, and gestational diabetes mellitus is associated with a higher risk of pre-eclampsia [Hapo Study Group, 2008, Persson & Hanson, 1998]. Infant exposed to maternal diabetes in uterus have and increased risk of diabetes and obesity in childhood and adulthood [Silverman et al., 1998]. Studies indicate that the magnitude of fetal-neonatal risk is proportional to the severity of maternal hyperglycemia [Langer & Conway, 2000]. Gestational diabetes is one of the most common complications in pregnancy occurring in 2,2% - 8,8% of each year, dependent on the ethnic mix of the population and the criteria used for diagnosis.

4.1.5 MODY

MODY (Maturity onset diabetes of young) is a monogenic and autosomal dominant form of diabetes mellitus. Disease was described in 1974 - 1975 and since then newer gene mutations and subgroups of MODY have been identified [Tattersall, 1974; Tattersall & Fajans, 1975]. To distinguish MODY from type 1 diabetes tests need to be done to establish the absence of diabetes antibodies (anti-insulin, anti-islet, anti-glutamic acid decarboxylase). In obese people, the absence of insulin resistance, will differentiate it from type 2 diabetes. MODY presents in children, adolescent or young adults and may account for up to 5% of diabetes cases [Johnson, 2007]. MODY patients have a strong family history of diabetes, suggestive of a primary genetic cause [Fajans et al., 2001; Mitchell & Frayling, 2002]. MODY is caused by changes to a single gene and if either one of the parents carriers this gene they have a 50% chance of passing it on to their child. Disease progression in MODY is though to be largely independent of nongenetic factors other than time. A primary physiological defect caused [Fajans et al., 2001; Mitchell & Frayling, 2002]. Nine of genetic forms of MODY have been identified to date, and these have been termed MODY 1 – 9. These rare diabetic disorders are associated with heterozygosity for mutations in single genes, including 7 transcription factors (MODY 1, 3, 4, 5, 6, 7 and 9) and 2 metabolic enzymes (MODY 2 and 8). In some cases, there are significant differences in the activity of the mutant gene product that contribute to variations in the clinical features of the diabetes.

4.1.6 Neonatal diabetes mellitus

Neonatal diabetes mellitus is defined as insulin-sensitive hyperglycemia occurring in the first months of life, lasting for more than 2 weeks and required insulin for management [Shield, 2000]. It is rare, with an incidence of approximately 1 in 500 000 births [von Muhlendahl & Herkenhoff, 1995]. Neonatal diabetes mellitus is considered distinct from autoimmune type 1 diabetes, which manifests after the first 3 to 6 months of life [Hathout et al., 2000]. In this disease, antibodies to insulin or islet cells and other markers of autoimmune type 1 diabetes are absent. There are two separate forms of neonatal diabetes mellitus that vary in the length of insulin dependency in the premature stage of disease. In about 50% of cases of neonatal diabetes mellitus, diabetes is transient and resolves at a median age of 3 months (Transient Neonatal Diabetes Mellitus). The other 50% of cases of neonatal diabetes mellitus are permanent (Permanent Neonatal Diabetes Mellitus) [Neve et al., 2005]. The etiology of neonatal diabetes mellitus is genetically heterogeneous, producing abnormal development or absence of pancreas or islets, decreased β-cell mass secondary to increased β-cell apoptosis, and β-cell dysfunction that limits insulin secretion [Aguilar-Bryan & Bryan, 2008]. Transient neonatal diabetes mellitus is a form of neonatal diabetes that appears in the first six weeks of life and usually ends by 18 months. It is characterized by intrauterine growth retardation, dehydration, small gestational age at birth, and failure to thrive. Permanent neonatal diabetes mellitus can occur alone or as a larger genetic syndrome. In permanent neonatal diabetes mellitus, diabetes develops within days to months after birth and persists throughout life. Intrauterine growth retardation, hyperglycemia, sever dehydration, osmotic polyuria, and failure to thrive are all associated with permanent neonatal diabetes mellitus.

4.2 Hypoglycemia

4.2.1 Definition of hypoglycemia

Normally, the body maintains the levels of sugar in the blood within a range of about 70 to 110 mg/dL, depending on when a person last ate. In the fasting state, blood sugar can occasionally fall below 60 mg/dL and even to below 50 mg/dL and not indicate a serious abnormality or disease. This can be seen in healthy women, particularly after prolonged fasting. Hypoglycemia, also called low blood glucose or low blood sugar, occurs when glucose drops below normal levels. Hypoglycemia is defined arbitrarily as blood glucose of less than 50 mg/dL (2.8 mmol/L) with neuroglycopenic symptoms or less than 40 mg/dL (2.2 mmol/L) in the absence of symptoms [Carroll et al., 2003]. The clinical manifestations of hypoglycemia are nonspecific. Therefore, clinically significant hypoglycemia is characterized by Whipple's triad: 1) symptoms of neuroglycopenia, 2) simultaneous blood glucose lower than 40 mg/dL (2.2 mmol/L), 3) relief of symptoms with the administration of glucose. All 3 criteria should be met to establish a diagnosis of hypoglycemia. Asymptomatic hypoglycemia with glucose levels as low as 30 mg/dL (1.7 mmol/L) can be seen during fasting in normal women and during pregnancy [Merimee & Tyson, 1974].

Asymptomatic patients may have artifactural hypoglycemia due to *in vitro* consumption of glucose by blood cell elements such as in leukemia or polycythemia [Carroll et al., 2003].

4.2.2 Signs and symptoms of hypoglycemia

Because of the effectiveness of the normal defenses against falling plasma glucose concentrations, hypoglycemia is an uncommon clinical event, except in persons who use drugs that lower plasma glucose levels, to treat diabetes mellitus [Cryer, 2004; Cryer et al., 2009; Guettier & Gorden, 2006]. According to Cryer and colleagues [Cryer et al., 2009], in healthy individuals, symptoms of hypoglycemia develop at a mean plasma glucose concentration of approximately 55 mg/dL (93.0 mmol/L). However, the glycemic threshold for this and other responses to hypoglycemia shift to lower plasma glucose concentrations in patients with recurrent hypoglycemia [Cryer, 2001 a, Cryer, 2009]. Documentation of Whipple's triad established that a hypoglycemic disorder exists. In a person who does not have diabetes mellitus an unequivocally normal plasma glucose concentration during a symptomatic episode indicates that symptoms are not the result of hypoglycemia [Cryer et al., 2009]. The clinical manifestations of hypoglycemia are nonspecific. The central nervous system relies primarily on glucose for generation of cellular energy, but has reserves sufficient for only a few minutes and cannot synthesize glucose. Furthermore, studies have demonstrated that glucose is an obligate metabolic fuel for the brain under physiological conditions. It is to note, that glucose is not the only fuel that can be utilized by the brain. The noninjured brain can also utilize ketone bodies, particularly during starvation [Robinson & Williamson, 1980]. On the other hand, the brain cannot use fuels others than glucose during acute hypoglycemia [Cryer, 2001 a; Cryer, 2007; Wahren et al., 1999]. When the brain is deprived of its supply of glucose, serious neurological dysfunction occurs [Carroll et al., 2003]. During severe hypoglycemia, glycogen stores appear to play a special role in maintaining brain function. Studies suggest that increasing brain glycogen stores protects neuronal activity [Wender et al., 2000]. Results obtained from human and animal studies showed that the most sensitive neuronal populations are the superficial layers of the cortex, the hippocampus, the caudate nucleus, and the subiculum [Auer et al., 1984; Auer et al., 1985]. Hypoglycemia induces neuronal death [Lacherade et al., 2009]. The neuronal death resulting from hypoglycemia is not a straightforward result of energy failure but instead results from a sequence of events initiated by hypoglycemia [Such et al., 2007]. These events include activation of neuronal glutamate receptors [Nellgard & Wieloch, 1992], production of mitochondrial reactive oxygen species [Singh et al., 2004], neuronal zinc release [Assaf & Chung, 1984], and extracellular release of excitatory amino acids (glutamate and aspartate) [Engelsen et al., 1986]. Activation of postsynaptic glutamate receptor and postsynaptic zinc accumulation induce a variety of mechanisms leading to neuronal death [Patockova et al., 2003; Singh et al. 2004]. According to Carroll and colleagues [Carroll et al., 2003], there are 4 pathophysiologic mechanisms capable of exceeding the body's counterregulatory capacity and causing severe hypoglycemia: excessive insulin effect, diffuse hepatic dysfunction, limited substrate for gluconeogenesis and excessive glucose consumption. More than one mechanism may be responsible, especially in ill patients. Symptoms of hypoglycemia are categorized as neuroglycopenic and neurogenic or autonomic. Symptoms of hypoglycemia may be nonspecific but tend to be similar for repeated episodes in the same individual. The symptoms associated with hypoglycemia are sometimes mistaken for symptoms caused by conditions not related to blood sugar. Unusual stress and anxiety can cause excess production of catecholamines, resulting in symptoms similar to those caused by hypoglycemia but having no relation to blood sugar levels. Symptoms can being slowly or suddenly, progressing from mild discomfort to severe confusion or panic within minutes. If left untreated, hypoglycemia can get worse and cause confusion, clumsiness, or fainting. Severe hypoglycemia can lead to seizures, coma, and even death. General symptoms of hypoglycemia are: nausea, dizziness, collapse, weight gain. Neurogenic symptoms result from sympathoadreanl discharge triggered by hypoglycemia. They include sweating, tremor, palpitations, tachycardia, agitation, nervosity, hunger [Towler et al., 1993]. Symptoms linked to neuroglycopenia are direct result of the lack of brain metabolic energy. Neuroglycopenic symptoms occur at glucose levels of approximately 45 mg/dL and impair the ability of affected individual to take corrective action to abort severe hypoglycemia [Carroll et al., 2003]. These symptoms include impairment of consciousness, mental concentration, vision, speech, memory. Blurred vision, fatigue, seizures, paralyses, ataxia, loss of consciousness, unusual or bizarre behavior, and emotional liability [Cryer, 2008 a; Guettier & Gorden, 2006; McAulay et al., 2001; Ng, 2010; Towler et al., 1993]. Coma may result from values below 40 - 50 mg/dL [Ben-Ami et al., 1999], and death in extreme cases. Hypoglycemia can also happen during sleep. Some signs of hypoglycemia during sleep include crying out or having nightmares, finding pajamas or sheets damp from perspiration, feeling tired, irritable, or confused after waking up. The symptoms of hypoglycemia rarely develop until the level of sugar in the blood falls below 60 mg/dL of blood. Some people develop symptoms at slightly higher levels, especially when blood sugar levels fall quickly, and some do not develop symptoms until the sugar levels in their blood are much lower. The body first responds to a fall in the level of sugar in the blood by releasing noradrenaline (epinephrine) from the adrenal glands. Hormone stimulates the release of sugar from body stores but also causes symptoms similar to those of an anxiety attack: sweating, nervousness, shaking, faintness, palpitations, and hunger. Sometimes people who are hypoglycemic are mistakenly thought to be drunk. In adults and children older than 10 years, hypoglycemia is uncommon except as a side effect of diabetes treatment. Hypoglycemia in people who not have diabetes is far less common than once believed [Cryer, 2008; Guettier & Gorden, 2006; Service, 1995; Service, 1999]. It can occur in some people under certain conditions such as early pregnancy, prolonged fasting, and long periods of strenuous exercise. Hypoglycemia can also result, however, from other medications or diseases, hormone or enzyme deficiencies, or tumors.

4.2.3 Causes and types of hypoglycemia

Two types of hypoglycemia can occur in people who do not have diabetes: reactive hypoglycemia, also called postprandial hypoglycemia, occurs within 4 hours after meals and fasting hypoglycemia, also called postabsorptive hypoglycemia, is often related to an underlying disease [Cryer, 2008]. This classification has been criticised for being unhelpful diagnostically. According to Servise [1995] some causes of hypoglycemia can present with both postabsorptive and postprandial (e.g. insulinoma). Other disorders can present with erratically occuring symptoms independent of food ingestion (e.g. factitous hypoglycemia). Patients with an insulinoma, who typically have postabsorptive hypoglycemia, may experience postprandial hypoglycemia, and post-gastric-bypass patients, who typically have postprandial hypoglycemia, may have symptoms when fasting. Indeed, some disorders, e.g. factitous hypoglycemia, are not readily classified as either postabsorptive or postprandial [Cryer et al., 2009]. Therefore, a more useful approach for clinicans is a classification based on clinical characteristics [Ng, 2010]. Symptoms of the both reactive and fasting hypoglycemia are similar to diabetes-related hypoglycemia. Symptoms may include hunger, sweating, shakiness, dizziness, light-headedness, sleeping, confusion, dificulty speaking, anxiety, and weaknes. The average age of a patient diagnosed with an insulinoma is the early 40s, but cases have been reported in patients ranging from birth to age 80 years [Garza, 2008].

4.2.3.1 Reactive hypoglycemia (postprandial hypoglycemia)

A diagnostic of reactive hypoglycemia is considered only after possible causes of low blood sugar have been rulet out. Reactive hypoglycemia with no known cause is a condition in which the symptoms of low blood sugar appear 2 to 5 hours after eating foods, especially when meals contain high levels of simple carbohydrates (as for example glucose). Reactive hypoglycemia refers to hypoglycemia caused by external influences, like diet and medication use. This type is more amenable to management or cure. Reactive hypoglycemia can be seen in patients who have had surgical removal of the stomach and in patients who had other surgigal procedures (gastrojejunostomy, vagotomy, pyloroplast). This type of hypoglycemia, alimentary hypoglycemia, is another form of hypoglycemia. In the absence of stomach, glucose in the meal is rapidly absorbed into the blood stream through the intestines, causing sudden hyperglycemia. In order to correct this sudden hyperglycemia, excessive amounts of insulin are released by the pancreas, which drives the blood glucose down, causing hypoglycemia. The reactive hypoglycemia in gastrectomy patients occurs early, usually within 1 hour after a meal. In heredity fructose intolerance and galactosemia, an inherited deficiency of a heaptic enzyme causes acute inhibition of hepatic glucose output when fructose or galactose is ingested. In patients with leucine sensitivity in childhood leucine provokes an exaggerated insulin secretory response to a meal and reactive hypoglycemia. Reactive hypoglycemia can occur when blood glucose falls, stores of glucose from the liver are exhausted and an individual chooses not to eat. The body gradually adjusts to this situation by using muscle protein to feed glucose to brain and fat to fuel the other body cells, tissues and organs, but before this adjustment takes place, an individual may experience symptoms of glucose deprivation to the brain. Reactive hypoglycemia seldom causes glucose levels to drop low enough to induce severe neuroglycopenic symptoms; therefore, a history of true loss of consciousness is highly suggestive of an etiology other than reactive hypoglycemia. Reactive hypoglycemia has been suggested to be more common in people who are insulin-resistant, and it may be a frequent precursor to type 2 diabetes. Therefore patients who have a family history of type 2 diabetes or insulin-resistance syndrome, may be at higher risk of developing hypoglycemia. Reactive hypoglycemia often is treated successfully with dietary changes and is associated with minimal morbidity. Mortality is not observed. Reactive hypoglycemia is reported most frequently by women. It typically is in women aged 25 - 35 years. The average age of a patients diagnosed with an insulinoma is the early 40s, but cases have been reported in patients ranging from birth to age 80 years [Garza, 2009]. Idiopathic postprandial hypoglycemia is another form of reactive hypoglycemia [Ng, 2010]. It is a disorder in which autonomic and neuroglycopenic symptoms develop postprandially, accompanied by low plasma glucose [Brun et al., 2000]. This disease is due to various mechanisms, as for example: 1) high insulin sensitivity, 2) an exaggerated insulin response, either related to insulin resistance or to increased glucagon-like peptide 1, 3) renal glycosuria, 4) defects in glucagon response [Brun et al., 2000]. In idiopathic postprandial syndrome, autonomic symptoms, appear 2 - 5 hours after a meal. It is to note that plasma glucose concentration is normal [Charles et al., 1981]. This phenomenon is due to enhanced catecholamine release following a meal or enhanced sensitivity to normal postprandial noradrenaline (norepinephrine) and adrenaline (epinephrine) release. This condition is also known as pseudohypoglycemia [Foster & Rubenstein, 1998].

4.2.3.2 Fasting hypoglycemia (postabsorptive hypoglycemia)

Fasting hypoglycemia, also called postabsorptive hypoglycemia, is diagnosed from a blood samples that shows a blood glucose level below 50 mg/dL after an overnight fast, between meals, or after physical activity. Fasting hypoglycemia occurs when the stomach is empty. It usually develops in the early morning when a person awakens. In otherwise healthy people, prolonged fasting (even up to several days) and prolonged strenuous exercise (even after a period of fasting) are unlikely to cause hypoglycemia. However, there are several conditions or diseases in which the body fails to maintain adequate levels of sugar in the blood after a period without food. Causes of fasting hypoglycemia include certain medications, alcoholic beverages, critical illnesses, hormonal dificiences, some kinds of tumors, and certain conditions occurring in infancy and childhood. Drugs, including some used to treat diabetes, are the most common cause of hypoglycemia. Many other drugs have been reported to cause hypoglycemia, as for example: salicylates, sulfa medications, pentamidine, quinine [Cryer, 2008; Malouf & Brust, 1985; Murad et al, 2009]. In people who drink heavily without eating, alcohol can block the release of stored sugar from the liver. The body's break-down of alcohol interferes with the liver's efforts to raise blood glucose. The alcohol directly interferes with heaptic gluconeogenesis, but not glycogenolysis. The energy required for metabolism of alcohol is diverted from the energy needed to take up lactate. Patients who drink alcohol may become hypoglycemic after 12 - 24 hour when the glycogen stores are depleted. Hypoglycemia caused by excessive drinking can be serious and even fatal. Some illnesses that affect the liver, heart, or kidneys can cause hypoglycemia. Liver insufficiency/failure from any cause may result in deficient glycogen stores or inadequate gluconeogenesis. In advanced liver failure, the defects may be severe enough to cause hypoglycemia. The kidneys have the capacity to produce glucose by gluconeogenesis. Isolated renal failure is rarely associated with hypoglycemia. More often, renal failure is associated with hupoglycemia in patients who are on insulin or insulin secretagogues as insulin is cleared by the kidney. Sepsis is other cause of hypoglycemia. In this case, hypoglycemia can occur due to decreased gluconeogenesis. Hormonal deficiencies may cause hypoglycemia in very young children, but rarely in adults. Certain endocrine deficiencies are associated with poor gluconeogenesis, poor glycogenolysis, or both. These include: adrenal insufficiency, hypopituitarism, isolated growth hormone deficiency, hypothyroidism, isolated glucagon deficiency, and sympathetic nervous system defects. Shortages of cortisol, growth hormone, glucagon or epinephrine can lead to fasting hypoglycemia. Mesenchymal tumors, hepatocellular carcinoma, adrenocortical tumors, carcinoid tumors, leukemia and lymphomas are nonislet cell tumors most commonly associated with hypoglycemia [Diaz et al., 2008; Guettier & Gorden, 2006; Jayaprasad et al., 2006; Ng, 2010]. Although the pathogenesis is incompletely understood, it is belived that these tumors may secrete an insulin like substance that may be biologically active. An alternative hypothesis is that these tumors are so large that they require a significant amount of glucose the liver/kidney are unable to match. Insulinomas can cause hypoglycemia by raising insulin levels too high in relation to the blood glucose level. These tumors are rare and do not normally spread to other parts of the body. The estimated incidence is 1 case per 250 000 patients-years [Service et al., 1991]. It is characterized by neuroglycopenia spells and occurs primarily in a fasting state, and only occasionally in a postprandial period [Kar et al., 2006]. Approximately 60% of patients with insulinoma are female. Insulinomas are uncommon in persons younger than 20 years and are rare in those younger than 5 years. The median age at diagnosis is about 50 years. In some people, an autoimmune disorder lowers sugar levels in the body by changing insulin secretion or by some other means. Hypoglycemia due to anti-insulin antibody is a rare disorder occurring in people often with a history of autoimmune disease [Ng, 2010]. Pregnancy is associated with lower glucose level because of decreased gluconeogenesis due to decreased substrate supply [Pugh et al., 2009]. Inborn errors of carbohydrate metabolism are rare and present during the first days of life [Gustafsson, 2009; Menhesha et al., 2007]. Infants present with fasting hypoglycemia, especially at night. Children rarely develop hypoglycemia and causes may include the following: brief intolerance to fasting, often during an illness that disturbs regular eating patterns, hyperinsulinism, which can result in temporary hypoglycemia in newborns, which is commons in infants of mather with diabetes, enzyme deficiencies that affet carbohydrate metabolism and hormone deficiencies.

5. Hypoglycemia in diabetes mellitus

Hypoglycemia occurring as a complication of therapy for diabetes is common [Chen, 2010; Ito et al., 2010; Swinnen et al., 2010]. Mild hypoglycemia occurs in more than half of all patients with diabetes who are in therapy. Hypoglycemia can occur as a side effect of some diabetes medications, including insulin and oral diabetes medications that increase insulin production. Rapid-acting insulin analogues may decrease the frequency of hypoglycemia associated with regular insulin administration. Insulin lispro has been shown to decrease postprandial glucose excursions and to result in less hypoglycemia in the postabsorptive state [Holleman et al., 1997]. Long-acting analogues, such as glargine, may decrease the frequency of hypoglycemia in both type 1 and type 2 diabetic patients [Pieber et al., 2000; Rosenstock et al., 2001]. Several studies have demonstrated a reduction in hypoglycemic events during continuous subcutaneous insulin infusion using a portable electromechanical pump when compared with multiple injection regimens [Pickup & Keen, 2002]. The effect of normal aging may contribute to the risk for severe hypoglycemia in older diabetic patients treated with sulfonylureas and insulin. Glycemic control in the pregnant diabetic women has major consequence on maternal and fetal morbidity and mortality. The strict control that is recommended during pregnancy leads to a high risk for hypoglycemia, the incidence reported as high as 72% in several studies [Coustan et al., 1986; Rosenn et al., 1995]. The majority of episodes occur during the first 20 weeks of gestation [Kimmerle et al., 1992]. Factors that may contribute to the occurrence of hypoglycemia during pregnancy include anorexia, changes in hormonal counterregulation or the development of altered hypoglycemic awareness [Bjorklund et al., 1998; Dagogo-Jack et al., 1993]. Exercise is an important mode of therapy in both type 1 and type 2 diabetes. High levels of insulin resulting from therapy may prevent the increased mobilization of glucose normally induced by exercise, and hypoglycemia may ensure. Exercise may cause immediate, early, and delayed hypoglycemia, particularly in type 1 diabetic patients and in patients with type 2 diabetes on insulin or sulfonylurea therapy. In general, hypoglycemia during exercise tends to be less of problem in this population. Injection of insulin into the arm or abdomen decreases the hypoglycemic effect of exercise by 57% and 89%, respectively, in comparison with injection of insulin into the leg [Koivisto & Felig, 1978]. Nonselective β-blockers attenuate some components of the autonomic response to hypoglycemia and could increase the risk of hypoglycemia. In study with elderly diabetic patients, no significant impact on the rate of hypoglycemia could be associated with any particular class of antihypertensives [Shorr et al., 1997]. Although in general in type 2 diabetes mellitus there is less hypoglycemia risk versus type 1 diabetes mellitus, the frequency of hypoglycemia increases with increased diabetes and insulin treatment duration in type 2 diabetes mellitus [Cryer, 2008 b]. Recent clinical trials have better quantified the risk of hypoglycemia in both type 1 and type 2 diabetes [Leese et al., 2003; Pramming et al., 2000]. Severe hypoglycemia is operationally defined as an episode that the patient cannot self-treat, so that external help is required, regardless of the glucose concentration. Mild or moderate hypoglycemia refers to episodes that the patient can self-treat, regardless of the severity of symptoms, or when blood glucose levels are noted to be lower than 60 mg/dL. The incidence of mild or moderate hypoglycemia episodes is difficult to determine accurately because they are rarely reported, although they are common in insulin-treated patients [Gabriely & Shamoon, 2004]. Representative event rates for severe hypoglycemia in type 1 diabetes mellitus are from 62 to 170 episodes per 100 patient-years [MacLeod et al., 1993]. These reported during aggressive insulin therapy of type 2 diabetes mellitus range from 3 to 73 episodes per 100 patient-years [MacLeod et al., 1993]. When glucagon responses to hypoglycemia are deficient, epinephrine and autonomic warning symptoms become critical for the integrity of glucose counterregulation. Iatrogenic hypoglycemia attenuates the magnitude of adrenaline and autonomic symptom responses to a subsequent hypoglycemic episode [de Galan et al., 2006]. Any hypoglycemia can provoke this phenomenon [Bolli et al., 1984; Davis & Shamoon, 1991; White et al., 1983]. Consequently, a downward vicious cycle of worsening counterregulation and recurrent hypoglycemia may ultimately lead to hypoglycemia unawareness. Clinical syndrome of hypoglycemia unawareness is defined as onset of neuroglycopenia before the appearance of autonomic warning symptoms and typified clinically by the inability to perceive hypoglycemia by symptoms [de Galan et al., 2006]. Patients with hypoglycemia unawareness are unable to manifest adequate behavioral defenses against developing hypoglycemia, therefore, hypoglycemia unawareness is also associated with a high frequency of severe iatrogenic hypoglycemia [Gold et al., 1994]. These patients are at a specifically high risk for severe disabling hypoglycemia (e. g. complicated by coma or seizures) that requires external assistance [Gold et al., 1994]. Hypoglycemia unawareness is generally though to be the result of reduced sympathoadrenal responses and the resultant reduced neurogenic symptom responses to a given level of hypoglycemia [Cryer, 2002; Hepburn et al., 1991]. According to de Galan and colleagues [de Galan et al., 2006], various terms are used for the combination of defective hormonal counterregulation and hypoglycemia unawareness, as for example: counterregulatory failure, hypoglycemia-associated autonomic failure (HAAF), and hypoglycemia unawareness syndrome. A reduced sympathoadrenal response is the key feature of hypoglycemia-associated autonomic failure and, thus, the pathogenesis of iatrogenic hypoglycemia in diabetes [Cryer, 2006]. According to suggestion described by Cryer [Cryer, 2005] "The concept of HAAF in type 1 [Dagogo-Jack et al., 1993] and advanced type 2 [Segel et al., 2002] diabetes posits that recent antecedent iatrogenic hypoglycemia causes both defective glucose counterregulation (by reducing epinephrine responses to a given level of subsequent hypoglycemia in the setting of absent decrements in insulin and absent increments in glucagon) and hypoglycemia unawareness (by reducing sympathoadrenal and the resulting neurogenic symptom responses to a given level of subsequent hypoglycemia) a thus a vicious cycle of recurrent hypoglycemia". Reduced sympathoadrenal actions play a key role in the pathogenesis of both defective counterregulation and hypoglycemia unawareness and thus HAAF in diabetes [Cryer, 2004]. The mediators and mechanisms of HAAF are largely unknown [Cryer, 2005]. Different hypotheses are discussed [Cryer, 2001; Cryer, 2005; Cryer, 2006; Cryer et al., 2003; Cryer et al., 2009]. It is suggested that there are three causes of HAAF in diabetes: the originally recognized hypoglycemia-related HAAF, exercise-related HAAF, and sleep-related HAAF [Cryer, 2004]. The clinical impact of HAAF is well established in type 1 diabetes and it is less established in type 2 diabetes [Cryer, 2004]. Patients with iatrogenic hypoglycemia causes recurrent morbidity in most people with type 1 diabetes and many with type 2 diabetes, and it is sometimes fatal. Iatrogenic hypoglycemia often causes recurrent physical morbidity, recurrent or persistent psychosocial morbidity, or both and sometimes causes death [Cryer et al., 2003]. A direct relation between hypoglycemia and death has been proposed in the "dead-in-bed" syndrome [de Galan et al., 2006]. According to Maran et al. [1994] and Veneman et al. [1994], the dead-in-bed syndrome is rare disorder characterized by an unexpected death in young, previously healthy, tightly controlled patients with type 1 diabetes. Death in this syndrome is thought to be result of a fatal ventricular arrhythmia caused by hypoglycemia-induced lengthening of the QT interval [Bischof et al., 2004]. Corrected QT interval prolongation and increased QT dispersion have been demonstrated during acute-insulin-induced hypoglycemia in healthy subjects [Laitinen et al., 2008], in patients with type 1 and type 2 diabetes [Landstedt-Hallin et al., 1999; Rothenbuhler et al., 2008] or during nocturnal hypoglycemia in patients with type 1 diabetes [Murphy et al., 2004]. Myocardial cells can use either fatty acids or glucose oxidation as their source of energy [Stanley & Chandler, 2002]. Under normal conditions, the oxidation of fatty acids is prominent and in diabetic patients, the use of fatty acids is predominant [Lacherade et al., 2009]. During acute insulin-induced hypoglycemia or during nocturnal hypoglycemia in type 1 diabetes have been observed: cardiac rate and rhythm disturbances (tachycardia and brachycardia), and ventricular and atrial ectopy [Fisher et al., 1990; Gill et al., 2009; Laitinen et al., 2008]. Ventricular repolarization abnormalities appear to be the main feature observed during episodes of hypoglycemia [Lacherade et al., 2009]. It is not yet known to what extent hypoglycemia contributes to mortality in type 2 diabetes mellitus [Lacherade et al. 2009]. Hospitalization is required in a minority of patients, usually for observation of neurologic signs during hypoglycemia, such as seizures, obtundation, coma, or focal neurologic signs. The need for hospitalization arises most commonly in diabetic patients, although hypoglycemia is frequently identified in patients with malnutrition and associated alcohol consumption, mental illness, or severe underlying medical illness [Hart & Frier, 1998]. Hypoglycemia occurs in 1.2% of hospitalized patients and is of somewhat more diverse etiology [Fischer et al., 1986]. Hypoglycemia in diabetes is fundamentally the result of treatments that raise insulin levels and thus lower plasma glucose concentration.

5.1 Recommendations and prevention

Cryer and colleagues [Cryer et al., 2009] recommend "1) that both the conventional risk factors and those indicative of compromised defenses against hypoglycemia be considered in a patient with recurrent treatment-induced hypoglycemia, and 2) with a history of hypoglycemia unawareness, a 2- to 3-wk period of scrupulous evidence of avoidance of hypoglycemia". Patients with diabetes become concerned about the possibility of developing hypoglycemia when the self-monitored blood glucose concentration is falling rapidly or is no greater than 70 mg/dL [Cryer et al., 2009]. Therefore diabetic patients need to be well informed about: the symptoms of hypoglycemia, the physiologic factors that come into play, the time course of the drugs they use; how to prevent and treat episodes of hypoglycemia, how to monitor their blood glucose levels, and the warning symptoms of hypoglycemia [Gabriely & Shamoon, 2004]. One of the most important things to prevent hypoglycemia is to educate the patient. Patients should always have a rapidly available source of glucose with them to treat hypoglycemia at the first sign of low glucose. Briscoe & Davis [2006] suggest that: 1) if blood glucose is < 70 mg/dL, give 15 - 20 g of quick-acting carbohydrate; 2) if test blood glucose 15 minutes after treatment is still < 70 mg/dL, re-treat with 15 g of additional carbohydrate; 3) if blood glucose is not < 70 mg/dL but is > 1 hour until the next meal, have a snack with starch and protein; 4) keep glucagon injection kit available for patients who are unconscious or unable to take in oral carbohydrate. It is to note, that insulin preparations have different onsets of action, times of peak effect, and effective duration of action. These differences affect both glycemic control and hypoglycemic episodes. Therefore, these factors must be considered when adjusting the treatment. A history of recurrent hypoglycemia should be investigated.

5.2 Hypoglycemia in type 1 diabetes mellitus

5.2.1 Pathophysiology

Secretion of the three main counterregulatory hormones normally responsible for rapid reversal of hypoglycemia is severely disrupted in type 1 diabetes. Insulin secretion is either insignificant or absent and glucagon release during hypoglycemia is also impaired soon after the onset of diabetes. The plasma glucagon concentration does not increase as it should during hypoglycemia [Gerich et al., 1973]. This is because the pancreatic α-cell glucagon secretory response to hypoglycemia is irreversibly lost [Cryer, 2001 b; Cryer et al., 2003]. The mechanism of the absent glucagon response to hypoglycemia that characterizes established type 1 diabetes is not known [Cryer et al., 2003]. Epinephrine is the main defense against hypoglycemia in patients with type 1 diabetes of > 5 years duration [Briscoe & Davis, 2006]; however, epinephrine release during hypoglycemia becomes progressively defective in type 1 diabetes [Amiel et al., 1988; Bolli et al., 1983]. It is to note, that epinephrine secretory response to falling glucose levels is typically attenuated in type 1 diabetes [Amiel et al., 1988; Dagogo-Jack et al., 1993]. HAAF in type 1 diabetes apparently results from antecedent episodes of mild hypoglycemia that further degrade the counterregulatory response [Dagogo-Jack et al., 1993]. Patients with type 1 diabetes already have a reduced counterregulatory response, therefore HAAF may play a role in the vicious circle of hypoglycemia begetting hypoglycemia. It is to note, that avoidance of hypoglycemia in type 1 diabetes can improve the epinephrine response [Crauston et al., 1994]. Iatrogenic hypoglycemia in diabetes is the result of treatments that raise insulin levels and thus lower plasma glucose concentration. In type 1 diabetes iatrogenic hypoglycemia is the result of the interplay of relative or absolute insulin excess and compromised glucose counterregulation [Cryer, 2001]. It is suggested [Cryer, 2001] that absolute or relative insulin excess occurs when insulin or insulin secretagogue or sensitizer doses are excessive, exogenous glucose delivery is decreased, endogenous glucose production is decreased, glucose utilization is increased, sensitivity to insulin is increased, and insulin clearance is decreased. It is to note, that the conventional risk factors for iatrogenic hypoglycemia are based on the premise that absolute or relative insulin excess is the sole determinant of risk [Cryer, 2001]. In patients with type 1 diabetes, treated with insulin, insulin levels are unregulated and do not decrease until the subcutaneous depot is depleted, even though the plasma glucose levels may have started to fall. Insulin injected subcutaneously enters the circulation much slower and therefore elevated insulin levels persist considerably longer. Differences in insulin absorption may explain why a dose of insulin to maintain normoglycemia at one time may be too much at other times and creating a risk for hypoglycemia.

5.2.2 Frequency

In type 1 diabetes, the Diabetes Control and Complications Triad reported 62 severe hypoglycemic episodes per 100 patient-years [The DCCT Research Group, 1993]. Population-based studies in northern Europe reported 100 to 160 patient-years [Leese et al., 2003]. The average patient with type 1 diabetes suffers two episodes of symptomatic hypoglycemia per week, and one episode of temporarily disabling hypoglycemia (often with seizure or coma) per year [Cryer et al., 2009]. An estimated 2 to 4% of patients with type 1 diabetes die from hypoglycemia [Cryer et al., 2009]. In most instances, death cannot be attributed directly to hypoglycemia, but relates to the circumstances under which the hypoglycemic event envolved, e.g. in traffic, during swimming etc.

5.3 Hypoglycemia in type 2 diabetes mellitus

5.3.1 Pathophysiology

Type 2 diabetes is characterized by a range of metabolic disorders: chronic hyperglycemia, declining β-cell effectiveness resulting in the absence of first-phase insulin response to nutrient ingestion, insulin insensitivity in fat and muscle cells, and hepatic glucose production in the prandial state [Aronoff, 2004; DeFronzo, 2004]. The traditional primary defects responsible for the development and progression of type 2 diabetes are impaired insulin secretion, increased hepatic glucose production and decreased peripheral glucose utilization. Insulin secretion may be increased early in the course of type 2 diabetes, as the pancreas attempts to compensate for the elevated fasting plasma glucose concentration and underlying insulin resistance. Insulin resistance is a key pathologic defect that is characteristic feature of type 2 diabetes [DeFronzo, 2009]. The liver, muscle and adipose tissue are severely resistant to the action of insulin. The current type 2 diabetes disease model supports more aggressive treatment later in the course of disorder and less aggressive treatment in its earlier stages [Stolar, 2010]. Hypoglycemia is a major barrier to care for physicians and their patients with type 2 diabetes. Certain agents prescribed for type 2 diabetes significantly increase the risk of hypoglycemia, whereas others are associated with a lower occurrence of hypoglycemia [DeFronzo, 2010; Kushner, 2011]. Exogenous insulin preparations have all been associated with hypoglycemia. Injected insulin can produce absolute or relative insulin excess largely because of dosing and pharmacokinetics[Briscoe & Davis, 2006; Gabriely & Shamoon, 2004]. Oral antidiabetic medications can be a source of iatrogenic hypoglycemia in patients with type 2 diabetes. Sulfonylurea drugs enhance insulin secretion and are associated with hypoglycemia, especially in the elderly [Nathan et al., 2009]. Most reported cases of severe hypoglycemia were in patients taking chlorpropamide or glyburide [Gordon et al., 2009; Nathan et al., 2009]. Sulfonylurea drugs can interact with other agents to cause severe hypoglycemia. For example, the additive or possibly synergistic effects during combined insulin and sulfonylurea therapy account for an increasing number of such episodes. Metformin monotherapy is usually not associated with hypoglycemia. The frequency of severe hypoglycemia is lower with metformin than with sulfonylureas or insulin [Kushner, 2011; Gabriely & Shamoon, 2004]. Thiazolidinediones, that increase sensitivity of muscle, fat, and liver to endogenous and exogenous insulin, are associated with a low occurrence of hypoglycemia [Kushner, 2011]. However, these drugs, as monotherapy do not increase the risk for hypoglycemia, may cause hypoglycemia when insulin is used concomitantly [Gabriely & Shamoon, 2004]. α-Glucosidase inhibitors slow the rate of polysaccharide digestion in the small intestine, are not associated with hypoglycemia [Nathan et al., 2009]. The incretins and dipeptidyl peptidase-4 (DPP-4) inhibitors increase insulin secretion via a glucose-dependent mechanism. These agents do not increase the risk for hypoglycemia. Nonsulfonylurea insulin secretagogues, such as glinide, stimulate insulin secretion, and are known to increase the risk of hypoglycemia [Kushner, 2011]. Counterregulatory responses to hypoglycemia have been investigated less systematically in type 2 diabetes than in type 1 diabetes [Cryer, 2002; Gerich, 1988; Zammitt & Frier, 2005]. Although various counterregulatory hormone deficiencies have been described in type 2 diabetes, these were mostly mild, and epinephrine secretion was invariably preserved. The studies have shown that counterregulatory hormonal release occurs at higher blood glucose levels than in non-diabetic subjects and patients with type 1 diabetes [Levy et al., 1998; Spyer et al., 2000]. On the other hand, in type 2 diabetes, residual β-cell function largely preserves the first-line defence against hypoglycemia. Consequently, the glucagon response is retained, hypoglycemic risk is limited and further counterregulatory defects are prevented [Veneman et al., 1993].

5.3.2 Frequency

Episodes of severe hypoglycemia are much less frequent in patients with intensively treated type 2 diabetes than with type 1 diabetes [MacLeod et al., 1993]. Obtained results indicate that 8 to 31% of insulin-treated patients with type 2 diabetes report having trouble in correctly identifying hypoglycemic events [Hepburn et al., 1990]. These patients have a nine fold higher risk for severe iatrogenic hypoglycemia than patients with normal hypoglycemic awareness [Bottini et al., 1997]. A study of patients with sulfonylureas and/or metformin observed that 20% of those taking sulfonylureas had experience symptoms of hypoglycemia in the preceding 6 months [Jennings et al., 1989]. Frequency of hypoglycemia in type 2 diabetic patients in dependence on age, mode of therapy, nationality, sex etc. is described in details by Zammitt & Frier [2005]. To note, according to Rodbard and colleagues [Rodbard et al., 2009] "For some patients, the risk of hypoglycemia may warrant specific choices of therapy and reevaluation of therapeutic goals. These patients include those who have a duration of diabetes greater than 15 years and advanced macrovascular disease, hypoglycemia unawareness, limited life expectancy, or other serious comorbities".

6. References

Aguilar-Bryan L., & Bryan J. (2008). Neonatal diabetes mellitus. *Endocrine Reviews,* Vol.29, No.3, pp. 265-291, ISSN 0163-769X

Amiel S.A., Sherwin R.S., Simons D.C. & Tamborlane W.V. (1988). Effect of intensive insulin therapy on glycemic threshold for counterregulatory hormone release. *Diabetes,* Vol.37, No.3, pp. 901-907, ISSN 0012-1797

Aronoff S.L. (2004). Glucose metabolism and regulation: beyond insulin and glucagon. *Diabetes Spectrum,* Vol.17, No.3, pp. 183-189, ISSN 1040-9165

Aronoff S.L., Berhowitz K., Shreiner B. & Want L. (2004). Glucose metabolism and regulation: beyond insulin and glucagon. *Diabetes Spectrum,* Vol.17, No.3, pp. 183-190, ISSN 1040-9165

Assaf S.Y. & Chung S.H. (1984). Release of endogenous Zn^{2+} from brain tissue during activity. *Nature,* Vol.308, No.5961, pp. 734-736, ISSN 0028-0836

Atkinson M.A. & Eisenbarth G.S. (2001). Type 1 diabetes: new perspectives on disease pathogenesis and treatment. *Lancet,* Vol.358, No.9277, pp. 221-229, ISSN 1040-6736

Auer R., Hugh J., Cosgrove E. & Curry B. (1989). Neuropathologic findings in three cases of profound hypoglycemia. *Clinical Neuropathology,* Vol.8, No.2, pp. 63-68, ISSN 0722-5091, Kalimo H., Olsson Y. & Siesjo B.K. (1985). The temporal evolution of hypoglycemic brain damage. I. Light- and electro-microscopic findings in the rat cerebral cortex. *Acta Neuropathologica,* Vo.67, No.1-2, pp. 13-24, ISSN 0001-6322

Auer R.N., Kalima H., Olsson Y. & Siesjo B.K. (1984). Hypoglycemic brain injury in the rat. Correlation of density of brain damage with EEG isoelectric time: a quantitative study. *Diabetes,* Vol.33, No.1, pp. 1090-1098, ISSN 0012-1797

Avery M.D. & Rossi M.A. (1994). Gestational diabetes. *Journal of Nurse-Midwifery,* Vol.39, No.2, Suppl., pp. 9S-19S, ISSN 0730-7659

Bell G.I., Horita S. & Karam J.H. (1984). A polymorphic locus near the insulin gene is associated with insulin-dependent diabetes mellitus. *Diabetes,* Vol.33, No.2, pp. 176-183, ISSN 0012-1797

Ben-Ami H., Nagachandran P., Mendelson A. & Edoute Y. (1999). Drug-induced hypoglycemic coma in 102 diabetic patients. *Archives of Internal Medicine.* Vol.159, No.3, pp. 281-284, ISSN 0003-9926

Bischof M.G., Mlynarik V., Brehm A. et al. (2004). Brain energy metabolism during hypoglycemia in healthy and type 1 diabetic subjects. *Diabetologia,* Vol.47, No.4, pp. 648-651, ISSN 0012-186X

Bjorklund A., Adamson U., Andreasson K. et al. (1998). Hormonal counterregulation and subjective symptoms during induced hypoglycemia in insulin-dependent diabetes mellitus patients during and after pregnancy. *Acta Obstetricia et Gynecologica Scandinavica,* Vol.77, No.6, pp. 625-634, ISSN 0001-6349

Bjornholm M. & Zierath J. (2005). Insulin signal transduction in human skeletal muscle: identifying the defects in type 2 diabetes. *Biochemical Society Transactions,* Vol.33, No.Pt2, pp. 354-357, ISSN 0300-5127

Black E.E., Wagenmakers A.J., Glatz J.F. et al. (2000). Plasma FFA utilization and fatty acid-binding protein content are diminished in type 2 diabetic muscle. *American Journal of Physiology - Endocrinology and Metabolism,* Vol.279, No.1, pp. E146-E154, ISSN 0193- 1849

Boden G. (1999). Free fatty acids, insulin resistance, and type 2 diabetes mellitus. *Proceedings of the Association of American Physicians,* Vol.111, No.3, pp. 241-248, ISSN 1081-650X

Bolli G., de Feo P., Compagnucci P. et al. (1983). Abnormal glucose counterregulation in insulin-dependent diabetes mellitus: interaction of anti-insulin antibodies and impaired glucagon and epinephrine secretion. *Diabetes,* Vol.32, No.2, pp. 134-141, ISSN 0012-1797

Bolli G.B., De Feo P., Cosmo S. et al. (1984). A reliable and reproducible test for adequate glucose counterregulation in type 1 diabetes. *Diabetes,* Vol.33, No.8, pp. 732-737, ISSN 0012-1797

Bottini P., Boschetti E., Pampanelli S. et al. (1997). Contribution of autonomic neuropathy to reduced plasma adrenaline responses to hypoglycemia in IDDM: evidence for a nonselective defect. *Diabetes,* Vol.46, No.5, pp. 814-823, ISSN 0012-1797

Briscoe V.J. & Davis S.N. (2006). Hypoglycemia in type 1 and type 2 diabetes: physiology, pathophysiology, and management. *Clinical Diabetes,* Vol.24, No.3, pp. 115-121, ISSN 0891-8929

Brun J.F., Fedou C. & Mercier J. (2000). Postprandial reactive hypoglycemia. *Diabetes and Metabolism (Paris),* Vol.26, No.5, pp.337-351, ISSN 1262-3636

Butte N.F. (2000). Carbohydrate and lipid metabolism in pregnancy: normal compared with gestational diabetes mellitus. *The American Journal of Clinical Nutrition,* Vol.71, 5Suppl, pp. 1256S-1261S

Carroll M.F., Burge M.R. & Schade D.S. (2003). Severe hypoglycemia in adults. *Reviews in Endocrine and Metabolic Disorders,* Vol.4, No.2, pp. 149-157, ISSN 1389-9155

Charles M.A., Hofeldt F., Shackelford A. et al. (1981). Comparison of oral glucose tolerance tests and mixed meals in patients with apparent idiopathic postabsorptive hypoglycemia. *Diabetes,* Vol.30, No.6, pp.465-470, ISSN 0012-1797

Chen L.A. (2010). A literature review of intensive insulin therapy and mortality in critically ill patients. *Clinical Nurse Specialist,* Vol.24, No.2, pp. 80-86, ISSN 0887-6274

Cheung N.W. (2009). The management of gestational diabetes. *Vascular Health and Risk Management,* Vol.5, pp. 153-164, ISSN 1178-2048

Concannon P., Gogolin-Ewans K.J., Hinds D.A. et al (1998). A second-generation screen of the human genome for susceptibility to insulin-dependent diabetes mellitus. *Nature Genetics,* Vol.19, No.3, pp. 292-296, ISSN 1061-4036

Couston D.R., Reese E.A., Sherwin R.S. et al. (1986). A randomized clinical trial of insulin pump vs. intensive conventional therapy in diabetic pregnancies. *Journal of the American Medical Association,* Vol.255, No.5, pp. 631-636, ISSN 0002-9955

Cox N.J., Wapelhorst B., Morrison V.A. et al. (2001). Seven regions of the genome show evidence of linkage to type 1 diabetes in a consensus analysis of 767 multiplex families. *American Journal of Human Genetics,* Vol.69, No.4, pp. 820-830, ISSN 0002-9297

Cranston I., Lomas J., Maran A., Macdonald I. & Amiel S.A. (1994). Restoration of hypoglycemia unawareness in patients with long-duration insulin-dependent diabetes mellitus. *The Lancet,* Vol.344, No.8918, pp. 283-287, ISSN 0140-6736

Cryer P.E. (1992). Glucose homeostasis and hypoglycemia, In: *William's Textbook of Endocrinology.* J.D. Wilson, D.W. Foster (Ed.), 1223-1253, ISBN 0-7216-9514-0, Philadelphia, Pa

Cryer P. (2001 a). The prevention and correction of hypoglycemia. In: *Handbook of physiology: Section 7, the endocrine system. Vol.II. The endocrine pancreas and regulation of metabolism.* Jefferson L., Cherrington A., Goodman H. (Eds.), 1057-1092, ISBN 0195113268, New York: Oxford University Press

Cryer P.E. (2001 b). Hypoglycemia risk reduction in type 1 diabetes. *Experimental and Clinical Endocrinology & Diabetes,* Vol.109, Suppl.2, pp. S412-S423, ISSN 0947-7349

Cryer P.E. (2002). Hypoglycemia: the limiting factor of Type I and Type II diabetes. *Diabetologia,* Vol.45, No.7, pp. 937-948, ISSN 0012-186X

Cryer P.E. (2004). Diverse causes of hypoglycemia-associated autonomic failure in diabetes. *The New England Journal of Medicine,* Vol.350, No.22, pp. 2272-2279, ISSN 0028-4793

Cryer P.E. (2005). Mechanisms of hypoglycemia-associated autonomic failure and its component syndromes in diabetes. *Diabetes,* Vol.54, No.12, pp. 3592-3601, ISSN 0012- 1797

Cryer P.E. (2006). Mechanisms of sympathoadrenal failure and hypoglycemia in diabetes. *The Journal of Clinical Investigation,* Vol.116, No.6, pp. 14701473, ISSN 0021-9738

Cryer P.E. (2007). Hypoglycemia, functional brain failure, and brain death. *The Journal of Clinical Investigation,* Vol.117, No.4, pp. 868-870, ISSN 0021-9738

Cryer P. (2008 a). Glucose homeostasis and hypoglycemia. In: *Williams Textbook of Endocrinology* Kronenberg H., Melmed S., Polonsky K. et al (Eds.), 1503-1533, ISBN 978-1-4160-2911-3, Philadelphia: Saunders Elsevier

Cryer P.E. (2008 b). Hypoglycemia: still the limiting factor in the glycemic management of diabetes. *Endocrine Practice,* Vol.14, No.6, pp. 750-756, ISSN 1530-891X

Cryer P.E., Axelrod L., Grossman A.B. et al. (2009). Evaluation and management of adult hypoglycemic disorders: and endocrine society clinical practice guideline. *The Journal of Clinical Endocrinology and Metabolism,* Vol.94, No.3, pp. 709-728, ISSN 0021-972X

Cryer P.E., Davis S.N. & Shamoon H. (2003). Hypoglycemia in diabetes. *Diabetes Care,* Vol.26, No.6, pp. 1902-1912, ISSN 0149-5992

Dagogo-Jack S.E., Craft S. & Cryer P.E. (1993). Hypoglycemia-associated autonomic failure in insulin-dependent diabetes mellitus. *The Journal of Clinical Investigation,* Vol.91, No.3, pp. 819-828, ISSN 0021-9738

Davis M.R. & Shamoon H. (1991). Counterregulatory adaptation to recurrent hypoglycemia in normal humans. *Journal of Clinical Endocrinology and Metabolism,* Vol.73, No.5, pp. 995-1001, ISSN 0021-972X

DeFronzo R.A. (1988). The triumvirate: beta cell, muscle, liver - a conclusion responsible for NIDDM. *Diabetes,* Vol. 37, No.6, pp. 667-684, ISSN 0012-1797

DeFronzo R.A. (2004). Pathogenesis of type 2 diabetes mellitus. *Medical Clinics of North America,* Vol.88, No.4, pp. 787-835, ISSN 0025-7125

DeFronzo R.A. (2009). From the triumvirate to the ominous octet: a new paradigm for the treatment of type 2 diabetes mellitus [Banting Lecture]. *Diabetes,* Vol. 58, No.4, pp. 773-795, ISSN 0012-1797

DeFronzo R.A. (2010). Overview of newer agents: where treatment is going. *The American Journal of Medicine,* Vol.123, No.3A, pp. S38-S48, ISSN 0002-9343

de Galan B.E., Schouwenberg B.J.J.W., Tack C.J. & Smits P. (2006). Pathophysiology and management of recurrent hypoglycaemia and hypoglycaemia unawareness in diabetes. *The Netherlands Journal of Medicine,* Vol.64, No.8, pp. 269-279, ISSN 0300-2977

Diaz R., Aparicio J., Mendizábal A., Faus M. et al. (2008). Paraneoplastic hyperinsulinism and secondary hypoglycemia in a patient with advanced colon cancer: A rare association. *World Journal of Gastroenterology,* Vol.14, No.12, pp. 1952-1954. ISSN 1007- 9327

Doria A., Patti M-E. & Kahn C.R. (2008). The emerging genetic architecture of type 2 diabetes. *Cell Metabolism,* Vol.8, No.3, pp. 186-200, ISSN 1550-4131

Dorman J.S. & Bunker C.H. (2000). HLA-DQ locus of the human leucocyte antigen complex and type 1 diabetes mellitus: a HUGE review. *Epidemiological Reviews,* Vol.22, No.2, pp. 218-227, ISSN 0193-936X

Drucker D.J. (2007). The role of gut hormones in glucose homeostasis. *The Journal of Clinical Investigation,* Vol.117, No.1, pp. 24-30, ISSN 0021-9738

Ecker J.L., Greenberg J.A., Norwitz E.R. et al. (1997). Birth weight as a predictor of brachial plexus injury. *Obstetrics and Gynecology,* Vol.89, No.5Pt1, pp. 643-647, ISSN 0029-7844

Engelsen B., Westerberg E., Fonnum F. & Wieloch T. (1986). Effect of insulin-induced hypoglycemia on the concentrations of glutamate and related amino acids and energy metabolism in the intact and decorticated rat neostriatum. *Journal of Neurochemistry,* Vol.47, No.5, pp. 1634-1641, ISSN 0022-3042

Fajans S.S., Bell G.I. & Polonsky K.S. (2001). Molecular mechanisms and clinical pathophysiology of maturity-onset diabetes of the young. *The New England Journal of Medicine,* Vol.345, No.13, pp. 971-980, ISSN 0028-4793

Fischer K.F., Lees J.A. & Newman J.H. (1986). Hypoglycemia in hospitalized patients. Causes and outcomes. *The New England Journal of Medicine,* Vol.315, No.20, pp. 1245- 1250, ISSN 0028-4793

Fisher J.M., Gillen G., Hepburn D.A., Dargie H.J. & Frier B.M. (1990). Cardiac responses to acute insulin-induced hypoglycemia in humans. *American Journal of Physiology. Heart and Circulatory Physiology,* Vol.258, No.6 Pt 2, pp. H1775-H1779, ISSN 0363-6135

Foster D.W. & Rubenstein A.H. (1998). Hypoglycemia. In: *Harrison's Principles of Internal Medicine* 14th ed. Fauci A.S., Braunwald E., Isselbacher K.J. (Eds.), 2081-2087, ISBN 0-07-020291, New York: McGraw-Hill

Foulis A.K., Mc Gill M. & Farquharson M.A. (1991). Insulitis in type 1 (insulin-dependent) diabetes mellitus in man - macrophages, lymphocytes, and interferon-gamma containing cells. *The Journal of Pathology,* Vol.165, No.2, pp. 97-103, ISSN 1096-9896

Gabriely I. & Shamoon H. (2004). Hypoglycemia in diabetes: common, often unrecognized. *Cleveland Clinic Journal of Medicine,* Vol.71, No.4, pp. 335-347, ISSN 0891-1150

Garner P. (1995). Type 1 diabetes mellitus and pregnancy. *Lancet,* Vol.346, No.8968, pp. 157-161, ISSN 0140-6736

Garza H. (2009). Minimizing the risk of hypoglycemia in older adults: a focus on long-term care. *The Consultant Pharmacist,* Vol.24, Suppl.B, pp. 18-24, ISSN 0888-5109

Gerich J.E. (1988). Glucose counterregulation and its impact on diabetes mellitus. *Diabetes,* Vol.37, No.12, pp. 1608-1617, ISSN 0012-1797

Gerich J.E. (1993). Control of glycemia. *Baillier's Best Practice and Research in Clinical Endocrinology & Metabolism,* Vol.7, No.3, pp.551-586, ISSN 0145-7217

Gerich J.E., Langlois M., Noacco C., Karam J.H. & Forsham P.H. (1973). Lack of glucagon response to hypoglycemia in diabetes: evidence for an intrinsic pancreatic alpha cell defect. *Science,* Vol.182, No.4108, pp. 171-173, ISSN 0036-8075

Gilespie K.M. (2006). Type 1 diabetes: pathogenesis and prevention (Review). *Canadian Medical Association Journal,* Vol.175, No.2, pp. 165-170, ISSN 0820-3946

Gill G.V., Woodward A., Casson J.F. & Weston P.J. (2009). Cardiac arrhythmia and nocturnal hypoglycemia in type 1 diabetes - the "dead in bed" syndrome revisited. *Diabetologia,* Vol.52, No.1, pp. 42-45, ISSN 0012-186X

Gold A.E., MacLeod K.M. & Frier B.M. (1994). Frequency of severe hypoglycemia in patients with type 1 diabetes with impaired awareness of hypoglycemia. *Diabetes Care,* Vol.17, No.7, pp. 697-703, ISSN 0149-5992

Gordon M.R., Flockhart D., Zawadzki J.K., Taylor T., Ramey J.N. & Eastman R.C. (1988). Hypoglycemia due to inadvertent dispensing of chlorpropamide. *The American Journal of Medicine,* Vol.85, No.2, pp. 271-272, ISSN 0002-9343

Guettier J.M. & Gorden P. (2006). Hypoglycemia. *Endocrinology and Metabolism Clinics of North America,* Vol.35, No.4, pp. 753-766, ISSN 0889-8529

Gustafsson J. (2009). Neonatal energy substrate production. *Indian Journal of Medical Research,* Vol.130, No.5, pp. 618-623, ISSN 0019-5340

Haller M.J., Atkinson M.A. & Schatz D. (2005) Type 1 Diabetes Mellitus: Etiology, presentation and management. *Pediatric Clinics of North America,* Vol.52, No.6, pp. 1553-1578, ISSN 0031-3955

Hapo Study Cooperative Research Group. (2008). Hyperglycemia and adverse pregnancy outcomes. *The New England Journal of Medicine,* Vol.358, pp. 1991-2002, ISSN 0028-4793

Hart S.P. & Frier B.M. (1998). Causes, management and morbidity of acute hypoglycemia in adults requiring hospital admission. *QJM: An International Journal of Medicine,* Vol.91, No.7, pp. 505-510, ISSN 1460-2725

Hathout E.H., Sharkey J., Racine M. et al. (2000). Diabetic autoimmunity in infants and preschoolers with type 1 diabetes. *Pediatric Diabetes,* Vol.1, No.3, pp. 131-134, ISSN 1399-543X

Hepburn D.A., Patrick A.W., Brash H.M., Thomson L. & Frier B.M. (1991). Hypoglycemia unawareness in type 1 diabetes: a lower plasma glucose is required to stimulate sympathoadrenal activation. *Diabetic Medicine,* Vol.8, No.10, pp. 934-945, ISSN 1464-5491

Hepburn D.A., Patrick A.W., Eadington D.W., Ewing D.J. & Frier B.M. (1990). Unawareness of hypoglycaemia in insulin-treated diabetic patients: prevalence and relationship to autonomic neuropathy. *Diabetic Medicine,* Vol.7, No.8, pp. 711-7117, ISSN 0742-3071

Hod M., Merlob P., Friedman S. et al. (1991). Gestational diabetes mellitus: A survey of perinatal complications in the 1980s. *Diabetes,* Vol.40, Suppl.2, pp. 74-78, ISSN 0012-1797

Holleman F., Schmitt H., Rottiers R., Rees A., Symanowski S. & Anderson J.H (1997). Reduced frequency of severe hypoglycemia and coma in well-controlled IDDM patients treated with insulin lispro. The Benelux-UK Insulin Lispro Study Group. *Diabetes Care,* Vol.20, No.12, pp. 1827-1832, ISSN 0149-5992

Ito T., Otsuki M., Igarashi H. et al. (2010). Epidemiological study of pancreatic diabetes in Japan in 2005: A nationwide study. *Pancreas,* Vol.39, No.6, pp. 829-835, ISSN 0885-3177

Jayaprasad N., Anees T., Bijin T. & Madhusoodanan S. (2006). Severe hypoglycemia due to poorly differentiated hepatocellular carcinoma. *The Journal of the Association of Physicians of India,* Vol.54, pp. 413-415, ISSN 0004-5772

Jennings A.M., Wilson R.M. & Ward J.D. (1989). Symptomatic hypoglycemia in NIDDM patients treated with oral hypoglycemic agents. *Diabetes Care,* Vol.12, No.3, pp. 203-207, ISSN 0149-5992

Johnson J.D. (2007). Pancreatic beta-cell apoptosis in maturity onset diabetes of the young. *Canadian Journal of Diabetes,* Vol.31, No.1, pp. 67-74, ISSN 1499-2671

Kar P., Price P., Sawers S., Bhattacharya S., Reznek R.H. & Grossman A.B. (2006). Insulinomas may present with normoglycemia after prolonged fasting but glucose-stimulated hypoglycemia. *The Journal of Clinical Endocrinology and Metabolism,* Vol.91, No.12, pp. 4733-4736, ISSN 0021-972

Kimmerle R., Heinemann L., Delecki A. et al. (1992). Severe hypoglycemia incidence and predisposing factors in 85 pregnancies of type I diabetic women. *Diabetes Care,* Vol.15, No.8, pp. 1034-1037, ISSN 0149-5992

Koivisto V.A. & Felig P. (1978). Effects of leg exercise on insulin absorption in diabetic patients. *The New England Journal of Medicine,* Vol.298, pp. 79-83, ISSN 0028-4793

Koukkou E., Watts G.F. & Lowy C. (1996). Serum lipid, lipoprotein and apolipoprotein changes in gestational diabetes mellitus: a cross-sectional and prospective study. *Journal of Clinical Pathology,* Vol.49, pp. 634-637, ISSN 0021-9746

Kushner P. (2011). Minimizing the risk of hypoglycemia in patients with type 2 diabetes mellitus. *Diabetes, Metabolic Syndrome and Obesity: Targets and Therapy,* Vol.3, pp. 49-53, ISSN 1178-7007

Lacherade J-C, Jacqueminet S. & Preiser J-C. (2009). An overview of hypoglycemia in the critically ill. *Journal of Diabetes Science and Technology,* Vol.3, No.6, pp. 1242-1249, ISSN 1932-2968

Laitinen T., Lyyra-Laitinen T., Huopio H. et al. (2008). Electrocardiographic alterations during hyperinsulinemic hypoglycemia in healthy subjects. *Annals of Noninvasive Electrocardiology,* Vol.13, No.2, pp. 97-105, ISSN 1082-720X

Landstedt-Hallin L., Euglund A., Adamson U. & Lins P.E. (1999). Increased QT dispersion during hypoglycemia in patients with type 2 diabetes mellitus. *Journal of Internal Medicine,* Vol.246, No.3, pp. 299-307, ISSN 1365-2796

Langer O. & Conway D.L. (2000). Level of glycemia and perinatal outcome in pregestational diabetes. *Journal of Maternal-Fetal Medicine,* Vol.9, No.1, pp. 35-41, ISSN 1476-4954

Langer O. & Mazze R. (1988). The relationship between large-for-gestational age infants and glycemic control in women with gestational diabetes. *American Journal of Obstetrics and Gynecology,* Vol.159, No.6, pp. 1478-1483, ISSN 0002-9378

Leese G.P., Wang J., Broomhall J. et al. (2003). Frequency of severe hypoglycemia requiring emergency treatment in type 1 and type 2 diabetes: a population based study of health service resource use. *Diabetes Care,* Vol.26, No.4, pp. 1176-1180, ISSN 0149-5992

Levy C.J., Kinsley B.T., Bajaj M. & Simons D.C. (1998). Effect of glycemic control on glucose counterregulation during hypoglycemia in NIDDM. *Diabetes Care,* Vol.21, No.8, pp. 1330-1338, ISSN 0149-5992

Lin Y. & Sun Z. (2010). Current views on type 2 diabetes. *Journal of Endocrinology,* Vol. 204, pp. 1-11, ISSN 0022-0795

MacLeod K.M., Hepburn D.A. & Frier B.M. (1993). Frequency and morbidity of severe hypoglycemia in insulin-treated diabetic patients. *Diabetic Medicine,* Vol.10, No.3, pp. 238-245, ISSN 0742-3071

Majithia A.R. & Florez C.J. (2009). Clinical translation of genetic predictors for type 2 diabetes. *Current Opinion in Endocrinology, Diabetes and Obesity,* Vol.16, No.2, pp. 100- 106, ISSN 1072-296X

Malouf R. & Brust J.C.M. (1985) Hypoglycemia: causes, neurological manifestations, and outcome. *Annals of Neurology,* Vol.17, No.5, pp. 421-430, ISSN 0364-5134

Maran A., Cranston I., Lomas J., Macdonald I. & Amiel S.A. (1994). Protection by lactate of cerebral function during hypoglycemia (see comments). *The Lancet,* Vol.343, No.8888, pp. 16-20, ISSN 0140-6736

Martin A.O., Simpson J.L., Ober C. & Freinkel N. (1985). Frequency of diabetes mellitus in mothers of probands with gestational diabetes: possible maternal influence on the predisposition to gestational diabetes. *American Journal of Obstetrics and Gynecology,* Vol.151, No.4, pp. 471-475, ISSN 0002-9378

Mauvais-Jarvis F. & Kahn C.R. (2000). Understanding the pathogenesis and treatment of insulin resistance and type 2 diabetes mellitus: what can we learn from transgenic and knockout mice? *Diabetes Metabolism (Paris),* Vol.26, No.6, pp. 433-448, ISSN 0338- 1684

McAulay V, Deary I.J. & Frier B.M. (2001). Symptoms of hypoglycaemia in people with diabetes. *Diabetic Medicine,* Vol.18, No.9, pp. 690-705, ISSN 0742-3071

McLellan J.A., Barrow B.A., Levy J.C. et al. (1995). Prevalence of diabetes mellitus and impaired glucose tolerance in parents of women with gestational diabetes. *Diabetologia,* Vol. 38, No.6, pp. 693-698, ISSN 0012-186X

Mengesha Y., Frezghi E. & Gebremichael A. (2007). A neonate with persistent hypoglycemia and seizures. *Journal of the Eritrean Medical Association,* Vo.2, No.1, pp. 35-37, ISSN 1998-6017

Merimee T.J. & Tyson J.E. (1974). Stabilization of plasma glucose during fasting. Normal variation in two separate studies. *The New England Journal of Medicine,* Vol.291, No.24, pp. 1275-1278, ISSN 0028-4793

Metzger B.E. (1991). 1920 overview of GDM. Accomplishment of the last decade-challenges for the future. *Diabetes,* Vol.40, Suppl.2, pp. 1-2, ISSN 0012-1797

Mitchell S.M. & Frayling T.M. (2002). The role of transcription factors in maturity-onset diabetes of the young. *Molecular Genetics and Metabolism,* Vol.77, No.1-2, pp. 35-43, ISSN 1096-7192

Murad M.H., Coto-Yglesias F., Wang A.T. et al. (2009). Drug-induced hypoglycemia: a systematic review. *The Journal of Clinical Endocrinology and Metabolism,* Vol.94, No.3, pp. 741-745, ISSN 0021-972

Murphy N.P., Ford-Adams M.E., Ong K.K. et al. (2004). Prolonged cardiac repolarisation during spontaneous nocturnal hypoglycemia in children and adolescent with type 1 diabetes. *Diabetologia,* Vol.47, No.11, pp. 1940-1947, ISSN 0012-186X

Nathan D.M., Buse J.B., Davidson M.B. et al. (2009). Medical management of hypoglycemia in type 2 diabetes: A consensus algorithm for the initiation and adjustment of therapy: A consensus statement of the American Diabetes Association and the European Association for the Study of Diabetes. *Diabetes Care,* Vol.32, No.1, pp. 193-203, ISSN 0149-5992

Nellgard B. & Wieloch T. (1992). Cerebral protection by AMPA- and NMDA-receptor agonists administered after severe insulin-induced hypoglycemia. *Experimental Brain Research,* Vol.92, pp. 259-266, ISSN 0014-4819

Neve B., Fernandez-Zapico M.E., Ashkenazi-Katalan V. et al. (2005). Role of transcription factor KLF11 and its diabetes-associated gene variants in pancreatic beta cell function. *Proceedings of the National Academy of Sciences, USA,* Vol.102, No.13, pp. 4807-4812, ISSN 0027-8424

Ng C.L. (2010). Hypoglycemia in nondiabetic patients. *Australian Family Physician,* Vol.39, No.6, pp. 399-404, ISSN 0300-8495

Patockova J., Marhol P, Tumova E. et al. (2003). Oxidative stress in the brain tissue of laboratory mice with acute post insulin hypoglycemia. *Physiological Research,* Vol.52, No.1, pp. 131-135, ISSN 0862-8408

Peakman M. (2001). Advance in understanding the immunopathology of type 1 diabetes mellitus. *CPD Bulletin of Immunology and Allergy,* Vol.2, No.1, pp. 23-26, ISSN 1367-8949

Perkins J.M., Dunn J.P. & Jagasia S.M. (2007). Perspectives in gestational diabetes mellitus: a review of screening, diagnosis, and treatment. *Clinical Diabetes,* Vol.25, No.2, pp. 57-62, ISSN 0891-8929

Perley M.J. & Kipnis D.M. (1967). Plasma insulin response to oral and intravenous glucose studies in normal and diabetic studies. *The Journal of Clinical Investigation,* Vol.46, No.12, pp. 1954-1962, ISSN 0021-9738

Persson B. & Hanson U. (1998). Neonatal morbidities in gestational diabetes mellitus. *Diabetes Care,* Vol.21, Suppl.2, pp. B79-B84, ISSN 0149-5992

Phielix E., & Mensink M. (2008). Type 2 diabetes mellitus and skeletal muscle metabolic function. *Physiology & Behavior,* Vol.94, No.2, pp. 252-258, ISSN 0031-9384

Pickup J. & Keen H. (2002). Continuous subcutaneous insulin infusion at 25 years: evidence base for the expanding use of insulin pump therapy in type 1 diabetes. *Diabetes Care,* Vol.25, No.3, pp. 593-598, ISSN 0149-5992

Pieber T.R., Eugene-Jolchine I. & Derobert E. (2000). Efficacy and safety of HOE 901 versus NPH insulin in patients with type 1 diabetes. The European Study Group of HOE 901 in type 1 diabetes. *Diabetes Care,* Vol.23, No.2, pp. 157-162, ISSN 0149-5992

Poulsen P., Kyvik K.O., Vaag A. & Beck-Nielsen H. (1999). Heritability of type II (non- insulin-dependent) diabetes mellitus and abnormal glucose tolerance - a population-based twin study. *Diabetologia,* Vol.42, No.2, pp. 139-145, ISSN 0012-186X

Pramming S., Pedersen-Bjergaard U., Heller S.P. et al. Severe hypoglycemia in unselected patients with type 1 diabetes: a cross sectional multicentre survey. *Diabetologia,* Vol.43, Suppl.1, A194, ISSN 0012-186X

Pugh S.K., Doherty D.A., Maganu E.F., Chauhan S.P., Hill J.B. & Morrison J.C. (2009). Does hypoglycemia following a glucose challenge test identity a high risk pregnancy. *Reproductive Health,* Vol.6, No10, ISSN 1742-4755

Rabinovitch A. (2000). Autoimmune diabetes mellitus. *Science and Medicine,* Vol.7, No.3, pp. 18-27, ISSN 1087-3309

Ridderstrale M. & Groop L. (2009). Genetic dissection of type 2 diabetes. *Molecular and Cellular Endocrinology,* Vol.297, No.1-2, pp. 10-17, ISSN 0303-7207

Risch N. (1987). Assessing the role of HLA-linked and unlinked determinants of disease. *American Journal of Human Genetics,* Vol.40, No.1, pp. 1-14, ISSN 0002-9297

Robinson A.M. & Williamson D.H. (1980). Physiological roles of ketone bodies as substrate and signals in mammalian tissues. *Physiological Reviews,* Vol.60, No.1, ISSN 0031-9333

Rodbard H.W., Jellinger P.S., Davidson J.A. et al. (2009). Statement by an American Association of Clinical Endocrinologists/American College of Endocrinology Consensus Panel on Type 2 Diabetes Mellitus: and algorithm for glycemic control. *Endocrine Practice,* Vol.15, No.6, pp. 540-558, ISSN 1530-891X

Rosenn B., Miodovnik M., Holcberg G., Khoury J.C. & Siddigi T.A. (1995). Hypoglycemia: the price of intensive insulin therapy for pregnant women with insulin dependent diabetes mellitus. *Obstetrics and Gynecology,* Vol.85, No.3, pp. 417-422, ISSN 0029-7844

Rosenstock J., Schwartz S.L., Clark C.M. et al. (2001). Basal insulin therapy in type 2 diabetes: 28-week comparison of insulin glargine (HOE 901) and NPH insulin. *Diabetes Care,* Vol.24, No.4, pp. 631-636, ISSN 0149-5992

Rothenbuhler A., Bibal C.P., Le Fur S. & Bougneres P. (2008). Effects of controlled hypoglycemia test on QTc in adolescent with Type 1 diabetes. *Diabetic Medicine,* Vol.25, No.12, pp. 1483-1485, ISSN 0742-3071

Scollan-Kolippoulos M., Guadagno S. & Walker E. (2006). Gestational diabetes management: guidelines to a healthy pregnancy. *Nurse Practitioner,* Vol.31, No.6, pp. 14-19, ISSN 0361-1817

Segel S.A., Paramore D.S. & Cryer P.E. (2002). Hypoglycemia-associated autonomic failure and advanced in type 2 diabetes. *Diabetes,* Vol.51, No.3, pp. 724-733, ISSN 0012-1797

Sepe S.J., Connell F.A., Geiss L.S. et al. (1985). Gestational diabetes: Incidence maternal characteristics and perinatal outcome. *Diabetes,* Vol.34, Suppl.2, pp. 13-16, ISSN 0012- 1797

Service F.J. (1995). Hypoglycemic disorders. *The New England Journal of Medicine,* Vol.332, No.17, pp. 1144-1152, ISSN 0028-4793

Service F.J. (1999). Classification of hypoglycemic disorders. *Endocrinology and Metabolism Clinics of North America,* Vol.28, No.3, pp. 501-517, ISSN 0889-8529

Service F.J., McMahon M.M., O'Brien P.C. et al. (1991). Functioning insulinoma: incidence, recurrence, and long-term survival of patients. *Mayo Clinic Proceedings,* Vol.66, No.7, pp. 711-719, ISSN 0025-6196

Shield J.P. (2000). Neonatal diabetes: new insights into aetiology and implications. *Hormone Research,* Vol.53, Suppl.1, pp. 7-11, ISSN 0301-0163

Shorr R.I., Ray W.A., Daugherty J.R., Griffin M.R. (1997). Antihypertensives and the risk of serious hypoglycemia in older persons using insulin and sulfonylureas. *Journal of the American Medical Association,* Vol.278, No.1, pp. 40-43, ISSN 0002-9955

Singh P., Jain A. & Kaur G. (2004). Impact of hypoglycemia and diabetes on CNS: correlation of mitochondrial oxidative stress with DNA damage. *Molecular and Cellular Biochemistry,* Vol.260, No.1-2, pp. 153-159, ISSN 0300-8177

Spyer G., Hattersley A., Macdonald I.A., Amiel S. & MacLeod K.M. (2000). Hypoglycemic counterregulation at normal blood glucose concentrations in patients with well controlled type 2 diabetes. *The Lancet,* Vol.356, No.9246, pp. 1970-1974, ISSN 1470- 2045

Staiger H., Machicao F., Fritsche A. & Häing H-U. (2009). Pathomechanisms of type 2 diabetes genes. *Endocrine Reviews,* Vol.30, No.6, pp. 557-585, ISSN 0163-769X

Stanley W.C. & Chandler M.P. (2002). Energy metabolism in the normal and failing heart: potential for therapeutic interventions. *Heart Failure Reviews,* Vol.7, No.2, pp. 115-130, ISSN 1382-4147

Stolar M. (2010). Glycemic control and complications in type 2 diabetes mellitus. *The American Journal of Medicine,* Vol.123, No.3A, pp. S3-S11, ISSN 0002-9343

Suh S.W., Gum E.T., Hamby A.M., Chan P.H. & Swanson R.A. (2007). Hypoglycemic neuronal death is triggered by glucose reperfusion and activation of neuronal NADH oxidase. *The Journal of Clinical Investigation,* Vol.117, No.4, pp. 910-918, ISSN 0021-9738

Swinnen S.G., Dain M.P., Aronson R. et al. (2010). A 24-week, randomized, treat-to-target trial comparing initiation of insulin glargine once-daily with insulin detemir twice-daily in patients with type 2 diabetes inadequately controlled on oral glucose-lowering drugs. *Diabetes Care,* Vol.33, No.6, pp. 1176-1178, ISSN 0149-5992

Szablewski L. (2011). *Glucose homeostasis and insulin resistance,* Bentham E-Books, eISBN 978-1-60805-189-2, 2011

Tattersal R.B. (1974). Mild familial diabetes with dominant inheritance. *Quarterly Journal of Medicine,* Vol.43, No.170, pp. 339-357, ISSN 1460-2725

Tattersal R.B. & Fajans S.S. (1975). A difference between the inheritance of classical juvenile-onset and maturity-onset type diabetes of young people. *Diabetes,* Vol.24, No.1, pp. 44-53, ISSN 0012-1797

The DCCT Research Group. (1993). The effect of intensive treatment of diabetes on the development and progression of long-term complications in insulin-dependent diabetes mellitus. *The New England Journal of Medicine,* Vol.329, No.14, pp. 977-986, ISSN 0028-4793

Todd J.A. (1999). From genome to aetiology in a multifactorial disease type-1 diabetes. *BioEssays,* Vol.21, No.2, pp. 164-173, ISSN 0265-9247

Todd J.A. & Wicker L.S. (2001) Genetic protection from the inflammatory disease type 1 diabetes in humans and animal models. *Immunity,* Vol.15, No.3, pp. 387-395, ISSN 1074-7613

Towler D.A., Havlin C.E., Craft S. et al. (1993). Mechanisms of awareness of hypoglycemia: perception of neurogenic predominately cholinergic rather than neuroglycopenic symptoms. *Diabetes,* Vol.42, No.12, pp. 1791-1798, ISSN 0012-1787

Van Staa T., Abenhaim L. & Monette J. (1997). Rates of hypoglycemia in users of sulfonylureas. *Journal of Clinical Epidemiology,* Vol.50, No.6, pp. 735-741, ISSN 0895- 4356

Veneman T., Mitrakou A., Mokan M., Cryer P. & Gerich J. (1993). Induction of hypoglycemia unawareness by asymptomatic nocturnal hypoglycemia. *Diabetes,* Vol.42, No.9, pp. 1233-1237, ISSN, 0012-1797

Veneman T., Mitrakou A., Mokan M., Cryer P. & Gerich J. (1994). Effect of hyperketonemia and hyperlacticacidemia on symptoms, cognitive dysfunction, and counterregulatory hormone response during hypoglycemia in normal humans. *Diabetes,* Vol.43, No.11, pp. 1311-1317, ISSN, 0012-1797

von Muhlendahl K.E. & Herkenhoff H. (1995). Long-term course of neonatal diabetes. *The New England Journal of Medicine,* Vol. 333, No.11, pp. 704-708, ISSN 0028-4793

Wagaarachchi P.T., Fernand L., Premachadra P. & Fernand D.J.S. (2001). Screening based on risk factors in an Asian population. *Journal of Obstetrics and Gynecology,* Vol.21, No.1, pp. 32-34, ISSN 0144-3615

Wahren J., Ekberg K., Fernquist-Forbes E. & Nair S. (1999). Brain substrate utilization during acute hypoglycemia. *Diabetologia,* Vol.42, No.7, pp. 812-818, ISSN 0012-186X

Warram J.H., Krolewski A.S. & Kahn C.R. (1988). Determinants of IDDM and perinatal mortality in children of diabetic mothers. *Diabetes,* Vol.37, No.10, pp. 1328-1334, ISSN 0012-1797

Watanabe R.M., Black M.H., Xiang A.H., Allayee H., Lawrance J.M. & Buchanan T.A. (2007). Genetics of gestational diabetes mellitus and type 2 diabetes. *Diabetes Care,* Vol.30, Suppl.2, pp. S134-S140, ISSN 0149-5992

Wender R., Brown A.M., Fern R., Swanson R.A., Farrell K. & Ransom B.R. (2000). Astrocytic glycogen influences axon function and survival during glucose deprivation in central white matter. *The Journal of Neuroscience,* Vol.20, No.18, pp. 6804-6810, ISSN 0270- 6474

White N.H., Skor D.A., Cryer P.E., Levandoski L.A., Bier D.M. & Santiago J.V. (1983). Identification of type I diabetic patients at increased risk for hypoglycemia during intensive therapy. *The New England Journal of Medicine,* Vol. 308, No.9, pp. 485-491, ISSN 0028-4793

Zammitt N.N. & Frier B.M. (2005). Hypoglycemia in type 2 diabetes. Pathophysiology, frequency and effects of different treatment modalities. *Diabetes Care,* Vol.28, No.12, pp. 2948-2961, ISSN 0149-5992

Part 5

Section E

13

Neurologic Manifestations of Hypoglycemia

William P. Neil and Thomas M. Hemmen
University of California, San Diego
United States of America (USA)

1. Introduction

Unlike most other body tissues, the brain requires a continuous supply of glucose. It has very limited endogenous glycogen stores, and does not produce glucose intrinsically.[1] Although it accounts for 2% of body weight, the brain utilizes 25% of the body's glucose due to its high metabolic rate.[2, 3] Evidence for the brains sole reliance on glucose came from obtaining a respiratory quotient of one after measuring differences between arterial and venous content of oxygen and carbon dioxide in blood traveling through the brain.[4]

In the past, neurons were thought to directly metabolize glucose, however, more recent studies suggest astrocytes may play an important role in glucose metabolism.[5] Astrocytic foot processes surround brain capillaries, which deliver glucose to the brain. With this, they form the first cellular barrier for entering glucose.[5] Astrocytes contain the non-insulin dependent GLUT1 transporter, as well as the insulin dependent GLUT4 transporter, suggesting a possible role for astrocytes in regulating and storing brain glucose in an insulin dependent and independent manner (see figure 1).[6-8]

In addition to glucose, the brain contains a very limited store of glycogen, (between 0.5 and 1.5 g, or about 0.1% of total brain weight). Unlike peripheral tissue, where glycogen is readily mobilized during hypoglycemia, the brain can only function normally for a limited duration. Glycogen content seems to fall in areas of highest brain metabolic rate, suggesting at least some, albeit limited role as fuel during hypoglycemia.[7]

Although the brain relies primarily on glucose during normal conditions, it can use ketone bodies during starvation. These ketone bodies cannot however meet all of the metabolic demands of the brain.[9]

2. Pathophysiology

The brain areas most vulnerable to hypoglycemia are (in order) the subiculum, small and medium sized caudate neurons, area CA1 of the hippocampus, the dentate gyrus and superficial cortical layers, specifically layers 2 and 3.[10] Damage induced by hypoglycemia in the rat brain was not limited to a particular type of neuron, but those near the cerebrospinal fluid (CSF) spaces seemed to be more vulnerable.[10] Similar distribution of injury was shown in autopsy of three human subjects with hypoglycemia.[11]

Excitatory amino acids such as glutamate and aspartate were found in larger than normal quantities in the CSF space of hypoglycemic animals.[12, 13] These increases occur as a result of less glucose as a substrate for the tricarboxylic acid (TCA) cycle during hypoglycemia. Lower glucose levels ultimately lead to lower acetate levels. This, in turn causes oxaloacetate

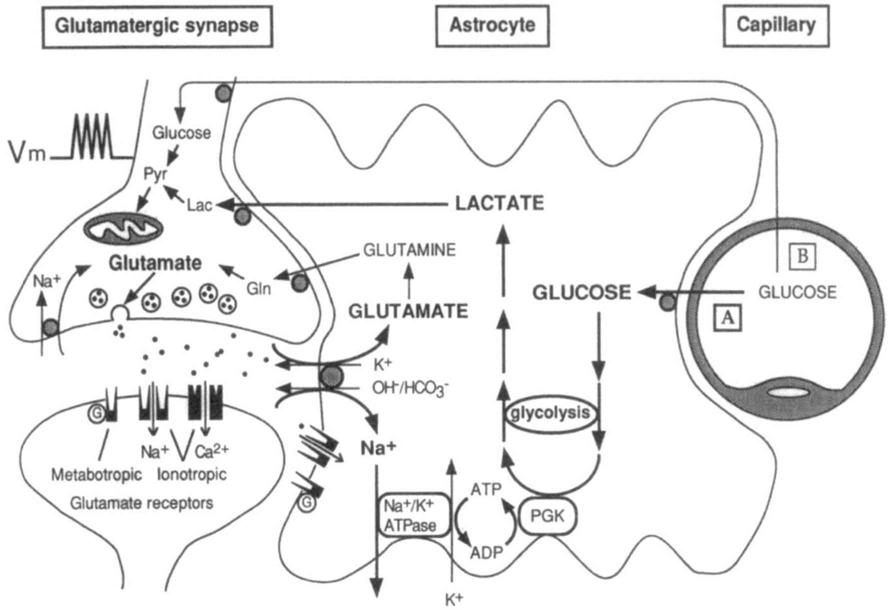

from Pellerin 1994

Fig. 1. Schematic of the mechanism for glutamate-induced glycolysis in astrocytes during physiological activation. At glutamatergic synapses, glutamate depolarizes neurons by acting at specific receptor subtypes. The action of glutamate is terminated by an efficient glutamate uptake system located primarily in astrocytes. Glutamate is cotransported with Na^+, resulting in an increase in$[Na^+]$i, leading to activation of Na^+/K^+-ATPase. The pump, fuled by ATP provided by membrane-bound glycolytic enzymes[possibly phosphoglycerate kinase(PGK); see ref. 22], activates glycolysis-i.e., glucose utilization and lactate production- in astrocytes. Lactate, once released, can bi taken up by neurons and serve as an adequate energy substrate. For graphic clarity, only lactate uptake into presynaptic terminals is indicated. However, this process could also occur at the postsynaptic neuron. Based on recent evidence, glutamate receptors are also shown on astrocytes(12). This model, which summarizes in vitro experimental evidence indicating glutamate-induced glycolysis, is taken to reflect cellular and molecular events occurring during activation of a given cortical area[arrow labeled A(activation)]. Direct glucose uptake into neurons under basal conditions is also shown[arrow labeled B(basal conditions)]. Pyr, pyruvate; Lac, lactate; Gln, glutamine; G, guanine nucleotide binding protein.

to form aspartate, and α ketoglutarate to form glutamate (see figure 2).[14, 15] Glutamate and aspartate build up in the tissue, then interstitial space and ultimately CSF space.[12] These findings suggest the possibility of an excitotoxic agent rather than insufficient glucose substrate as a cause for neuronal dysfunction and death during hypoglycemia.[10]

Glutamate and aspartate cause sustained glutamate receptor activation, particularly at the NMDA receptor.[16-19] The excess glutamate and aspartate activation leads initially to sodium and water influx which causes cellular edema.[20] This is followed by calcium (an important neuronal second messenger) influx into the cells, which causes dysfunction of many intracellular processes.[21-24] NMDA receptor activation leads to the production of reactive oxygen species which damage neuronal DNA.[25] The DNA damage in turn activates poly (ADP-ribose) polymerase-1 (PARP-1). Under normal conditions, PARP-1 acts to repair DNA, but with extensive damage, it can increase apoptosis inducing factor and stimulate cell death (see figure 3).[26, 27] Hypoglycemic neuronal death can be halted by severing glutamatergic axons, or by blocking glutamate receptors in animals.[17, 18]

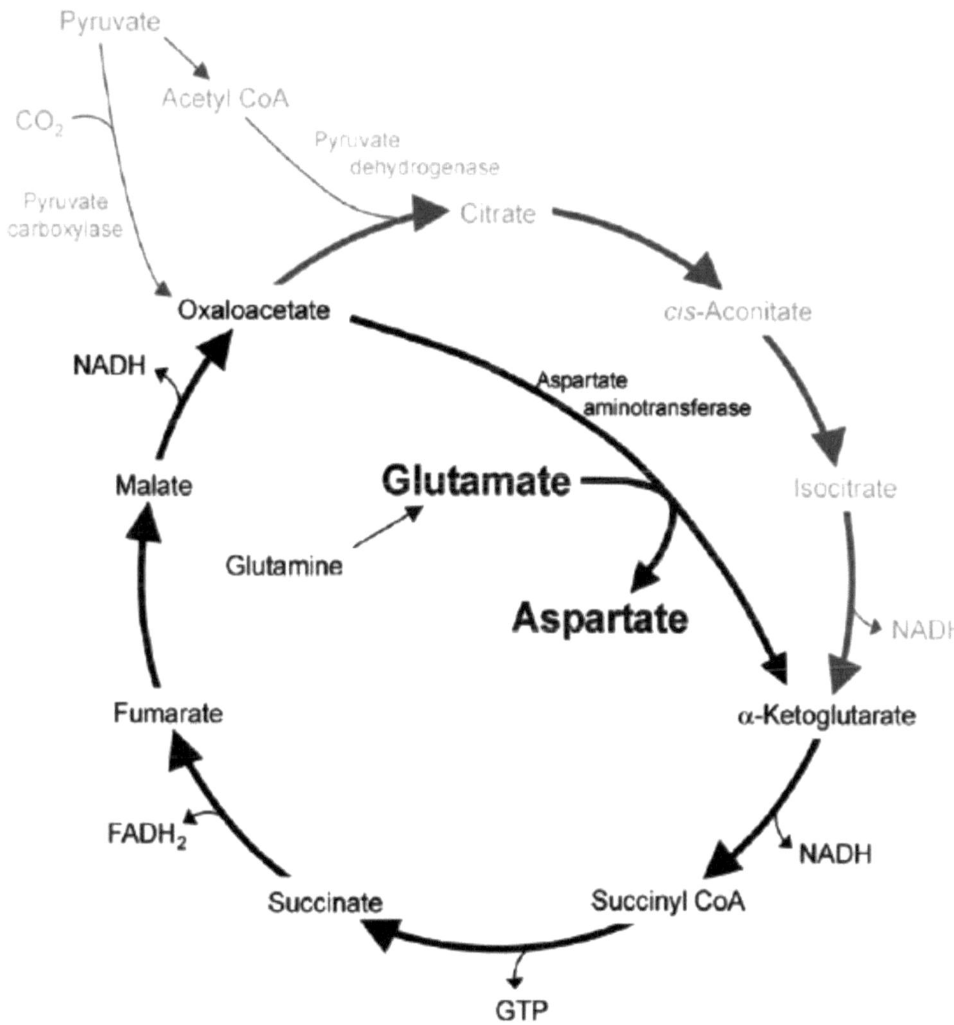

from Sutherland 2008

Fig. 2. Truncation of the Krebs Cycle during Hypoglycemia. Adapted from Sutherland: Medicinal Chemistry , 2008, 4; 379-85

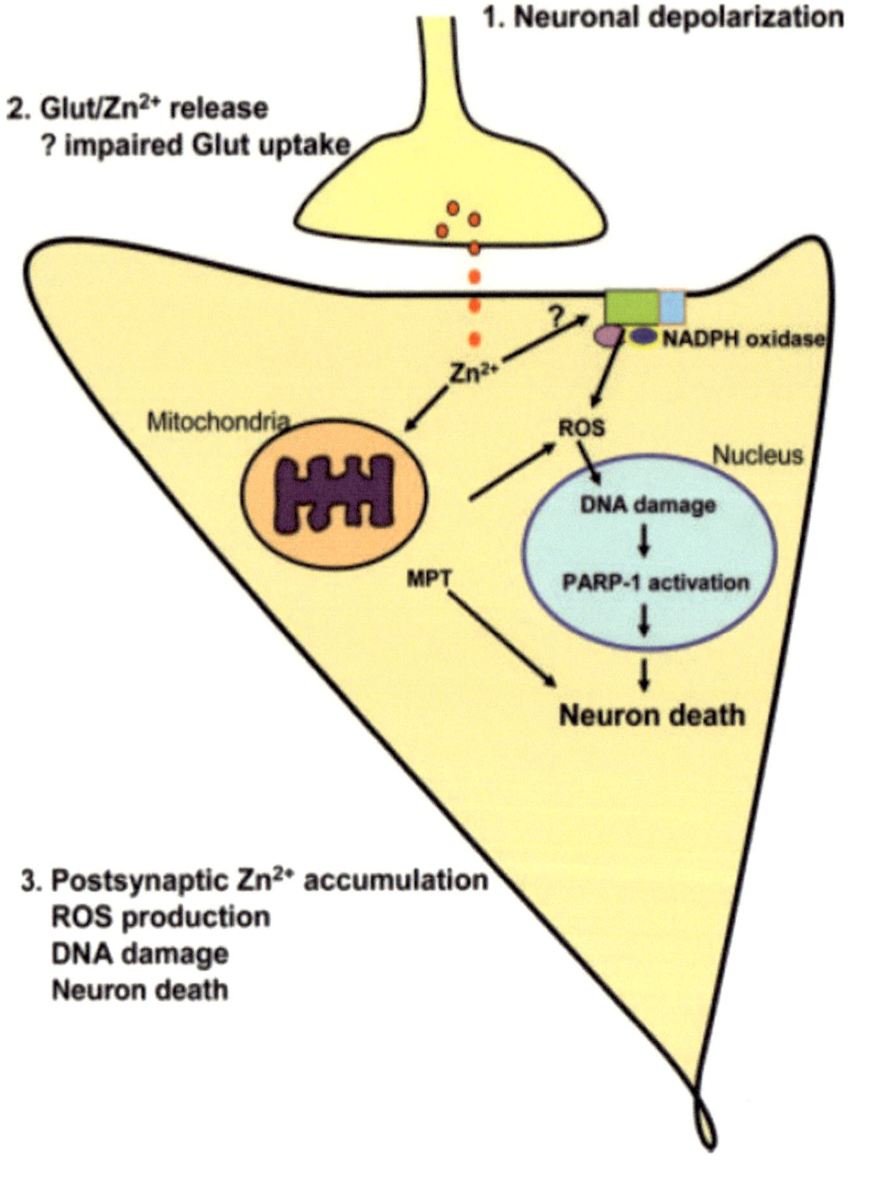

from Suh 2007

Key aspects of hypoglycemia-induced neuronal death. (1) Neuronal depolarization is induced by hypoglycemia. (2) Depolarization leads to release of glutamate, aspartate, and zinc. Impaired astrocyte uptake may contribute to increased glutamate extracellular levels. (3) Glutamate receptor activation and zinc influx induce production of reactive oxygen species (ROS) from mitochondria or NADPH oxidase, subsequent DNA damage and activation of poly(ADP-ribose) polymerase-1 (PARP-1), mitochondrial permeability transition (MPT), and cell death.

Fig. 3. Key Aspects of Hypoglycemia induced Neuronal Cell Death. From Suh : Glia55:1280–1286 (2007)

3. Clinical manifestations

Neuronal function is known to worsen at lower levels of blood glucose. Under normal conditions, endogenous insulin secretion ceases at levels of around 4.5mmol/l (81 mg/dL). Counterregulatory hormones such as glucagon and epinephrine are later secreted in response to a fall in blood glucose to 3.8 mmol/l (68 mg/dL). This causes autonomic symptoms such as sweating, irritability and tremulousness. At 2.8 mmol/l (50 mg / dl) profound neurologlycopenic symptoms such as seizure, cognitive disturbance and confusion occur. Below this level coma appears, electroencephalogram (EEG) becomes flat, and neuron death occurs below 1 mmol/L (18 mmol/dL)(see figure 4).[1]

Hypoglycemia has been recognized as a clinical syndrome since 1924.[28] In 1985, Malouf and Brust evaluated 125 patients with hypoglycemia presenting to a local hospital over a one year period.[29]Among their study cohort, sixty-five patients were obtunded, stuporous, or comatose. Another 38 had confusion or "bizarre" behavior, 10 were dizzy or tremulous, 9 had seizures, and 3 had hemiparesis. Diabetes mellitus, alcoholism, and sepsis, alone or in combination, accounted for 90% of predisposing conditions. Death occurred in 11%, but was only attributed directly to hypoglycemia in one patient. Four patients had residual neurologic symptoms after resolution of hypoglycemia.[29]

The neurological manifestations of thirty patients with hypoglycemia from insulinoma were described by Daggett and Nabarro.[30] They found that the most common presentation was confusion (20 cases), followed by coma (16 cases), seizures (8 cases) and weakness (8 cases).[30] Their review included information about 220 other patients with hypoglycemia and insulinoma from 7 series. Among these, 152 cases had confusion, 82 had coma, 58 had seizures, 18 had headache, and 6 had weakness.[30]

Recurrent exposure to hypoglycemia, particularly in insulin treated type 1 diabetes, but to a lesser extent in type 2 diabetes can chronically impair the counterregulatory response to hypoglycemia. Two recognized syndromes are hypoglycemia associated autonomic failure (HAAF), and impaired awareness of hypoglycemia (IAH). After 20 years, around half of patients with type 1 diabetes have an impaired response of glucagon and epinephrine to hypoglycemia.[31] Likely as a result of the blunted epinephrine response, IAH develops, as there are less of the typical clinical manifestations from epinephrine such as sweating and tremors.[32]

Various other neurological manifestations of hypoglycemia have been described. These include headache, cognitive disturbance, hemiplegia, coma, and seizures.

4. Headache

Since 1933, fasting and hunger have been understood to precipitate migraine attacks.[33-36] One of the largest studies to demonstrate fasting as a migraine precipitant included 1883 patients who responded to a questionnaire regarding dietary habits in the 24 hours before the migraine. Fasting was found to be a precipitating factor in 67% of patients.[37]

A headache as a direct result of fasting, and without the autonomic features of migraine has been described.[38] It is usually diffuse, nonpulsatile of moderate intensity, and should occur 16 hours after fasting, with resolution within 72 hours of food intake (see table 1). The lifetime prevalence of this type of headache is estimated to be 4.1%.[39]

Various other headache types have been attributable to fasting for religious reasons, and come under various names such as *Yom Kippur Headache* and *Ramadan Headache.* A study

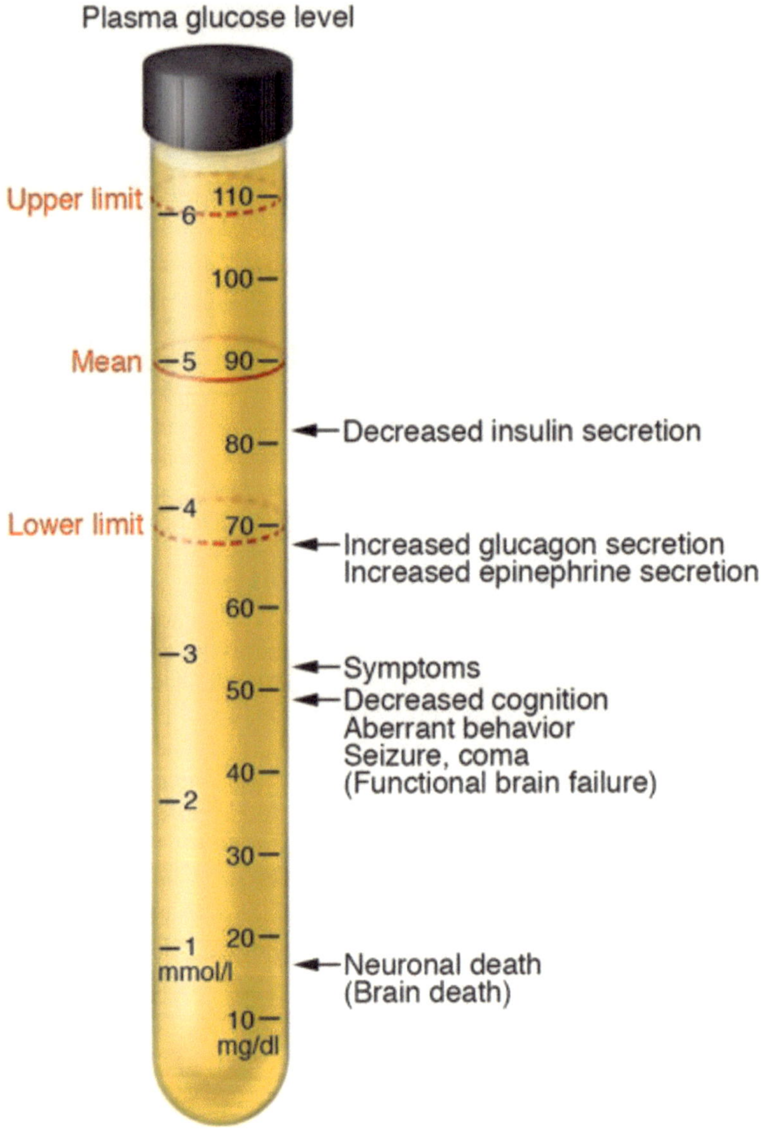

from Cryer, 2007

Fig. 4. Sequence of responses to falling arterial plasma glucose concentrations. The solid horizontal line indicates the mean and the dashed horizontal lines the upper and lower limits of physiological postabsorptive plasma glucoseconcentrations in humans. The glycemic thresholds for decrements in insulin secretion, increments in glucagon and epinephrine secretion, symptoms, and decrements in cognition. Have been defined in healthy humans (1) (see text). Those for seizure and coma and for neuronal death are extrapolated from clinical observations of humans (9) and studies in monkeys (12) as well as in other experimental animals (13–15). In this issue of the JCI, Suh and colleagues (13) report that glucose reperfusion increased brain neuronal death in their rodent model of profound hypoglycemia.

Diagnostic criteria for headache attributed to fasting (code 10.5)
A. Headache with at least one of the following characteristics and fulfilling criteria C and D:
1. Frontal location
2. Diffuse pain
3. Non-pulsating quality
4. Mild or moderate intensity
B. The patient has fasted for >16 h
C. Headache develops during fasting
D. Headache resolves within 72 h after resumption of food intake

Table 1. International HA classification

comparing 211 patients who observed a total fast for 25 hours during Yom Kippur to 136 patients who did not found 82 (39%) of the fasters complained of headache compared to 7% of non-fasters.[40] Although abstinence from caffeine and nicotine was observed in the fasting group, this did not appear to have an influence on headache. A questionnaire given to 91 participants who had observed a complete fast on the first day of Ramadan and 25 who had not found 41% of the fasting group complained of headache, compared to only 8% in the control group (p=0.002).[41] Although two of the subjects developed headache shortly after their last meal, suggesting to the author a possibility of reactive hypoglycemia, most of the headaches were attributable to caffeine withdrawal. Hypoglycemia was not formally evaluated in these studies.

Blau and Cumings attempted to identify a correlation between blood glucose and migraine. They had 12 migraine subjects fast for 19 hours, and measured blood sugar levels at regular intervals. Six of these subjects developed migraine, at an average of 11 to 14 hours after the beginning of the fast. The lowest blood sugar levels varied from 44 to 77 mg/dl.[42]

Pearce recorded serial blood glucose levels in 20 migraine patients, and 10 matched controls after injecting 0.15 units/kg body weight of insulin. Thirty minutes after the infusion, migraine patients had an average blood glucose level of 20.4 mg/dl. After 2 hours of observation, only one (5%) of the migraine patients developed a headache, and one (5%) developed aura without headache. None of the control subjects developed headache, and most patients complained of mild faintness, sweating and palpitations. The author concluded that hypoglycemia may be implicated only in a minority of migraine patients, and that more complex metabolic factors are likely implicated.[34]

5. Cognitive disturbance and dementia

Hypoglycemia can affect cognitive performance and learning acutely. There are well documented reports and experimental trials linking various cognitive disturbances with hypoglycemia. A link between long term development of dementia and repeated hypoglycemia is more controversial.

Memory and learning was tested among thirty-six type 1diabetics during an episode of controlled hypoglycemia with a target blood glucose of 2.5 mmol/l for 60 minutes. Subjects attempted to memorize instructions during euglycemia and recall was assessed during hypoglycemia. Word recall, story recall, visual recall was also assessed during hypoglycemia. Euglycemia was then restored and delayed memory for the conventional tasks was tested. Euglycaemic control subjects performed the same tasks at blood glucose of 4.5 mmol/l. Hypoglycemia impaired performance on the prospective memory task (p=0.004) as well as both immediate and delayed recall for the word (p<0.01) and story recall tasks (p<0.01). No difference was found among subject with normal or impaired glycemic awareness. There was no significant change on the visual memory task.[43]

McCrimmon et. Al. found diminished visual processing speed despite normal visual acuity in 20 non-diabetic subjects during controlled hypoglycemia.[44] Significant reductions in speed of naming and labeling skills at hypoglycemia without associated impairment in accuracy has been observed.[45] Immediate and delayed memory were impaired in 16 type 1 diabetic patients during controlled hypoglycemia of 2.5 mmol/l as assessed by the Trail Making B Test, and the Digit Symbol Test.[46] Similar tests have shown impairment in visuo-spatial ability during hypoglycemia.[47]

Tests of sensory perceptual processing, simple motor abilities, attention, learning, memory, language, and spatial and constructional abilities at plasma glucose levels of 2.2 mmol/l were diminished when compared to basal levels of performance at 8.9 mmol/L among 42 type 1 diabetics. Tests involving associative learning, attention, and mental flexibility were the most affected.[48] Others have shown similar disruptions in various cognitive domains during hypoglycemia, leading to little doubt of the acute effects of hypoglycemia on cognition.[49]

The role of hypoglycemic episodes on long term cognitive outcomes, and development of dementia is however more controversial. The 2007 Diabetes Control and Complications Trial (DCCT) and its follow-up Epidemiology of Diabetes Interventions and Complications (EDIC) followed 1144 diabetic patients for an average of 18 years.[50] Forty percent of these patients reported at least one episode of hypoglycemic seizure or coma. Despite this, there was no associated decline in any cognitive domain. Those with elevated glycated hemoglobin had moderate declines in motor speed (P=0.001) and psychomotor efficiency (P<0.001).[50]

More recently, a longitudinal cohort of 16,667 patients showed a greater risk of dementia among those with hypoglycemic episodes, with an attributable risk of dementia of 2.39% per year (95% CI 1.72%-3.01%).[51] This study was limited in that it was a retrospective review of electronic medical records. Furthermore, reverse causation may account for the association. Patients with dementia may have been more likely to have irregular food intake and make dosing errors in their glycemic medications. Further trials are needed to investigate a possible association between hypoglycemia and long term cognition.

6. Hypoglycemic hemiplegia

The clinical syndrome of hypoglycemic hemiplegia has been recognized for over 50 years.[52, 53] It appears to be rare, with case series reporting an incidence of 2% among those admitted with hypoglycemia.[29] Objective weakness was found in 7 patients with hypoglycemia from insulinoma; 3 had hemiparesis, 2 had paraparesis and 2 had monoparesis. On average the weakness resolved over a period of 1 hr to 3 days once normoglycaemia was maintained.[29, 30]

Wallis et. al. reviewed 16 patients presenting with weakness and blood glucose of less than 45 mg/dl.[54] Most patients were initially misdiagnosed as stroke, all but one were conscious during the attack, four had associated aphasia, most (12/16) had right sided weakness and all had resolution without recurrence within 15 minutes of glucose infusion. One of the patients had a total of four episodes of transient hemiplegia before hypoglycemia was diagnosed. He was left with permanent dysarthria and ataxia. One patient died after multiple recurrent hypoglycemic episodes and subsequent deep coma related to insulinoma. Autopsy of this patient showed diffuse cortical injury, but no focal lesions.[54]

Another review involving 29 patients found 72% were caused by insulin treatment, and mean serum glucose was 35 mg/dL. Most (78%) had recurrent attacks, and on average 3.5 attacks occurred before a diagnosis of hypoglycemic hemiparesis was made. Interestingly, the majority of patients (72%) had right sided weakness, most with aphasia.[55]

Hypoglycemia must be excluded in a patient presenting with symptoms consistent with transient ischemic attack or stroke. Current guidelines for the treatment of stroke patients with IV tissue plasminogen activator exclude those with a glucose level below 50 mg/dL if their symptoms are likely attributable to the hypoglycemia.[56] This presentation is however much more rare than ischemic stroke. During a one year period, three patients were admitted with hypoglycemic hemiplegia compared to 400 with ischemic stroke in an urban hospital.[29]

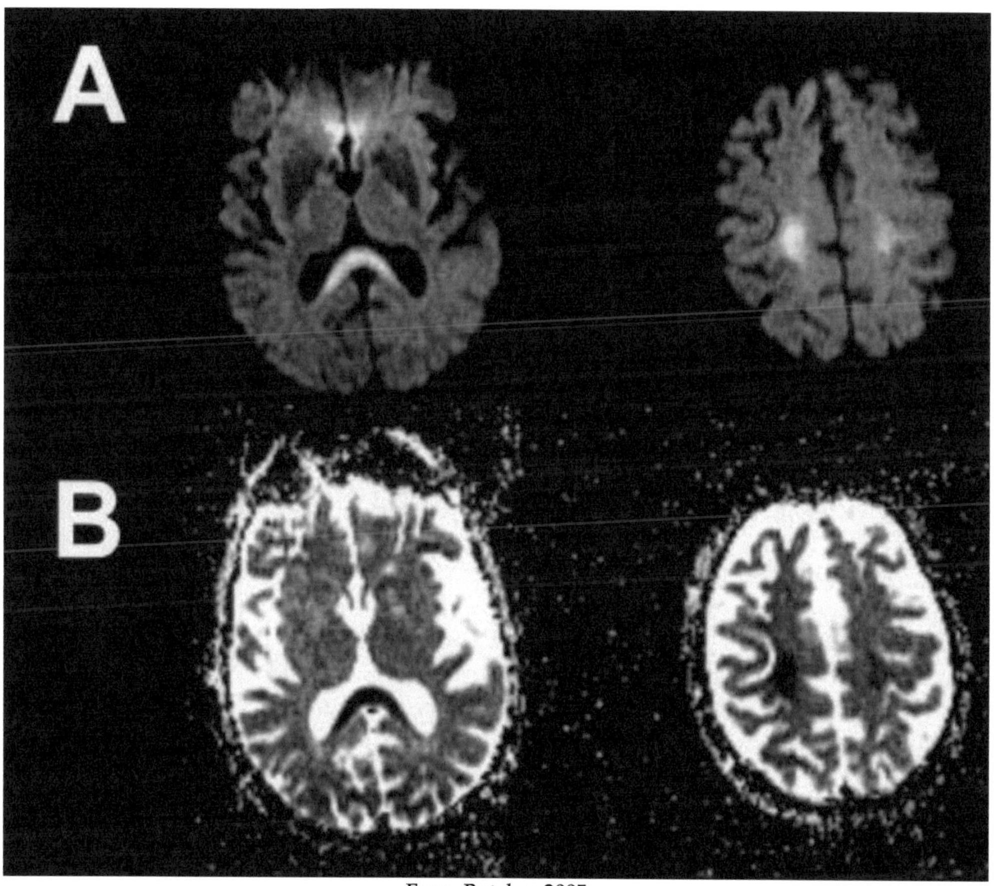

From Botcher 2005

Fig. 5. A, Initial DWI (repetition time/echo time/_ 4100/96/90;__1000 s/mm2; field of view 230 mm; matrix: 128_128) with increased signal intensities in bilateral corona radiata and splenium. B, Initial ADC maps with signal reduction also in bilateral corona radiata and splenium corresponding to DWI images.

Reports suggest that brain imaging during hypoglycemic hemiplegia, and coma may be similar to that observed during ischemic stroke. Specifically, in the setting of ischemic stroke, MRI shows restricted diffusion of water molecules due to ionic pump failure. This leads to restriction on diffusion weighted imaging (DWI) and prolongation of apparent diffusion coefficient (ADC). ADC changes were found to occur in association with the onset of EEG isoelectricity in insulin induced hypoglycemic rats.[57]

Case reports have shown ADC and DWI changes in patients with hypoglycemic hemiplegia. These changes usually reverse after clinical improvement with glucose recussitation.[58-60] Unlike ischemic stroke, hypoglycemic changes on MRI are often bilateral, affect the cortex, hippocampus and basal ganglia, and do not necessarily correspond to a vascular territory(see figure 5).[61]

Although hypoglycemic hemiplegia is initially clinically indistinguishable from an ischemic stroke, the pathophysiology is likely different. Autopsy studies have not demonstrated lesions in vascular territories, but rather diffuse damage.[11, 54] Hypoglycemia has been shown to produce vasodilatation in animals, unlike vasoconstriction seen in stroke.[62] Although case reports have shown patients with hypoglycemic hemiplegia and associated carotid artery stenosis, most others have not validated this observation.[54, 55, 63] The notion of underlying cerebrovascular disease as a cause for hypoglycemic hemiplegia does not seem to be supported.

Profound hypoglycemia causes tissue *alkalosis* resulting from ammonia formation and consumption of metabolic acids, unlike tissue acidosis seen in cerebral ischemia.[64] Hypoglycemic brain death preferentially affects neurons, whereas ischemia tends to affect glial and endothelial cells as well.[65] Hypoglycemia generally spares axons while damage from ischemia affects all parts of the neuron.[66]

7. Hypoglycemic coma

One of the most feared, and occasionally devastating effects of hypoglycemia is coma. The relationship between insulin treatment and coma was first recognized by Sakel in the 1930s.[67] He and others noticed that when treating schizophrenics with insulin (a now abandoned practice), a duration of treatment under 30 minutes allowed the patients to recover from the coma, but much longer, the coma would be irreversible.[67, 68] Insulin induced hypoglycemia to a level of 0.7 mmol/l (13 mg/dl) was found to produce significant brain damage after 5-6 hours in monkeys. [69]

A retrospective analysis over a 7 year period evaluated 102 patients admitted with coma and blood glucose of below 49 mg/dL, and improvement with glucose administration. Most patients were type 2 diabetics (92/102) taking glycemic agents. Risk factors included age over 60, renal dysfunction decreased energy intake or infection. Sixty two patients responded within 12 hours of treatment, while the others had no resolution for up to 72 hours. Death occur in 5 patients(4.9%).[70]

A prospective one year study found sixty five of 125 (52%) admissions for hypoglycemia presented with obtundation, stupor or coma.[29] While the length of time in coma could not always be determined, the one death related to hypoglycemia occurred in a patient with coma lasting over 20 hours. Of the 11 patients determined to be comatose for 12 hours or more, 10 remained comatose. Blood glucose level did not predict coma, as there was a wide range of blood glucose levels among these comatose patients, and similar results in those without coma.[29]

MR images of those in persistent vegetative state from hypoglycemia revealed lesions in the bilateral basal ganglia, cerebral cortex, substantia nigra, and hippocampus, which suggests the particular vulnerability of these areas.[61] Involvement of the basal ganglia seems to portend a worse outcome, though evidence is limited to case reports.[71]

Two markers of neuronal injury, NSE and S-100 may predict death or otherwise poor outcome in profound hypoglycemic coma. They showed no change in diabetics with mild hypoglycemic episodes, but were markedly elevated in 3 patients who died from hypoglycemic brain injury.[72, 73] The disappearance of EEG activity is a prerequisite for hypoglycemia induced brain damage.[66]

8. Seizures

In autopsy studies, the cortex and hippocampus were most frequently involved in hypoglycemic brain damage.[11] These areas are also commonly involved in seizures from other causes.

In a prospective study of symptomatic hypoglycemia admissions over one year, 9 of 125 (7.2%) patients presented with seizures related to hypoglycemia. Among the 9 seizure patients, 3 had comorbid epilepsy, and 6 were intoxicated with alcohol. The majority of the seizures were generalized tonic clonic, most recurred, and one patient had status epilepticus.[29]

The landmark Diabetes Control and Complications Trial found 16 episodes of coma or seizure per 100 patient-years in the aggressive glucose control group, compared to 5 in the moderate control group.[74] Another prospective study had a rate of severe events (the combination of seizure or coma) at 4.8/100 patient-years. Most of the severe events were seizures, and risk factors were age under 6 and glycosalated hemoglobin <7%.[75]

A prospective study of 1382 patients with new onset seizures found that hypoglycemia was never found to be the inciting cause.[76] This apparent discrepancy may be due to the fact that serum glucose was drawn after dextrose was given to presenting patients. Furthermore, this study focused on all those presenting with seizures, indicating hypoglycemia leading to seizures may be a rare event in non-diabetics.

The NLSTEPSS study evaluated causes of status epilepticus in children, and found 4% were from metabolic causes.[77] Metabolic causes of status epilepticus were found in 11% of adult patients.[78] Unfortunately, these studies did not separate blood glucose from other metabolic causes.[78]

Quantitative EEG recordings have shown that epileptiform activity (spikes) occurred at higher blood glucose levels in diabetic than non-diabetic children, and overall, occurred at higher glucose levels in children(3mmol/l) compared with adults (2 mmol/l)(see figure 6).[79, 80] In a case review of four children wearing a continuous glucose monitor, hypoglycemia occurred on average 2-4 hours before seizure onset.[73]

During hypoglycemia, multiple metabolic derangements occur. In particular, the excitatory amino acids glutamate and aspartate increase out of proportion to a slight rise in extracellurlar GABA. The resulting brain excitatory milieu may account for seizure activity.[64]

Investigators showed that fasting and insulin infusion in rats increased the incidence of barrel rotations, which is a characteristic phenotype of hypoglycemic seizures in the animal. In particular, they showed a decreased release of GABA in the substantia nigra pars reticulate in rats with seizures.[81]

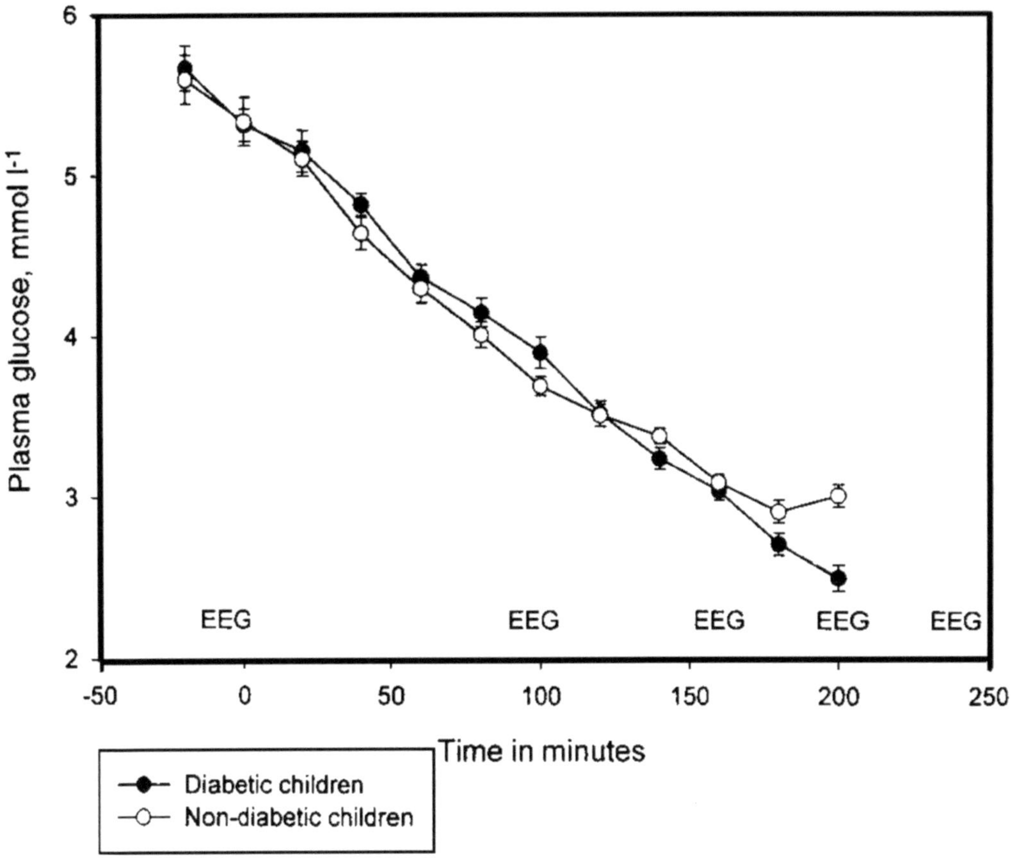

Fig. 6. Plasma glucose levels (mean ± SEM) during the hypoglycemic clamp, and approximate time at EEG regis- trations, in the 19 diabetic (solid circles) and 17 non-diabetic children (open circles) Bjorgaas 1998

9. Conclusion

Hypoglycemia has profound effects on the brain. At the cellular level, energy failure and excitotoxicity lead to interruptions of many critical cellular activities. Clinically, this can manifest as headache, seizure, stroke-like episodes, cognitive dysfunction, and coma.

10. References

[1] Cryer PE. Hypoglycemia, functional brain failure, and brain death. *The Journal of Clinical Investigation*. 2007;117:868

[2] Magistretti PJ, Pellerin L. Cellular mechanisms of brain energy metabolism. Relevance to functional brain imaging and to neurodegenerative disorders. *Ann N Y Acad Sci*. 1996;777:380-387

[3] Pellerin L. Food for thought: The importance of glucose and other energy substrates for sustaining brain function under varying levels of activity. *Diabetes & Metabolism*.36:S59

[4] Cooper JR BF, Roth RH. *The biochemical basis of neuropharmacology*. New York: Oxford University Press; 1974.
[5] Pellerin L, Magistretti PJ. Glutamate uptake into astrocytes stimulates aerobic glycolysis: A mechanism coupling neuronal activity to glucose utilization. *Proc Natl Acad Sci U S A*. 1994;91:10625-10629
[6] Vannucci SJ, Simpson IA. Synopsis of the workshop entitled "is lactate a nutrient for neurons" held at the brain energy meeting in trondheim, norway. *Journal of Neuroscience Research*. 2001;66:821
[7] Brown AM. Brain glycogen re-awakened. *Journal of Neurochemistry*. 2004;89:537
[8] Brown A. M. WRE, Baltan Tekkök S., and Ransom B. R. Functional insulin receptors are selectively expressed on cns astrocytes. *Soc Neurosci Abstr*. 2002;28:581
[9] Robinson AM, Williamson DH. Physiological roles of ketone bodies as substrates and signals in mammalian tissues. *Physiol Rev*. 1980;60:143-187
[10] Auer RN, Wieloch T, Olsson Y, Siesjö BK. The distribution of hypoglycemic brain damage. *Acta Neuropathologica*. 1984;64:177
[11] Auer RN, Hugh J, Cosgrove E, Curry B. Neuropathologic findings in three cases of profound hypoglycemia. *Clin Neuropathol*. 1989;8:63-68
[12] Sandberg M, Butcher SP, Hagberg H. Extracellular overflow of neuroactive amino acids during severe insulin-induced hypoglycemia: In vivo dialysis of the rat hippocampus. *J Neurochem*. 1986;47:178-184
[13] Engelsen B, Westerberg E, Fonnum F, Wieloch T. Effect of insulin-induced hypoglycemia on the concentrations of glutamate and related amino acids and energy metabolites in the intact and decorticated rat neostriatum. *J Neurochem*. 1986;47:1634-1641
[14] Suh SW, Hamby AM, Swanson RA. Hypoglycemia, brain energetics, and hypoglycemic neuronal death. *Glia*. 2007;55:1280-1286
[15] Sutherland GR, Tyson RL, Auer RN. Truncation of the krebs cycle during hypoglycemic coma. *Med Chem*. 2008;4:379-385
[16] Olney JW, Sharpe LG. Brain lesions in an infant rhesus monkey treated with monsodium glutamate. *Science*. 1969;166:386-388
[17] Wieloch T, Engelsen B, Westerberg E, Auer R. Lesions of the glutamatergic cortico-striatal projections in the rat ameliorate hypoglycemic brain damage in the striatum. *Neurosci Lett*. 1985;58:25-30
[18] Wieloch T. Hypoglycemia-induced neuronal damage prevented by an n-methyl-d-aspartate antagonist. *Science*. 1985;230:681-683
[19] Sandberg M, Nystrom B, Hamberger A. Metabolically derived aspartate--elevated extracellular levels in vivo in lodoacetate poisoning. *J Neurosci Res*. 1985;13:489-495
[20] Olney JW. Inciting excitotoxic cytocide among central neurons. *Adv Exp Med Biol*. 1986;203:631-645
[21] Choi DW. Ionic dependence of glutamate neurotoxicity. *J Neurosci*. 1987;7:369-379
[22] Choi DW. Glutamate neurotoxicity and diseases of the nervous system. *Neuron*. 1988;1:623-634
[23] Choi DW, Maulucci-Gedde M, Kriegstein AR. Glutamate neurotoxicity in cortical cell culture. *J Neurosci*. 1987;7:357-368
[24] MacDermott AB, Mayer ML, Westbrook GL, Smith SJ, Barker JL. Nmda-receptor activation increases cytoplasmic calcium concentration in cultured spinal cord neurones. *Nature*. 1986;321:519

[25] Dugan LL, Sensi SL, Canzoniero LM, Handran SD, Rothman SM, Lin TS, Goldberg MP, Choi DW. Mitochondrial production of reactive oxygen species in cortical neurons following exposure to n-methyl-d-aspartate. *J Neurosci.* 1995;15:6377-6388
[26] Yu SW, Wang H, Poitras MF, Coombs C, Bowers WJ, Federoff HJ, Poirier GG, Dawson TM, Dawson VL. Mediation of poly(adp-ribose) polymerase-1-dependent cell death by apoptosis-inducing factor. *Science.* 2002;297:259-263
[27] Ha HC, Snyder SH. Poly(adp-ribose) polymerase is a mediator of necrotic cell death by atp depletion. *Proc Natl Acad Sci U S A.* 1999;96:13978-13982
[28] Harris S. Hyperinsulinism and dysinsulinism. *Journal of the American Medical Association.* 1924;83:729-733
[29] Malouf R, Brust JCM. Hypoglycemia: Causes, neurological manifestations, and outcome. *Annals of Neurology.* 1985;17:421
[30] Daggett P, Nabarro J. Neurological aspects of insulinomas. *Postgraduate Medical Journal.* 1984;60:577-581
[31] Gerich JE BG. Counterregulatory failure. In: Frier BM FB, ed. *Hypoglycaemia and diabetes: Clinical and physiological aspects.* London: Edward Arnold; 1993:253-267.
[32] BM F. Impaired awareness of hypoglycaemia. In: Frier BM FM, ed. *Hypoglycaemia in clinical diabetes.* Chichester: John Wiley & Sons; 2007:141-170.
[33] Critchley M, Ferguson F. Migraine. *The Lancet.* 1933;221:123
[34] Pearce J. Insulin induced hypoglycaemia in migraine. *Journal of Neurology, Neurosurgery & Psychiatry.* 1971;34:154-156
[35] Jacome DE. Hypoglycemia rebound migraine. *Headache: The Journal of Head and Face Pain.* 2001;41:895
[36] Gray PA BH. Hypoglycemic headache. *Endocrinology.* 1935;19:549-560
[37] Dalton K. Food intake prior to a migraine attack--study of 2,313 spontaneous attacks. *Headache.* 1975;15:188-193
[38] The international classification of headache disorders: 2nd edition. *Cephalalgia.* 2004;24 Suppl 1:9-160
[39] Rasmussen BK, Olesen J. Symptomatic and nonsymptomatic headaches in a general population. *Neurology.* 1992;42:1225-1231
[40] Mosek A, Korczyn AD. Yom kippur headache. *Neurology.* 1995;45:1953-1955
[41] Awada A, al Jumah M. The first-of-ramadan headache. *Headache.* 1999;39:490-493
[42] Blau JN, Cumings JN. Method of precipitating and preventing some migraine attacks. *Br Med J.* 1966;2:1242-1243
[43] Warren R, Zammitt N, Deary I, Frier B. The effects of acute hypoglycaemia on memory acquisition and recall and prospective memory in type 1 diabetes. *Diabetologia.* 2007;50:178
[44] McCrimmon RJ, Deary IJ, Huntly BJP, MacLeod KJ, Frier BM. Visual information processing during controlled hypoglycaemia in humans. *Brain.* 1996;119:1277-1287
[45] Holmes CS, Koepke KM, Thompson RG, Gyves PW, Weydert JA. Verbal fluency and naming performance in type i diabetes at different blood glucose concentrations. *Diabetes Care.* 1984;7:454-459
[46] Sommerfield AJ, Deary IJ, McAulay V, Frier BM. Short-term, delayed, and working memory are impaired during hypoglycemia in individuals with type 1 diabetes. *Diabetes Care.* 2003;26:390-396
[47] Wright RJ, Frier BM, Deary IJ. Effects of acute insulin-induced hypoglycemia on spatial abilities in adults with type 1 diabetes. *Diabetes Care.* 2009;32:1503-1506

[48] Draelos MT, Jacobson AM, Weinger K, Widom B, Ryan CM, Finkelstein DM, Simonson DC. Cognitive function in patients with insulin-dependent diabetes mellitus during hyperglycemia and hypoglycemia. *The American Journal of Medicine.* 1995;98:135
[49] Widom B, Simonson DC. Glycemic control and neuropsychologic function during hypoglycemia in patients with insulin-dependent diabetes mellitus. *Ann Intern Med.* 1990;112:904-912
[50] Long-term effect of diabetes and its treatment on cognitive function. *New England Journal of Medicine.* 2007;356:1842-1852
[51] Whitmer RA, Karter AJ, Yaffe K, Quesenberry CP, Selby JV. Hypoglycemic episodes and risk of dementia in older patients with type 2 diabetes mellitus. *JAMA: The Journal of the American Medical Association.* 2009;301:1565-1572
[52] Wortis J BK, Orenstein L, Rosenbaum I. Further experiences at bellevue hospital with the hypoglycemic insulin treatment of schizophrenia. *American Journal of Psychiatry.* 1937;94:153-158
[53] JohnWortis KB, Larry Orenstein, Innis Rosenbaum. Further experiences at bellevue hospital with the hypoglycemic insulin treatment of schizophrenia. *American Journal of Psychiatry.* 1937;94:153-158
[54] Wallis WE, Donaldson I, Scott RS, Wilson J. Hypoglycemia masquerading as cerebrovascular disease (hypoglycemic hemiplegia). *Ann Neurol.* 1985;18:510-512
[55] Foster JW, Hart RG. Hypoglycemic hemiplegia: Two cases and a clinical review. *Stroke.* 1987;18:944-946
[56] Adams HP, Jr., del Zoppo G, Alberts MJ, Bhatt DL, Brass L, Furlan A, Grubb RL, Higashida RT, Jauch EC, Kidwell C, Lyden PD, Morgenstern LB, Qureshi AI, Rosenwasser RH, Scott PA, Wijdicks EF. Guidelines for the early management of adults with ischemic stroke: A guideline from the american heart association/american stroke association stroke council, clinical cardiology council, cardiovascular radiology and intervention council, and the atherosclerotic peripheral vascular disease and quality of care outcomes in research interdisciplinary working groups: The american academy of neurology affirms the value of this guideline as an educational tool for neurologists. *Circulation.* 2007;115:e478-534
[57] Hasegawa Y, Formato JE, Latour LL, Gutierrez JA, Liu K-F, Garcia JH, Sotak CH, Fisher M, Brayden JE. Severe transient hypoglycemia causes reversible change in the apparent diffusion coefficient of water. *Stroke.* 1996;27:1648-1656
[58] Bottcher J, Kunze A, Kurrat C, Schmidt P, Hagemann G, Witte OW, Kaiser WA. Localized reversible reduction of apparent diffusion coefficient in transient hypoglycemia-induced hemiparesis. *Stroke.* 2005;36:e20-22
[59] Cordonnier C, Oppenheim C, Lamy C, Meder JF, Mas JL. Serial diffusion and perfusion-weighted mr in transient hypoglycemia. *Neurology.* 2005;65:175
[60] Hasegawa Y, Formato JE, Latour LL, Gutierrez JA, Liu KF, Garcia JH, Sotak CH, Fisher M. Severe transient hypoglycemia causes reversible change in the apparent diffusion coefficient of water. *Stroke.* 1996;27:1648-1655; discussion 1655-1646
[61] Fujioka M, Okuchi K, Hiramatsu K-I, Sakaki T, Sakaguchi S, Ishii Y. Specific changes in human brain after hypoglycemic injury. *Stroke.* 1997;28:584-587
[62] Dieguez G, Fernandez N, Garcia JL, Garcia-Villalon AL, Monge L, Gomez B. Role of nitric oxide in the effects of hypoglycemia on the cerebral circulation in awake goats. *Eur J Pharmacol.* 1997;330:185-193

[63] Portnoy HD. Transient "ischemic" attacks produced by carotid stenosis and hypoglycemia. *Neurology*. 1965;15:830-832
[64] Auer RN. Progress review: Hypoglycemic brain damage. *Stroke*. 1986;17:699-708
[65] Helgason CM. Blood glucose and stroke. *Stroke*. 1988;19:1049-1053
[66] Auer RN. Hypoglycemic brain damage. *Forensic Science International*. 2004;146:105
[67] Sakel M. The methodical use of hypoglycemia in the treatment of psychoses. *American Journal of Psychiatry*. 1937;94:111-129
[68] Fazekas JF, Alman, R.W., Parrish A.E. Irreversible posthypoglycemic coma. *American Journal of Medical Science*. 1951;222:640-643
[69] Kahn KJ, Myers, R.E. Insulin-inducedhypoglycaemia in the non–human primate: Clinical consequences. *Brain hypoxia*. 1971:185–194
[70] Ben-Ami H, Nagachandran P, Mendelson A, Edoute Y. Drug-induced hypoglycemic coma in 102 diabetic patients. *Arch Intern Med*. 1999;159:281-284
[71] Finelli PF. Diffusion-weighted mr in hypoglycemic coma. *Neurology*. 2001;57:933
[72] Strachan MWJ, Abraha HD, Sherwood RA, Lammie GA, Deary IJ, Ewing FME, Perros P, Frier BM. Evaluation of serum markers of neuronal damage following severe hypoglycaemia in adults with insulin-treated diabetes mellitus. *Diabetes/Metabolism Research and Reviews*. 1999;15:5
[73] Buckingham B, Wilson DM, Lecher T, Hanas R, Kaiserman K, Cameron F. Duration of nocturnal hypoglycemia before seizures. *Diabetes Care*. 2008;31:2110-2112
[74] The effect of intensive treatment of diabetes on the development and progression of long-term complications in insulin-dependent diabetes mellitus. *New England Journal of Medicine*. 1993;329:977-986
[75] Davis EA, Keating B, Byrne GC, Russell M, Jones TW. Hypoglycemia: Incidence and clinical predictors in a large population-based sample of children and adolescents with iddm. *Diabetes Care*. 1997;20:22-25
[76] Singh RK, Stephens S, Berl MM, Chang T, Brown K, Vezina LG, Gaillard WD. Prospective study of new-onset seizures presenting as status epilepticus in childhood. *Neurology*.74:636-642
[77] Chin RFM, Neville BGR, Peckham C, Bedford H, Wade A, Scott RC. Incidence, cause, and short-term outcome of convulsive status epilepticus in childhood: Prospective population-based study. *The Lancet*. 2006;368:222
[78] Towne AR, Pellock JM, Ko D, DeLorenzo RJ. Determinants of mortality in status epilepticus. *Epilepsia*. 1994;35:27
[79] Bjorgaas M, Sand T, Vik T, Jorde R. Quantitative eeg during controlled hypoglycaemia in diabetic and non-diabetic children. *Diabet Med*. 1998;15:30-37
[80] Pramming S, Thorsteinsson B, Stigsby B, Binder C. Glycaemic threshold for changes in electroencephalograms during hypoglycaemia in patients with insulin dependent diabetes. *Br Med J (Clin Res Ed)*. 1988;296:665-667
[81] Velíšková J, Chudomel O, Poon KL, Marshall B, Velíšek L. The involvement of the substantia nigra pars reticulata in hypoglycemic seizures. *Epilepsia*. 2007;48:106

14

Hypoglycemia Associated with Type B Insulin Resistance

Hiroyuki Tamemoto, Shin-ichi Tominaga Hideo Toyoshima, San-e' Ishikawa and Masanobu Kawakami
Department of Biochemistry, Jichi Medical University
Department of Comprehensive Medicine, Saitama Medical Center Jichi Medical University
Department of Endocrinology and Metabolism, Saitama Medical Center Jichi Medical University
Japan

1. Introduction

Type B insulin resistance is a rare syndrome caused by anti-insulin receptor antibody. The anti-insulin receptor antibody inhibits binding of insulin to insulin receptor and severe insulin resistance results. Type B insulin resistance usually associates with systemic lupus erythematosus (SLE) or Sjögren syndrome (SjS). In United States, Patients are usually African American women with hyperandorogenism and acanthosis nigricans. To control abnormal autoantibody, predonisolone (PSL), cyclophosphamide, cyclosporine A, azathiopurine, methotrexate, plasmapheresis, mycophenolate mofetil and rituximab are used with various effects. In some cases, hypoglycemia follows after severe hyperglycemia is ameliorated with various therapies. Occasionally, the anti-insulin receptor antibody has partial agonist activity and hypoglycemia is the first symptom. We have experienced a case of hypoglycemia complicated with type B insulin resistance and polymyositis. We reviewed case reports of type B insulin resistance from Japan. The Japanese patients with type B insulin resistance are usually not obese and more men than women were found. Hypoglycemia was observed relatively frequently. Complication with SLE was common, however a rare case complicated with *Helicobacter pyroli* infection was also reported.

2. Case presentation

In Augst 2009, a 54-year-old man admitted to the hospital for muscle pain and weakness. One month before admission, he noticed edema on both feet and swelling of his fingers of both hands. He had no pain however the hotness of the fingers disturbed sleeping. Ten days before admission, he had difficulty in moving his fingers because of the edema and he had pain on the palmar side of his hands. Then, swelling of both thighs and muscle pain of both shoulders had developed. He found weakness of the legs but could still walk on the stairs. His family doctor found elevation of creatin kinase (1580 mU/ml) and thrombocytopenia (79000 /µl) and he was referred to this hospital. On admission, his body height was 167.6 cm, body weight was 69.6kg and the body mass index (BMI) was 24.0 kg/m^2. Pitting edema on lower legs and feet was found. His grasping power was difficult to measure because of the swelling of his fingers. However no apparent muscle weakness was observed by manual muscle testing. On his skin, no Gottron's sign or Heliotrope rash was observed. He had muscle pain in the thigh. He had history of left VIIth nerve palsy when he was 40. VIIth nerve palsy recurred on the right side in April and then he was diagnosed as diabetes mellitus. He smoked one pack of cigarette and drinks a can of beer every day. His mother had diabetes and otherwise no particular family history was noticed. The results of the laboratory tests are listed in Table 1.

WBC	6970 /µl	C3	53 mg/dl (65-135)
Hb	12.5 g/dl	C4	11 mg/dl
Ht	38.7%	D-dimer	2.9 µg/ml
Platelet	167000/µl	Anti-Jo-1 antibody	2
AST	163 mU/ml	Anti-RNP antibody	Negative
ALT	91 mU/ml	Anti-nuclear antibody	80 (diffuse, nuclear)
LDH	523 mU/ml	Anti-Scl-70 antibody	Negative
CK	3296 mU/ml	Anti-SSA antibody	16
CK-MM	97%	Anti-SSB antibody	Negative
CK-MB	3%	Anti-mitochondria M2 antibody	12
HbA1c	6.6%	KL-6	331 U/ml
Blood glucose after		SP-D	31.8 ng/ml
75 g oral glucose		SAA	10.8 µg/ml
0 min	54 mg/dl	CRP	0.35 mg/dl
60 min	186 mg/dl	CEA	3.1 ng/ml
120 min	249 mg/dl	CA19-9	3.3 U/ml
Plasma insulin after		Anti-insulin antibody	Negative
75 g oral glucose		Anti-insulin receptor antibody	Inhibition rate 41%
0 min	10 µU/ml	electromyogram	Low & short NMU in biceps, brachioradial, quadriceps femoris and tibialis anterior muscles
60 min	517µU/ml		
120 min	981µU/ml		

Table 1. Laboratory data of the case NMU: neuromuscular unit

He presented symptoms of fasting hypoglycemia and his fasting plasma glucose showed values between 50 and 70mg/dl repeatedly. His fasting plasma immunoreactive insulin (IRI) level was 21.2 µU/ml and was inappropriately high when the plasma glucose was 62mg/dl. At two hours after breakfast, his plasma glucose was 139mg/dl and the IRI at this time point was 379 µU/ml. The HbA1c at admission was 6.6%. To confirm diagnosis, 75 g oral glucose tolerance test was performed. The blood glucose level after 2 hours was 249 mg/dl. The IRI and C-peptide levels 2 hours after load were 981 µU/ml and 12.5 ng/ml respectively. Anti-insulin antibody was negative. Anti-insulin receptor antibody was present and the inhibition rate was 41%. During the course, serum creatine kinase level increased to over 7000 mU/ml and AST and ALT also moderately increased over 300 mU/ml. The antinuclear antibody, anti-SSA antibody and the Jo-1 antibody were positive, but not for anti-Scl70 or anti-SSB antibodies. Anti-mitochondria M2 antibody was also positive. The electromyogram was compatible with myopathy. A diagnosis of polymyositis complicated with type B insulin resistance was given. After that he was re-evaluated by a dermatologist for the presence of acanthosis nigricans and mild lesions were found in the axilla and the periumbilical region. Predonisolone therapy was started from 60 mg/day. The fasting plasma glucose increased to 198mg/dl and the plasma insulin level was 1399 μU/ml. To control the hyperglycemia, insulin therapy was started from 2 units of ultra-rapid insulin before each meal, then increased to 15 U/day. Severe hyperglycemia was ameliorated within one week and insulin therapy was stopped because fasting hypoglycemia recurred. Fasting hypoglycemia occurred repeatedly after discontinuation of insulin therapy but was manageable by oral glucose intake. The clinical course is presented in Figure 1.

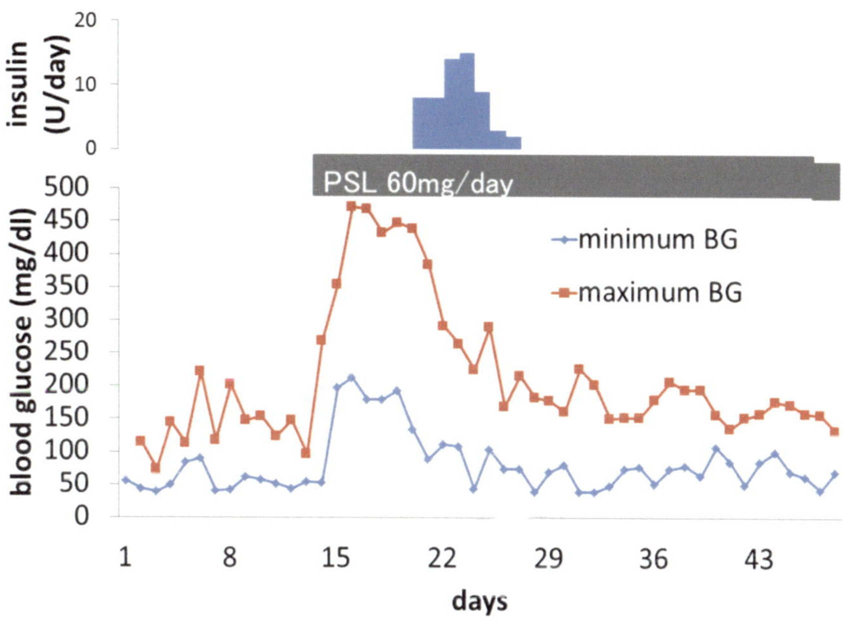

Fig. 1. Clinical course of the case

The creatine kinase and AST responded gradually, however the response was slow and methotrexate 10 mg/week was added to prednisolone therapy. After one month predonisolone was tapered to 50mg/day then 40mg/dl three weeks later. Thereafter tapering schedule was slowed to 2.5mg/day every two weeks. The creatine kinase level decreased to upper normal limit at two months after admission. The HbA1c at this time point was 6.0%.

Type B insulin resistance syndrome in Japan compared with that in the United States (US) have some differences.

Our case was positive for anti-insulin receptor antibody however his insulin resistance was weak and hyperglycemia after PSL therapy was easily controlled by short term insulin therapy. Relatively low inhibition rate of insulin binding (41%) may be the cause of this observation. The difference of clinical course compared with the typical case in US may be related to ethnicity. Therefore we screened case reports on type B insulin resistance in Japan (Table 2).

No	Age	sex	AN	BMI	Underlying disease	Hypoglycemia	OHA or insulin usage before hypoglycemia	Reference
1	54	M	Yes	24	polymyositis	Yes	No	This case
2	47	F	NR	NR	SLE	No		Takeda
3	48	F	NR	NR	SLE, depression	No		Sakai[1]
4	50	F	Yes	NR	SLE	Yes	Yes (IGF-1)	Yamasaki
5	59	M	NR	16	SLE	Yes	No	Kawashiri
6	55	M	NR	NR	SLE(possible)	Yes	No	Gojo
7	57	M	NR	NR	SLE	Yes	Yes	Ogata
8	56	M	No	22.7	SLE	Yes	No	Sato, Shigihara
9	23	F	Yes	20.4	SLE	Yes	No	Nagayama
10	61	F	NR	NR	SjS	No		Ito
11	72	F	No	21.2	SjS	No		Furukawa
12	44	F	Yes	Not obese	SjS, Hashimoto	No		Hirano
13	60	M	NR	NR	RA	Yes	No	Tokumori
14	67	M	NR	NR	UCTD	Yes	No	Yamagata
15	59	M	NR	NR	CH(C), PEG-IFN+ ribavirin	No		Miyamoto
16	74	M	Yes	18.4	IPMT	No		Uehara
17	48	F	Yes	19	T2DM only	Yes	Yes	Sakai[2]
18	68	M	NR	22.6	AP	No		Tashiro
19	84	M	No	23	ITP,	Yes	No	Imai
	86		NR	NR	ITP	Yes	No	Yamamiya

AN: acanthosis nigricans, BMI: body mass inex (kg/m^2), SLE: systemic lupus erythematosus, SjS: Sjögren's syndrome, RA: rheumatoid arthritis, UCTD: undifferentiated collagen tissue disease, CH(C): chronic hepatitis virus C infection, PEG-IFN: pegylated interferon, IPMT: intrapancreatic duct mucinous tumor, AP: angina pectoris, ITP: idiopathic thrombocytopenic purpura, IGF-1: insulin-like growth factor-1, NR: not reported

Table 2. Patients' profiles of type B insulin resistance in Japan

No	HbA1c (%)	Insulin dose (U/day)	FPG (mg/dl)	IRI (U/ml)	CPR (ng/ml)	PSL dose (mg/day)	Other treatments
1	6.0	15	62	21.2		60	MTX
2	13.4	80	NR	NR	NR	50	IGF-1, CyA, rituximab
3	NR	340		NR	NR	25	CyA 200mg/day, rituximab 500mg x2
4	NR	610	220	821	3.7 nM	30	IGF-1
5	9.5	68	67	316	3.08	30	Plasma exchange immunoadsorption CPA, CyA, IGF-1
6	NR	-	NR	NR	NR	NR	Bed time snack
7	NR	>300	NR	NR	# >450	Pulse	Plasma exchange
8	9.1	-	38	697.7	14.2	60	-
9	NR	-	116	2313	55	mPSL 0.5g x2 PSL 30	-
10	NR	NR	NR	NR	NR	50	IGF-1
11	11.1	160	NR	462	5.1	-	IGF-1
12	NR	300	131	699.5	NR	40	IGF-1
13	6.3	-	48	581	0.42	40	-
14	NR	NR	NR	NR	NR	50	*H.p.* eradication
15	NR	NR	NR	NR	NR	NR	-
16	13.8	138	NR	NR	#138.4		
17	11.2	>200	180	490	6.52	-	-
			111	NR	6.52		
			66	15.9	0.7		
18	8.5	-(OHA)	NR	>1000	NR	2.5	-
19	5.0	-	56	NR	NR	-	*H.p.* eradication
		-	NR	NR	NR	20	

FPG: fasting plasma glucose, IRI: immunoreactive insulin, CPR: C-peptide reactivity, PSL: predonisolone, mPSL: methyl predonisolone, MTX: methotrexate, IGF-1: insulin-like growth factor-1, CyA: cyclosporine A, CPA: cyclophosphamide, #: urinary excretion of C-peptide (μg/day), H.p.: Helicobactor pyroli, OHA: oral hypoglycemic agent

Table 3. Treatments of type B insulin resistance in Japan

In US, the majority of patients with type B insulin resistance are African American woman. Hyperandorogenism and acanthosis nigricans are common. Severe insulin resistance is the predominant symptoms and fasting or reactive hypoglycemia may follow after hyperglycemia is ameliorated by various treatments. Among reports on Japanese patients with type B insulin resistance, we found more men (11) than women (8). The description of acanthosis nigricans was not common. Among 9 cases with available report, 6 had acanthosis nigricans and 3 had not. Severe obesity was also rare. In the 24 cases of type B insulin resistance reported by Arioglu et al. three cases presented hypoglycemia after prolonged hyperglycemia (Arioglu 2002). Among the 19 cases in Japan, 11 cases had hypoglycemia somewhere during the course. Eight of these 11 cases were not using oral hypoglycemic agent or insulin when hypoglycemia was first noticed. Examples are briefly introduced below.

A 23-year-old Japanese woman with SLE and on hemodialysis developed severe general fatigue (Nagayama et al. 2008). Her fasting blood glucose was between 25 to 45mg/dl. Her serum insulin level was 2313.8 μU/ml and anti-insulin receptor antibody was positive by ^{125}I -insulin binding inhibition assay. She also presented with acanthosis nigricans. Her hypoglycemia was restored after steroid pulse followed by high dose steroid therapy.

A 56-year-old Japanese man was admitted to the hospital because of unconsciousness and hypoglycemia (Sato 2010). Anti-insulin antibody was positive. Episodes of hypoglycemia and hyperglycemia repeated despite predonisolone therapy (5-10 mg/day) Laboratory test revealed pancytopenia, positive antinuclear antibody and mild proteinuria. He also presented persistent discoid lesion of the skin. Renal biopsy was consistent with lupus nephritis. He was diagnosed as SLE and the dose of predonisolone was increased to 60 mg/day. After that his blood glucose improved along with proteinuria. The dose of predonisolone could be successfully tapered to 30 mg/day.

3. Underlying disease

Type B insulin resistance associates most frequently with SLE and related connective tissue diseases. Sjögren's syndrome and rheumatoid arthritis were also found. On the other hand, what is the prevalence of anti-insulin receptor antibody in SLE patients? Rosenstein et al. analyzed consecutive 38 patients with SLE or undifferentiated connective tissue disease (UCTD) for anti-insulin receptor antibody (Rosenstein et al. 2001). Within 26 SLE patients one was positive for anti-insulin receptor antibody and none in the 12 UCTD patients. None of their patients presented insulin resistance syndrome. In our case, polymyositis was the underlying disease. We searched PubMed for "polymyositis" and "insulin resistance" and found several reports on juvenile dermatomyositis (JDA) associated with lipodystrophy. In a report from Canada, 4 of 20 patients with JDA had lipodystrophy and severe insulin resistance (Huemer 2001). However anti-insulin receptor antibody was not detected by radioimmunoassay in these cases. Their pathophysiology was explained in the context of lipodystrophy. Lipodystrophy associated with dermatomyositis is not confined to pediatric patients. A case of 55-year-old woman with dermatomyositis complicated with lipodystrophy is reported (Lee and Hobbs). She developed hypertriglyceridemia 3 years after diagnosis of dermatomyositis and then lipodystrophy in the thigh appeared. Severe insulin resistance was not reported in this case. Our case did not have typical skin lesions suggestive of dermatomyositis nor lipodystrophy. Therefore our case is not categorized in these insulin resistance associated with dermatomyositis. There are also reports of type B insulin resistance associated with interferon-alpha treatment (Miyamoto). Unfortunately, the detail of this case was not described in the literature. A similar case is reported by Daniel et al. A 55-year-old African American man with hepatitis C developed severe hyperglycemia eight months after treatment with interferon-alpha and ribavirin. He needed up to 125 U/hr of insulin and anti-insulin receptor antibody was detected in his serum. After discontinuation of interferon-alpha and ribavirin, his insulin resistance resolved spontaneously. Type B insulin resistance associated with idiopathic thrombocytopenic purpura (ITP) is also reported. *Helicobactor pyroli* infection is one of the causes of ITP and eradication of *H. pyroli* by proton pump inhibitor and antibiotics may relieve the thrombocytopenia. In Japan a case of type B insulin resistance that was ameliorated after eradication of *H. pyroli* has been reported (Imai). Interestingly, three years after the first episode, hypoglycemia recurred in this patient (Yamamiya). This time his plasma insulin was below detection limit when he was hypoglycemic. Anti-insulin receptor antibody was not proved by ^{125}I-insulin binding inhibition assay. Unfortunately, other method to detect anti-insulin receptor antibody has not been performed. Imunoprecipitation of insulin receptor by the patient's serum may probe anti-insulin receptor antibody. The change of the epitope of the anti-insulin receptor antibody may result in agonistic activity without inhibiting insulin binding.

4. Treatment of abnormal glucose metabolism

The dose of insulin utilized to control hyperglycemia was substantially small compared with that in the US (Arioglu, Lupsa, Malek). The Japanese patients with type B insulin resistance were treated no more than several hundred units a day. In the cases reported by Arioglu, on average 5100 U/day was used. A case with type B insulin resistance and SLE reported by Bao et al. required up to 4500 U/day insulin to control hyperglycemia. She was treated with azathiopurine for 3 months. Another severe insulin resistance case reported by Ostwal et al. required up to 2800 U/day. She had SLE and anti-insulin receptor antibody was probed by immunoprecipitation assay. A steroid pulse therapy with mehylpredonisolone 1 g for 3 days was performed followed by maintenance dose of steroid and azathiopurine. Her insulin requirement decreased gradually and stopped. After that she required 3-hourly meals to avoid hypoglycemia. In the treatment of hyperglycemia, insulin like growth factor-I (IGF-I, Astellas Pharmaceutical Co. Ltd. Tokyo) injection was tried in several Japanese patients with varying effectiveness. The anti-insulin receptor antibody does not necessarily affect insulin-like growth factor receptor. Therefore IGF-1 injection is worth trying if there are no contraindications such as proliferative retinopathy or malignancy. Type B insulin resistance is potentially a self-limited disease. However to treat severe hyperglycemia in a certain time frame may require immunosuppressive medications and/or plasma exchange. In our patient, severe hyperglycemia developed only after initiation of predonisolone therapy. His hyperglycemia was controlled with relatively small dose of insulin in a short time and hypoglycemia repeated after discontinuation of insulin therapy. This may reflect the agonistic character of anti-insulin receptor antibody in his case. Because predonisolone is frequently used to treat underlying disease, hypoglycemia is relatively easy to control although timed snack may be required to avoid fasting hypoglycemia.

5. Treatment of autoimmunity

Attempt to control abnormal autoantibody is mainly through control over underlying disease. Because SLE is the most predominant underlying disease, predonisolone therapy with or without pulse therapy is most commonly attempted. Methotrexate, azathiopurine, cyclophosphamide and mycophenolate mofetil are also used in resistant cases. Plasmapheresis or immunoadsorption is used in some cases to remove anti-insulin receptor antibody in a short time. Recently rituximab is another choice to reduce B-cells producing autoantibodies. Because the case of type B insulin resistance is rare, randomized control study is difficult to perform. Therefore the comparison of effectiveness of these various therapies is difficult. The choice of treatment seems to be determined by the familiarity of the doctors to each treatment. Also the anti-insulin receptor antibody may disappear spontaneously at least in some cases. This complicates the analysis of result. Therefore it seems to be prudent to choose treatment based on the effectiveness to control the underlying disease.

6. Prognosis

Arioglu reported that the prognosis of type B insulin resistance may be poor especially in those with hypoglycemia. Among the 19 cases at least two was reported as deceased. One of the two, a 23 year-old woman was on hemodialysis complicated with SLE when her hypoglycemia developed. She had intractable lung infection during the treatment of exacerbated SLE. Another case, a 56 year-old man with severe SLE died of sepsis. Hypoglycemia was not the direct cause of death for these cases. We have no data for other cases.

7. Characterization of anti-insulin receptor antibody

The presence of anti-insulin receptor antibody is probed with various methods. Inhibition of binding of ^{125}I-labelled insulin to insulin receptor is the method commonly used by commercial laboratory in Japan. The result is reported as inhibition rate. One problem of binding inhibition is that we cannot know whether the anti-insulin receptor antibody has agonist activity to insulin receptor. Another problem is that insulin binding is interfered by anti-insulin antibody if it coexists. This is a rare occasion however there are several cases in whom both anti-insulin antibody and anti-insulin receptor antibody were probed. The anti-insulin receptor is polyclonal and the character of the antibody may change during the course. Yamasaki et al. analyzed the insulin-like activity of the patient's serum during the course from severe hyperglycemia to fasting hypoglycemia. At first, her hyperglycemia was resistant to insulin at maximum 610 μU/day. After treatment with PSL, fasting hypoglycemia occurred. The activity to stimulate 2-deoxyglucose uptake was most prominent in the serum during the hyperglycemic phase and the serum during the hypoglycemic phase showed weaker activity. The activity to stimulate insulin receptor autophosphorylation was also most strong in the serum during the hyperglycemic phase. Their data suggest that antibody with agonistic activity may also present in patients who show no hypoglycemia. Receptor down regulation caused by autoantibody may modify the patient's response.

8. Epitopes of the autoantibodies

The extracellular part of the insulin receptor is composed of leucine rich domain 1, cysteine rich domain, leucine rich domain 2 and three fibronectin type III domains (McKern). Analysis using chimeric receptor has provided clue to the epitope of the anti-insulin receptor antibodies. Chimeric IGF-I receptor containing residues 450-601 of the insulin receptor was recognized by 12 of 15 sera from type B insulin resistance (Zhang & Roth). Residues 471-593 is the first fibronectin type III domain and monoclonal antibody to this region can inhibit high affinity insulin binding (Surinya). The epitopes of anti-insulin receptor antibody were analyzed by recognition of peptides from human insulin receptor expressed in bacteria (Pritgent 1990). A monoclonal antibody (83-14) mimics insulin action and inhibits insulin binding. This antibody recognizes amino acids 469-592. Another monoclonal antibody (18-44) also mimics insulin action but does not inhibit insulin binding. This antibody recognizes amino acids 765-770 within the third fibronectin type III domain in the N-terminus of the beta subunit. Chrystallographic study of the ectodomain of human insulin receptor revealed that the insulin binding pocket is made of N-terminal leucine rich repeat and the first fibronectin type III domain (McKern). The third fibronectin type III domain is outside the insulin binding pocket. Therefore if antibody to amino acids 765-770 is predominant, hypoglycemia without insulin resistance will result. In such a case, anti-insulin receptor antibody cannot be proved by binding inhibition assay. In the case reported by Yamamiya, anti-insulin receptor antibody was not detected by insulin binding inhibition when hypoglycemia recurred. This may result from change in the epitopes of the autoantibody. We should recall the possibility of anti-insulin receptor antibody when we see hypoglycemia associated with very low insulin level.

9. References

Arioglu E., Andewelt A., Diabo C et al. Clinical course of the syndrome of autoantibodies to the insulin receptor (type B insulin resisitance): a 28 year prespective. Medicine 2002; 81: 87-100

Bao S., Root C., and Jagasia S. Type B insulin resistance syndrome associated with systemic lupus erythematosus. Endocr Pract. 2007; 13: 51-55

Coll AP. Thomas S., and Mufti GJ. Rituximab therapy for the type B syndrome of severe insulin resistance New Eng J Med 2004; 350: 310-311

Coll AP., Morganstein D., Jaynet D., Soos MA., O'Rahilly S. and Burke J. Successful treatment of type B insulin resistance in a patient with otherwise quiescent systemic lupus erythematosus Diabetic Medicine 2005; 22: 812-815

Daniel AL., Houlihan JL., Blum JS. And Walsh JP. Type B insulin resistance developing during interferon-alpha therapy. Endocri Pract 2009; 15: 153-157

Eriksson JW., Fowelin J., Bremeli T., Frederiksson L., Eliasson B and Yuu ZW. Successful treatment with plasmaphereis, cyclophosphamide, and cyclosporine A in type B syndrome of insulin resistance. Diabetes Care 1998; 21: 1217-1220

Fareau GG., Maldonado M., Oral E. and Balasubramanyam A. Regression of acanthosis nigricans correlates with disappearance of anti-insulin receptor autoantibodies and achievement of euglycemia in type B insulin resistance syndrome. Metabolism 2007; 56: 670-675

Fujita N., Yamasaki H., Yamakawa K., Uotani S., Kuwahara H., Degawa-Yamauchi M., Abe T., Ozaki M., Sera Y., Kawasaki E., Takino H., Yamaguchi Y. and Eguchi K. Decrease in the insulin receptor protein level by anti-inulin receptor antibodies: roles of tyrosine kinase activity and receptor internalization. Acta Diabetol 2002; 39:221-227

Furukawa T., Taniguchi Y., Okuno Y., Oohara T., Ogawa A., Shirakami A., Shibata Y. and Kasuga M. Journal of the Japan Diabetes Society 2008; 51: 629-634

Gehi A., Webb A., Nolte M. and Davis J. Treatment of systemic lupus erythematosus-associated type B insulin resistance syndrome with cyclophoophamide and mycophenolate mofetil. Arthritis & Rheumatism 2003; 48:1067-1070

Gojo J., Hayashi T., Sano K., Saito T., Sasaki H. and Tajima N. Journal of the Japan Diabetes Society 2008; 51:654

Hirano T. and Adchi M. Insulin-like growth factor 1 therapy for type B insulin resistance. Annals of Internal Medicine 1997; 127: 245-246

Huemer C., Kitson H., Malleson p.N., Sanderson S., Huemer M., Cabral D.A., Chanoine J.P. and Petty R.E. J Rheumatol 2001; 28: 610-615

Imai J., Yamada T., Saito T., Ishigaki Y., Hinokio Y., Kotake H., Oka Y. and Katagiri H. Eradication of insulin resistance. Lancet 2009; 374: 264

Ito R., Watanabe M., Maeda S., Namba H., Hayamizu Y. and Sakano S. Proceedings of the 54th Scientific Meeting of the Japanese Society of Rheumatology. 2010, 674

Kawashiri S., Kawakami A., Fujikawa K., Iwamoto N., Aramaki T., Tamai M., Nakamura H., Origuchi T., Ida H. and Eguchi K. Type B insulin resistance complicated with systemic lupus erythematosus Inter Med 2010; 49:487-490

Lee l.A. and Hobbs K.F. Lipodystrophy and metabolic abnormalities in a case of adult dermatomyositis. J Am Acd Dermatol 2007; 57: S85-87

Lupsa B.C., Chong A.Y, Cochran E.K., Soos M.A., Semple R.K. and Gorden P. Auoimmune forms of hypoglycemia. Medicine 2009; 88: 141-153

Miyamoto M. Journal of the Japan Diabetes Society 2008;51(supple1): S-231

Malek R., Chong A.Y., Lupsa b.C., Lungu A.O., Cochran E.K., Soos M.A., Semple R.K., Balow J.E. and Gorden P. Treatment of type B insulin resistance: a novel approach to reduce insulin receptor autoantibodies. J Clin Endocinol Metab 2010; 95: 3641-3647

McKern N.M., Lawrence M.C. et al. Structure of the insulin receptor ectodomain reveals a folded-over conformation. Nature 2006; 443:218-221

Nagayama Y., Morita H., Komukai D., Watanabe S. and Yoshimura A. Type B insulin resistance syndrome induced by increased activity of systemic lupus erythematosus in a hemodialysis patient. Clin Nephrol. 2008 69: 130-134

Ostwal V. and Oak J. Type B insulin resistance in a systemic lupus erythematosus patient. International J of Rheumatic Diseases 2009; 12: 174-176

Ogata H., Kawaguchi M., Kasai N., Tsuda K., Matsushita Y. and Inoue A. Journal of the Japan Diabetes Society 2007; 50: 457

Rosenstein ED., Advani S., Reits RE and Kramer N. The prevalence of insulin receptor antibodies in patients with systemic lupus erythematosus and related conditions. J Clin Rheumatol. 2001; 7: 371-373

Sakai Tomoyuki., Fukushima T., Sawaki T., Kounan T., Shimoyama K., Karasawa H., Masaki Y., Hirose Y., Ogawa N., Sugai S. and Umehara H. Nihon Rinsho Men-eki Gakkai Zasshi 2005; 28: 272

Page K.A., Dejardin S., Kahn C.R., Kulkarni R.N., Herold K.C. and Inzucchi S.E. A patient with type B insulin resistance syndrome, responsive to immune therapy. Nature Clinical Practice Endocrinology & Metabolism 2007; 3: 835-839

Prigent S.A., Stanley K.K. and Siddle K. Identificaiton of epitopes on the human insulin receptor reacting with rabbit polyclonal antisera and mouse monoclonal antibodies. J Biol Chem 1990; 265: 9970-9977

Sakai Toshimitsu, Okada M., Yamamoto A., Ohnishi M., Murakami T.,Kasuga H., Ogiwara N., Asaoka A., Hayashi H. and Arakawa Y. Journal of the Japan Diabetes Society 2005; 48: 745-749

Sato N., Ohsawa I., Takagi M., Gohda T., Horikoshi S., Shirato I., Yamaguchi Y. and Tomino Y. Type B insulin resistance syndrome with systemic lupus erythematosus Clin Nephrol 2010; 73: 157-162

Semple R.K., Halberg N.H., Burling K., Soos M.A., Schraw T., Luan J., Cochran E.K., Dunger D.B., Wareham N.J., Scherer P.E., Gorden P. and O'Rahilly S. Paradoxical elevation of high-molecular weight adiponectin in acquired extreme insulin resistance due to insulin receptor antibodies. Diabetes 2007; 56: 1712-1717

Shigihara N., Hirose T., Watanabe T., Ikeda F., Kanazawa A., Shimizu T., Uchino Y., Wataya H. and Kawamori R. A case of type B insulin resistance with severe hypoglycemia complicated systemic lupus erythematosus. Diabetes Journal 2009; 37: 104-108

Surinya K.H., Molina L., Soos M.A., Brandt J., Kristensen C. and Siddle K. Role of insulin receptor dimerization domains in ligand binding, cooperativity, and modulation by anti-receptor antibodies. J Biol Chem 2002; 277: 16718-16725

Takeda T., Nishizawa M., Fukuda M., Furuya K., Tsuda S., Satake H., Ito T., Nakagawa J., Nakano S. Kogoshi T. and Koya H. Journal of the Japan Diabetes Society 2006; 49:240

Tashiro K., Kosaki A., Fujitaka K., Jo H., Jo S., NomuraE., Hasegawa T., Toyoda N., Ukita C., Nishikawa M. and Iwasaka T. Journal of the Japan Diabetes Society 2009; 52: 406

Tokumori Y., Tsunoda H. and Kanbe T. Journal of the Japan Diabetes Society 2008; 51: 66

Uehara Y.,Ishizuka T., Tsuchiya A., Hashimoto K., Okada H., Shimizu H., Yamada M. and Mori M. Journal of Japanese Society of Endocrinology 2009; 85: 372

Yamagata M., Suzuki Y., Matsuura I, Furuta S., Iwamoto I and Yoshida S. Proceedings of the 54th Scientific Meeting of the Japanese Society of Rheumatology. 2010, 621

Yamamiya H., Kurita S., Nagaoka T. and Noto H. Journal of Japanese Society of Endocrinology 2011; 87:350

Yamasaki H., Yamaguchi Y., Fujita N., Kato C., Kuwahara H., Degawa-Yamauchi M., Yamakawa K., Abe T., Ozaki M., Sera Y., Uotani S., Kawasaki E., Takino H. and

Eguchi K. Anti-insulin receptor autoantibodies in a patient with type B insulin resistance and fasting hypoglycemia. Acta Diabetol. 2000; 37: 189-196

Zhang B and Roth R.A. A region of the inslin receptor important for ligand binding (residues 450-601) is recognized by patients' autoimmune antibodies and inhibitory monoclonal antibodies. Proc Natl Acad Sci U.S.A. 1991; 88: 9858-9862

Part 6

Section F

15

Role of Incretin, Incretin Analogues and Dipeptidyl Peptidase 4 Inhibitors in the Pathogenesis and Treatment of Diabetes Mellitus

Athanasia K. Papazafiropoulou,
Marina S. Kardara and Stavros I. Pappas
3rdDepartment of Internal Medicine and Center of Diabetes, General Hospital of Nikaia "Ag. Panteleimon" – Piraeus, Greece

1. Introduction

Type 2 diabetes mellitus (T2DM) is increasing in prevalence worldwide, and is expected to affect 440 million people by 2030 (IDF, 2009). Despite the development and use of several medications to control patients' blood glucose levels, the effective management of T2DM continues to be a challenge to physicians. In order to achieve HbA1c targets (<7.0%), patients must reach desirable fasting (90 mg/dL - 130 mg/dL) and postprandial glucose levels (<180 mg/dL) (American Diabetes Association, 2006). However, two thirds of patients with T2DM remain unable to reach the HbA1c targets (Koro, 1988; Fan, 2006).
Blood glucose levels are dependent on the dynamic processes of hepatic production of glucose and skeletal muscle use of glucose. Treatment strategies designed to improve these processes have as a result the improvement in patient's glycemic status. Different agents are currently available, providing physicians with several options for the management of T2DM. These clinical therapies include insulin and oral drugs that are classified as insulin sensitizers (e.g., biguanides and thiazolidinediones), insulin secretagogues (e.g., sulfonylureas and meglitinides), and alpha-glucosidase inhibitors. Newer treatment agents, incretin mimetics and dipeptidyl peptidase 4 (DPP-4) inhibitors, have been recently added to clinicians' therapeutic choices (Drucker, 2003; Drucker, 2006a).

2. The incretin effect

The concept that gut factors stimulate pancreatic endocrine secretion was hypothesized soon after secretin was discovered in 1902 (Kieffer, 1999). In 1906, this notion was tested by giving gut extracts to patients with diabetes, which reduced their glycosuria (Moore, 1906). In the 1920s, based on studies in dogs, the term incretins was introduced for the gastrointestinal hormones released in response to food ingestion (Zunz, 1929). These hormones are responsible for approximately 60% of the insulin secretion following a meal and for the so-called incretin effect. The incretin effect describes the phenomenon that oral glucose leads to a greater insulin response than an isoglycaemic intravenous glucose load (McIntyre, 1964; Nauck, 1986).

There are two major incretins: glucosedependent insulinotropic polypeptide (GIP) and glucagon-like peptide 1 (GLP-1). In this chapter we will focus on GLP-1 actions, since this molecule is preserved in patients with T2DM.

3. Physiological actions of GLP-1

GLP-1 is a product of the glucagons gene, which is expressed in pancreatic α-cells and in L-cells, located mostly in the lower small intestine and colon. GLP-1 concentrations increase as early as 5 to 10 minutes following ingestion of carbohydrates and lipids, well before the nutrients pass into the lower gut where most L-cells are located (Eissele, 1992; Deacon, 1995). Once released from L- cells, GLP-1 is rapidly metabolized by a widely distributed serine protease, DPP-4, resulting in a half-life of 1 to 2 minutes in the circulation. DPP-4, which is located on endothelial cells as well as in soluble form in plasma, cleaves the two N-terminal amino acids from GLP-1, causing a substantial loss of insulinotropic activity (Deacon, 1995; Vahl, 2003).

GLP-1 stimulates insulin secretion of the β-cells and inhibits glucagon secretion from the α-cells. Both actions occur in a glucose-dependent manner and lead to a normalisation of postprandial and fasting hyperglycaemia (Drucker, 2006b). In the gastrointestinal tract, GLP-1 has a direct effect on motility and slows gastric emptying. This effect contributes to a normalisation of postprandial hyperglycaemia and explains why long-term treatment with GLP-1 receptor agonists leads to weight loss (Drucker, 2006b). Under hypoglycaemic conditions the counter-regulation by glucagon is not affected and insulin secretion is not stimulated and, therefore, GLP-1 does not elicit hypoglycaemia (Drucker, 2006b).

Except for its antidiabetic actions, recent findings have shown that application of GLP-1 receptor agonists led to an improvement in cardiovascular parameters (reduction of systolic blood pressure, beneficial effects on myocardial ischaemia in animal models, positive effects on left ventricular function in heart failure) (Papazafiropoulou, 2011). In addition, animal studies in rodents and isolated human islets showed beneficial long-term actions of GLP-1 to β-cell mass (Fehmann, 1992; Brubaker, 2004). Whether these findings will have a positive effect on preventing T2DM progression is not known yet.

4. Incretins and the pathogenesis of T2DM

In T2DM patients the incretin effect is diminished. Incretins does not act as an insulinotropic hormones under chronic hyperglycaemia in T2DM. However, GLP-1 is still able to stimulate insulin secretion under hyperglycaemia in T2DM (Drucker, 2006). In addition, the effects of GLP-1 on gastric emptying and glucagon secretion are maintained in patients with T2DM (Nauck, 1993a).

A study confirmed that the incretin effect is reduced in patients with T2DM (Knop, 2007). Another study showed a significant reduction in the incretin effect and the GLP-1 response to oral glucose in T2DM patients compared with individuals with normal or impaired glucose tolerance (Muscelli, 2008). Notably, impaired actions of GLP-1 may be partially restored by improved glycemic control (Knop, 2007). The findings from a study of obese diabetic mice suggest that the effect of GLP-1 therapy may be caused by improvements in β-cell function and insulin sensitivity, as well as by a reduction in gluconeogenesis in the liver (Lee, 2007).

Several studies in T2DM patients have shown that synthetic GLP-1 administration induces insulin secretion, (Nathan, 1992; Nauck, 1993a) slows gastric emptying, and decreases inappropriately elevated glucagons secretion (Nauck, 1993a; Kolterman, 2003). Acute GLP-1 infusion studies showed that GLP-1 improved fasting and post prandial plasma glucose concentrations (Nathan, 1992; Nauck, 1993b). Long-term studies showed that this hormone exerts euglycemic effects, leading to improvements in HbA1c, and induces weight loss (Zander, 2002).

5. T2DM and incretin-based therapies

The incretin-based therapies offer a good alternative choice to the established antidiabetic compounds due to their satisfying antihyperglycaemic efficacy, their lack of risk of hypoglycaemia and their positive effects on body weight. In order to utilise GLP-1 action for T2DM, two options are presently available:

1. GLP-1-receptor agonists (or GLP-1 mimetics) as injectable compounds
2. DPP-4 inhibitors as orally active substances

6. GLP-1-receptor agonists

6.1 Exenatide

Exenatide is the synthetic form of exendin-4, a peptide first discovered in the saliva of the gila monster (heloderma suspectum) in 1992. It has a 53% amino acid sequence homology to human GLP-1 and is a GLP-1 receptor agonist (Eng, 1992). It is administered subcutaneously twice daily. A slow release formulation for once-weekly administration (Exenatide LAR [long-acting release]) is presently in clinical phase III studies (Drucker, 2008). Exenatide has a prolonged half-life in comparison to native GLP-1 of approximately 3.5 h. After subcutaneous injection sufficient plasma concentrations are reached for 4–6 hours (Kolterman, 2005).

In clinical studies exenatide lowered the HbA1c by 0.8–1.1% (Buse, 2004; DeFronzo, 2005). Exenatide in combination with metformin (Kendall, 2005), sulfonylurea (DeFronzo, 2005), or both (Buse, 2004) resulted in significant mean HbA1c reductions from baseline ranging from -0.77% to -0.86%. Patients also had statistically significant reductions in mean body weight from baseline (-1.6 kg to -2.8 kg). Comparative studies with insulin showed that effects of exenatide on glycaemic parameters are comparable to the improvement seen with insulin therapy (Heine 2005; Gallwitz, 2006; Barnett, 2007; Nauck, 2007). The comparative studies with insulin showed a difference in weight development of 4–5 kg in 30 weeks between the insulin and exenatide treated groups (Heine 2005; Barnett, 2007a; Nauck, 2007a).

An improvement of β-cell function [measured with HOMA-β (homeostatic modelling assessment of beta cell function) and the proinsulin: insulin ratio] was also observed in the clinical studies. First phase of insulin secretion was restored after an intravenous glucose bolus under treatment with exenatide (Gallwitz, 2006; Barnett, 2007b).

Severe hypoglycaemic events were only observed in exenatide-treated patients who had received combination therapy with sulfonylurea. For this reason a reduction in the dosage of sulfonylurea should be considered when initiating exenatide therapy. In the comparative studies comparing exenatide with insulin treatment, the incidence of nocturnal hypoglycaemic events was lower in the exenatide-treated patients (Gallwitz, 2006; Barnett, 2007).

The most frequent adverse events with exenatide were fullness and nausea. Nausea was the most common reason to stop therapy; with 2–6.4% drop-outs in the clinical studies with exenatide (Gallwitz, 2006; Barnett, 2007). Escalating the dose of exenatide from 5 µg to 10 µg after 4 weeks led to a transient increase in nausea which diminished with continued exposure to the higher dose (Gallwitz, 2006; Barnett, 2007).

In approximately 40% of exenatide-treated patients, anti-exenatide antibodies can be detected. However, over a time period of at least 3 years, these antibody titres did not have any obvious effect on glycaemic control (Drucker, 2008). Cases of acute pancreatitis have been reported since exenatide has been used (Ahmad, 2008; Cure, 2008). In total, the incidence of pancreatitis was low and similar to the elevated risk of pancreatitis that was observed in obese T2DM patients (Dore, 2009).

Exenatide is predominantly eliminated by glomerular filtration followed by proteolytic degradation (Yoo, 2006). Exenatide should not be used in patients with severe renal impairment (creatinine clearance <30 ml/min) or end stage renal disease. Additionally, caution should be applied when initiating or increasing doses of exenatide in patients with moderate renal impairment (creatinine clearance 30–50 ml/min) (Gallwitz, 2006; Barnett, 2007).

6.2 Liraglutide

Liraglutide is the first human GLP-1 analogue. It has two modifications in the amino acid sequence of native GLP-1 and an attachment of a fatty acid side chain to the peptide. It is injected subcutaneously once daily (Agerso, 2002). Liraglutide lowers blood glucose, body weight and food intake in animal models (Sturis, 2003). In clinical studies in approximately 4,200 T2DM patients liraglutide was efficacious and safe (Marre, 2009; Nauck, 2009; Zinman, 2009). In animal studies with diabetic rodents, liraglutide has been shown to increase β-cell mass.

Liraglutide in monotherapy in newly diagnosed T2DM patients led to HbA1c reduction of 0.9–1.1% in a dose of 1.2 or 1.8 mg once daily respectively, over a period of up to 2 years (Garber, 2008). In other studies, the same doses of liraglutide effectively lowered glycaemic parameters in various combinations with oral antidiabetic agents by approximately 1.0–1.5% (Garber, 2008; Garber, 2009).

Liraglutide treatment led to a significant weight loss (Deacon, 2009a; Vilsboll, 2009). The weight loss was accompanied by a more pronounced loss in visceral fat than subcutaneous fat (Deacon, 2009a; Vilsboll, 2009). Furthermore, systolic blood pressure was lowered by 2–6 mmHg in the liraglutide-treated patients. This effect was independent of the weight loss, as the reduction of blood pressure was already observed early on in therapy, when weight loss had not yet occurred (Garber, 2008; Garber, 2009; Zinman, 2009).

The incidence of hypoglycaemic episodes was comparable to placebo in all studies, where no sulfonylurea was used in the combination with liraglutide (Deacon, 2009a; Vilsboll, 2009). Gastrointestinal symptoms were also common, but nausea and vomiting were reported for a short period at the beginning of therapy (Buse, 2009). In the liraglutide clinical trials, there was no evidence of neutralizing antibodies (Garber, 2008; Garber, 2009; Zinman, 2009).

Animal studies showed that a rare type of thyroid cancer known as medullary thyroid cancer was associated with liraglutide in mice and rats, although the relevance of this finding to humans remains unknown. FDA has stipulated that liraglutide be contraindicated in patients

with a personal or family history of medullary thyroid cancer and in patients with multiple endocrine neoplasia syndrome type 2 (US Food and Drug Administration, 2010).
Data on the pharmacokinetic profile of liraglutide in mild to moderate renal impairment showed no alteration of the profile (Deacon, 2009a; Vilsboll, 2009).

7. DPP-4 Inhibitors

7.1 Sitagliptin

Sitagliptin was the first DPP-4 inhibitor approved for the T2DM treatment. The recommended dose of once-daily oral sitagliptin is 100 mg. At this dose, sitagliptin can inhibit ~80% of endogenous DPP-4 activity over a 24-hour period (Herman, 2005). Increases in HOMA-β ranging from 4% to 20% have been shown in the sitagliptin trials.
In the monotherapy trials, sitagliptin compared to placebo, resulted in statistically significant improvements in HbA1c and fasting glucose (Aschner, 2006; Raz, 2006; Scott, 2007). Sitagliptin given as add-on therapy to metformin (Charbonnel, 2006) resulted in similar HbA1c and fasting glucose reductions as in the monotherapy trials. The same result was observed, in a 24-week trial, when sitagliptin was added to pioglitazone vs pioglitazone and placebo (Rosenstock, 2006). In another study, reductions from baseline in HbA1c and fasting glucose were similar when sitagliptin was compared to glipizide, (Nauck, 2007). Increases in HOMA-β ranging from 4% to 20% have been shown in the sitagliptin trials.
Sitagliptin therapy has been shown to be weight neutral in all clinical trials except in one study in which sitagliptin given with metformin resulted in weight reduction of 1.5 kg after 52 weeks of treatment (Nauck, 2007b). The most common side effects of sitagliptin were headache, arthritis, nasopharyngitis, respiratory or urinary tract infections and rarely skin reactions (Aschner, 2006; Raz, 2006; Rosenstock, 2006). The incidence of hypoglycemia was low in these trials (<2%) and was similar to the placebo arms. Dose reduction of sitagliptin has been recommended for patients with moderate or severe renal insufficiency or end stage renal disease (Bergman, 2007).

7.2 Vildagliptin

Vildagliptin also acts by inhibiting circulating DPP-4 activity. It is available as a 50 mg twice-daily in combination with metformin, sulfonylurea or pioglitazone. Vildagliptin has been studied as monotherapy (Ristic, 2005; Pratley, 2006; Dejager, 2007), in combination with other oral antidiabetic agents (Ahren, 2004; Fonseca, 2007; Rosenstock, 2007), and against active comparator therapies including glitazones (Rosenstock, 2007) and metformin (Schweizer, 2007) Vildagliptin therapy was associated with an increase in HOMA-β (11% and 23%) in two monotherapy trials (Ristic, 2005; Pratley, 2006).
In placebo-controlled trials, vildagliptin monotherapy reduced HbA1c (range 0.5% to 0.9%) and fasting glucose (14.4 mg/dL to 19.8 mg/dL) from baseline. The HbA1c reductions observed with monotherapy were statistically significantly greater than placebo in all trials. In clinical studies testing vildaglitpin in monotherapy or combination therapy with metformin, glimepiride, pioglitazone or insulin, vildagliptin was able to decrease the HbA1c by approximately 0.5–1.0% (Ahren, 2008; Pratley, 2008; Barnett, 2009). Vildagliptin therapy was associated with an increase HOMA-β (11% and 23%) in two monotherapy trials (Ristic, 2005; Pratley, 2006), but improvement relative to placebo was only observed in one trial (Ristic, 2005).

Vildagliptin has a good safety and tolerability profile and the most common adverse events are flu-like symptoms, headache, dizziness, and rarely liver enzyme elevations. Vildagliptin, like the other DPP-4 inhibitors, is weight-neutral. The incidence of hypoglycemia was low in trials with vildagliptin and similar to the placebo (Fonseca, 2007; Rosenstock, 2007). No dose adjustment is required in patients with mild renal impairment (creatinine clearance ≥50 ml/min). Vildagliptin should not be used in patients with hepatic impairment, including patients with pre-treatment alanine aminotransferase or aspartate aminotransferase >3x the upper limit of normal.

7.3 Saxagliptin

Saxagliptin also acts by inhibiting circulating DPP-4 activity and is available as a 5 mg once-daily in combination with metformin, sulfonylurea or pioglitazone. Saxagliptin causes a reduction in HbA1c by 0.7–0.9%. Fasting plasma glucose is also lowered dose dependently lowered by saxagliptin (Rosenstock, 2008). In a study with drug-naïve patients, saxagliptin lowered all glycaemic parameters significantly (Rosenstock, 2009). As an add-on medication to a therapy with either metformin or glitazone, saxagliptin also led to significant metabolic improvements (Chacra, 2009; Deacon, 2009b; DeFronzo, 2009).
Saxagliptin did not cause hypoglycaemia, was well-tolerated and was weight-neutral. A meta-analysis of clinical phase III studies with saxagliptin showed favourable data on the development of cardiovascular events (Wolf, 2009).

8. In conclusion

Incretin-based therapies offer an alternative treatment option for T2DM patients by targeting pancreatic β-cell dysfunction. Both GLP-1 receptor agonists and DPP-4 inhibitors have been shown to be effective in improving glycemic control in patients with T2DM. They appear to be well tolerated, have a low risk of hypoglycaemia, lead to weight reduction or have a neutral effect on weight.
Choice of therapy should be based on a patient's profile and preference, with consideration given to the unique characteristics of the GLP-1 receptor agonists and DPP-4 inhibitors. The most patient-relevant and striking difference between the incretin-based therapies is that GLP-1 receptor agonists are injectable agents, while DPP-4 inhibitors are effective orally. GLP-1 receptor agonists offer more robust HbA1c level reductions and the potential for weight loss. Nausea, the most common adverse event observed with GLP-1 receptor agonist therapy is not observed in treatment with DPP-4 inhibitors. Advances in the investigation of incretin therapies will further improve treatment outcomes for patients with T2DM and help them reach target goals.

9. References

Agerso H, Jensen LB, Elbrond B, Rolan P, Zdravkovic M (2002). The pharmacokinetics, pharmacodynamics, safety and tolerability of NN2211, a new long-acting GLP-1 derivative, in healthy men. *Diabetologia,* 45,195–202

Ahmad SR, Swann J (2008). Exenatide and rare adverse events. *N Engl J Med,* 358,1970–1971

Ahren B (2008). Emerging dipeptidyl peptidase-4 inhibitors for the treatment of diabetes. *Expert Opin Emerg Drugs,* 13, 593–607

American Diabetes Association (2006). Diagnosis and classification of diabetes mellitus. *Diabetes Care,* 29(Suppl 1), S43-S48

Aschner P, Kipnes MS, Lunceford JK, Sanchez M, Mickel C, Williams-Herman DE (2006). Effect of the dipeptidyl peptidase-4 inhibitor sitagliptin as monotherapy on glycemic control in patients with type 2 diabetes. *Diabetes Care,* 29, 2632-2637

b. Barnett A (2007) Exenatide. *Expert Opin Pharmacother,* 8, 2593–2608

Barnett AH (2009). New treatments in type 2 diabetes: a focus on the incretin-based therapies. *Clin Endocrinol (Oxf),* 70, 343–353

a. Barnett AH, Burger J, Johns D, Brodows R, Kendall DM, Roberts A, Trautmann ME (2007). Tolerability and efficacy of exenatide and titrated insulin glargine in adult patients with type2 diabetes previously uncontrolled with metformin or a sulfonylurea: a multinational, randomized, open-label, two-period, crossover noninferiority trial. *Clin Ther,* 29, 2333–2348

Bergman AJ, Cote J, Yi B, Marbury T, Swan SK, Smith W, Gottesdiener K, Wagner J, Herman GA (2007). Effect of renal insufficiency on the pharmacokinetics of sitagliptin,a dipeptidyl peptidase-4 inhibitor. *Diabetes Care,* 30, 1862-1864

Brubaker PL, Drucker DJ (2004). Minireview: glucagon-like peptides regulate cell proliferation and apoptosis in the pancreas, gut, and central nervous system. *Endocrinology,* 145, 2653–2659

Buse JB, Henry RR, Han J, Kim DD, Fineman MS, Baron AD (2004). Effects of exenatide (exendin-4) on glycemic control over 30 weeks in sulfonylurea-treated patients with type 2 diabetes. *Diabetes Care,* 27, 2628–2635

Buse JB, Rosenstock J, Sesti G, Schmidt WE, Montanya E, Brett JH, Zychma M, Blonde L (2009). Liraglutide once a day versus exenatide twice a day for type 2 diabetes: a 26-week randomised, parallel-group, multinational, open-label trial (LEAD-6). *Lancet,* 374, 39–47

Chacra AR, Tan GH, Apanovitch A, Ravichandran S, List J, Chen R (2009). Saxagliptin added to a submaximal dose of sulphonylurea improves glycaemic control compared with uptitration of sulphonylurea in patients with type 2 diabetes: a randomised controlled trial. *Int J Clin Pract,* 63, 1395–1406

Charbonnel B, Karasik A, Liu J, Wu M, Meininger G (2006). Efficacy and safety of the dipeptidyl peptidase-4 inhibitor sitagliptin added to ongoing metformin therapy in patients with type 2 diabetes inadequately controlled with metformin alone. *Diabetes Care,* 29, 2638-2643

Cure P, Pileggi A, Alejandro R (2008). Exenatide and rare adverse events. *N Engl J Med,* 358, 1969–1970

a. Deacon CF (2009). Potential of liraglutide in the treatment of patients with type 2 diabetes. *Vasc Health Risk Manag,* 5, 199–211

b. Deacon CF, Holst JJ (2009). Saxagliptin: a new dipeptidyl peptidase-4 inhibitor for the treatment of type 2 diabetes. *Adv Ther,* 26, 488–499

Deacon CF, Johnsen AH, Holst JJ (1995). Degradation of glucagon-like peptide-1 by human plasma in vitro yields an N-terminally truncated peptide that is a major endogenous metabolite in vivo. *J Clin Endocrinol Metab,* 80, 952–957

DeFronzo RA, Hissa MN, Garber AJ, Luiz Gross J, Yuyan Duan R, Ravichandran S, Chen RS (2009). The efficacy and safety of saxagliptin when added to metformin therapy in patients with inadequately controlled type 2 diabetes with metformin alone. *Diabetes Care*, 32, 1649–1655

DeFronzo RA, Ratner RE, Han J, Kim DD, Fineman MS, Baron AD (2005). Effects of exenatide (exendin-4) on glycemic control and weight over 30 weeks in metformin-treated patients with type 2 diabetes. *Diabetes Care*, 28, 1092–1100

Dejager S, Razac S, Foley JE, Schweizer A (2007). Vildagliptin in drug-naive patients with type 2 diabetes: a 24-week, doubleblind, randomized, placebo-controlled, multiple-dose study. *Horm Metab Res*, 39, 218-223

Dore DD, Seeger JD, Arnold Chan K (2009). Use of a claimsbased active drug safety surveillance system to assess the risk of acute pancreatitis with exenatide or sitagliptin compared to metformin or glyburide. *Curr Med Res Opin*, 25,1019–1027

Drucker DJ, Buse JB, Taylor K, Kendall DM, Trautmann M, Zhuang D, Porter L (2008). Exenatide once weekly versus twice daily for the treatment of type 2 diabetes: a randomised, openlabel, non-inferiority study. *Lancet*, 372, 1240–1250

Drucker DJ, Nauck MA (2006). The incretin system: glucagonlike peptide-1 receptor agonists and dipeptidyl peptidase-4 inhibitors in type 2 diabetes. *Lancet*, 368, 1696–1705

b. Drucker DJ, Nauck MA (2006). The incretin system: glucagon-like peptide-1 receptor agonists and dipeptidyl peptidase-4 inhibitors in type 2 diabetes. *Lancet*, 368,1696–1705

Drucker DJ (2003). Enhancing incretin action for the treatment of type 2 diabetes. *Diabetes Care*, 26, 2929-2940

a. Drucker DJ (2006). Incretin-based therapies: a clinical need filled by unique metabolic effects. *Diabetes Educ*, 32(Suppl 2), 65S-71S

Eissele R, Göke R, Willemer S, Harthus HP, Vermeer H, Arnold R, Göke B (1992). Glucagon-like peptide-1 cells in the gastrointestinal tract and pancreas of rat, pig and man. *Eur J Clin Invest*, 22, 283–291

Eng J, Kleinman WA, Singh L, Singh G, Raufman JP (1992). Isolation and characterization of exendin-4, an exendin-3 analogue, from Heloderma suspectum venom. Further evidence for an exendin receptor on dispersed acini from guinea pig pancreas. *J Biol Chem*, 267, 7402–7405

Fan T, Koro CE, Fedder DO, Bowlin SJ (2006). Ethnic disparitiesand trends in glycemic control among adults with type 2 diabetes in the U.S. from 1988 to 2002. *Diabetes Care*, 29, 1924-1925

Fehmann HC, Habener JF (1992). Insulinotropic hormone glucagon-like peptide-I(7–37) stimulation of proinsulin gene expression and proinsulin biosynthesis in insulinoma beta TC-1 cells. *Endocrinology*, 130,159–166

Fonseca V, Schweizer A, Albrecht D, Baron MA, Chang I, Dejager S (2007). Addition of vildagliptin to insulin improves glycaemiccontrol in type 2 diabetes. *Diabetologia*, 50, 1148-1155.

Gallwitz B (2006). Exenatide in type 2 diabetes: treatment effects in clinical studies and animal study data. *Int J Clin Pract*, 60,1654–1661

Garber A, Henry R, Ratner R, Garcia-Hernandez PA, Rodriguez-Pattzi H, Olvera-Alvarez I, Hale PM, Zdravkovic M, Bode B (2008). Liraglutide versus glimepiride monotherapy for type 2 diabetes (LEAD-3 Mono): a randomised, 52-week, phase III, double-blind, parallel-treatment trial. *Lancet*, 373, 473–481

Garber A, Henry RR, Ratner RE, Hale P, Chang CT, Bode B (2009). Monotherapy with liraglutide, a once-daily human GLP-1 analog, provides sustained reductions in A1C, FPG, and weight compared with glimepiride in type 2 diabetes: LEAD-3 mono 2-year results. *Diabetes,* 58(Suppl 1), 162, OR

Heine RJ, van Gaal LF, Johns D, Mihm MJ, Widel MH, Brodows RG (2005). Exenatide versus insulin glargine in patients with suboptimally controlled type 2 diabetes: a randomized trial. *Ann Intern Med,* 143, 559–569

Herman GA, Stevens C, Van Dyck K, Bergman A, Yi B, De Smet M, Snyder K, Hilliard D, Tanen M, Tanaka W, Wang AQ, Zeng W, Musson D, Winchell G, Davies MJ, Ramael S, Gottesdiener KM, Wagner JA (2005). Pharmacokinetics and pharmacodynamics of sitagliptin, an inhibitor of dipeptidyl peptidase IV, in healthy subjects: results from two randomized, double-blind, placebo-controlled studies with single oral doses. *Clin Pharmacol Ther,* 78, 675-688

International Diabetes Federation (IDF) (2009). Diabetes Atlas. Available at http://www.diabetesatlas.org

Kendall DM, Riddle MC, Rosenstock J, Zhuang D, Kim DD, Fineman MS, Baron AD (2005). Effects of exenatide (exendin-4) on glycemic control over 30 weeks in patients with type 2 diabetes treated with metformin and a sulfonylurea. *Diabetes Care,* 28,1083–1091

Knop FK, Vilsbøll T, Højberg PV, Larsen S, Madsbad S, Vølund A, Holst JJ, Krarup T (2007). Reduced incretin effect in type 2 diabetes: cause or consequence of the diabetic state? *Diabetes,* 56, 1951–1959

Kolterman OG, Buse JB, Fineman MS, Gaines E, Heintz S, Bicsak TA, Taylor K, Kim D, Aisporna M, Wang Y Baron AD (2003). Synthetic exendin-4 (exenatide) signifi cantly reduces postprandial and fasting plasma glucose in subjects with type 2 diabetes. *J Clin Endocrinol Metab,* 88, 3082–3089

Kolterman OG, Kim DD, Shen L, Ruggles JA, Nielsen LL, Fineman MS, Baron AD (2005). Pharmacokinetics, pharmacodynamics, and safety of exenatide in patients with type 2 diabetes mellitus. *Am J Health Syst Pharm,* 62, 173–181

Koro CE, Bowlin SJ, Bourgeois N, Fedder DO (2004). Glycemic control from 1988 to 2000 among US adults diagnosed with type 2 diabetes: a preliminary report. *Diabetes Care,* 27,17-20

Lee YS, Shin S, Shigihara T, Hahm E, Liu MJ, Han J, Yoon JW Jun HS (2007). Glucagon-like peptide-1 gene therapy in obese diabetic mice results in long-term cure of diabetes by improving insulin sensitivity and reducing hepatic gluconeogenesis. *Diabetes,* 56, 1671–1679

Marre M, Shaw J, Brandle M, Bebakar WM, Kamaruddin NA, Strand J, Zdravkovic M, Le Thi TD, Colagiuri S (2009). Liraglutide, a once-daily human GLP-1 analogue, added to a sulphonylurea over 26 weeks produces greater improvements in glycaemic and weight control compared with adding rosiglitazone or placebo in subjects with Type 2 diabetes (LEAD-1 SU). *Diabet Med,* 26, 268–278

McIntyre N, Holdsworth CD, Turner DS (1964). New interpretation of oral glucose tolerance. *Lancet,* 41, 20–21

Moore B, Edie E, Abram J (1906). On the treatment of diabetes mellitus by acid extract of duodenal mucous membrane. *Biochem J,* 1, 28–38

Muscelli E, Mari A, Casolaro A, Camastra S, Seghieri G, Gastaldelli A, Holst JJ, Ferrannini E (2008). Separate impact of obesity and glucose tolerance on the incretin effect in normal subjects and type 2 diabetic patients. *Diabetes*, 57, 1340–1348

Nathan DM, Schreiber E, Fogel H, Mojsov S, Habener JF (1992). Insulinotropic action of glucagonlike peptide-I-(7-37) in diabetic and nondiabetic subjects. *Diabetes Care*, 15, 270–276

Nauck M, Frid A, Hermansen K, Shah NS, Tankova T, Mitha IH, Zdravkovic M, During M, Matthews DR (2009). Efficacy and safety comparison of liraglutide, glimepiride, and placebo, all in combination with metformin, in type 2 diabetes: the LEAD (liraglutide effect and action in diabetes)-2 study. *Diabetes Care*, 32, 84–90

A. Nauck MA, Duran S, Kim D, Johns D, Northrup J, Festa A, Brodows R, Trautmann M (2007). A comparison of twicedailyexenatide and biphasic insulin aspart in patients with type 2 diabetes who were suboptimally controlled with sulfonylurea and metformin: a non-inferiority study. *Diabetologia*, 50, 259–267

A. Nauck MA, Heimesaat MM, Orskov C, Holst JJ, Ebert R, Creutzfeldt W (1993). Preserved incretin activity of glucagon-like peptide 1 [7-36 amide] but not of synthetic human gastric inhibitory polypeptide in patients with type-2 diabetes mellitus. *J Clin Invest*, 91, 301–307

Nauck MA, Homberger E, Siegel EG, Allen RC, Eaton RP, Ebert R, Creutzfeldt W (1986). Incretin effects of increasing glucose loads in man calculated from venous insulin and C-peptide responses. *J Clin Endocrinol Metab*, 63, 492–498

B. Nauck MA, Kleine N, Orskov C, Holst JJ, Willms B, Creutzfeldt W (1993). Normalization of fasting hyperglycaemia by exogenous glucagon-like peptide 1 (7-36 amide) in type 2 (non-insulin-dependent) diabetic patients. *Diabetologia*, 36, 741–744

B. Nauck MA, Meininger G, Sheng D, Terranella L, Stein PP (2007). Efficacy and safety of the dipeptidyl peptidase-4 inhibitor, sitagliptin, compared with the sulfonylurea, glipizide, in patients with type 2 diabetes inadequately controlled on metformin alone: a randomized, double-blind, non-inferiority trial. *Diabetes Obes Metab*, 9, 194-205

Papazafiropoulou A, Pappas S, Papadogiannis D, Tentolouris N (2011). Cardiovascular Effects of Glucagon-like Peptide 1. *Mini Rev Med Chem,* 11, 97-105

Pratley RE (2008). Overview of glucagon-like peptide-1 analogs and dipeptidyl peptidase-4 inhibitors for type 2 diabetes. *Medscape J Med*, 10, 171

Pratley RE, Jauffret-Kamel S, Galbreath E, Holmes D (2006). Twelveweek monotherapy with the DPP-4 inhibitor vildagliptin improves glycemic control in subjects with type 2 diabetes. *Horm Metab Res*, 38, 423-428

Raz I, Hanefeld M, Xu L, Caria C, Williams-Herman D, Khatami H (2006). Efficacy and safety of the dipeptidyl peptidase-4 inhibitorsitagliptin as monotherapy in patients with type 2 diabetes mellitus. *Diabetologia*, 49, 2564-2571.

Retterstol K (2009). Taspoglutide: a long acting human glucagonlike polypeptide-1 analogue. *Expert Opin Investig Drugs* 18, 1405–1411

Ristic S, Byiers S, Foley J, Holmes D (2005). Improved glycaemic control with dipeptidyl peptidase-4 inhibition in patients with type2 diabetes: vildagliptin (LAF237) dose response. *Diabetes Obes Metab*, 7, 692-698

Rosenstock J, Aguilar-Salinas C, Klein E, Nepal S, List J, Chen R (2009). Effect of saxagliptin monotherapy in treatment-naivepatients with type 2 diabetes. *Curr Med Res Opin*, 25, 2401–2411

Rosenstock J, Baron MA, Camisasca RP, Cressier F, Couturier A, Dejager S (2007). Efficacy and tolerability of initial combination therapy with vildagliptin and pioglitazone compared with component monotherapy in patients with type 2 diabetes. *Diabetes Obes Metab*, 9, 175-185

Rosenstock J, Brazg R, Andryuk PJ, Lu K, Stein P (2006). Efficacy and safety of the dipeptidyl peptidase-4 inhibitor sitagliptin added to ongoing pioglitazone therapy in patients with type 2 diabetes: a 24-week, multicenter, randomized, double-blind, placebocontrolled, parallel-group study. *Clin Ther*, 28, 1556-1568

Rosenstock J, Reusch J, Bush M, Yang F, Stewart M (2009). The potential of albiglutide, a long-acting GLP-1 receptor agonist, in type 2 diabetes: a randomized controlled trial exploring weekly, biweekly, and monthly dosing. *Diabetes Care*, 32, 1880–1886

Rosenstock J, Sankoh S, List JF (2008). Glucose-lowering activity of the dipeptidyl peptidase-4 inhibitor saxagliptin indrug-naive patients with type 2 diabetes. *Diabetes Obes Metab*, 10, 376–386

Scott R, Wu M, Sanchez M, Stein P (2007). Efficacy and tolerability of the dipeptidyl peptidase-4 inhibitor sitagliptin as monotherapy over 12 weeks in patients with type 2 diabetes. *Int J Clin Pract*, 61, 171-180

Sturis J, Gotfredsen CF, Romer J, Rolin B, Ribel U, Brand CL, Wilken M, Wassermann K, Deacon CF, Carr RD, Knudsen LB (2003). GLP-1 derivative liraglutide in rats with beta-cell deficiencies: influence of metabolic state on beta-cell mass dynamics. *Br J Pharmacol*, 140:123–132

US Food and Drug Administration. Questions and answers—safety requirements for Victoza (liraglutide). http://www.fda.gov/Drugs/DrugSafety/PostmarketDrugSafetyInformationforPatients andProviders/ucm198543.htm. Accessed August 9, 2010.

Vahl TP, Paty BW, Fuller BD, Prigeon RL, D'Alessio DA (2003). Effects of GLP-1-(7-36) NH2, GLP-1-(7-37), and GLP-1- (9-36)NH2 on intravenous glucose tolerance and glucose-induced insulin secretion in healthy humans. *J Clin Endocrinol Metab*, 88, 1772–1779

Vilsboll T (2009). Liraglutide: a new treatment for type 2 diabetes. *Drugs Today (Barc)*, 45, 101–113

Vilsboll T, Brock B, Perrild H, Levin K, Lervang HH, Kolendorf K, Krarup T, Schmitz O, Zdravkovic M, Le-Thi T, Madsbad S (2008). Liraglutide, a once-daily human GLP-1 analogue, improves pancreatic B-cell function and arginine-stimulated insulin secretion during hyperglycaemia in patients with Type 2 diabetes mellitus. *Diabet Med*, 25,152–156

Werner U (2008). Preclinical pharmacology of the new GLP-1 receptor agonist AVE0010. *Ann Endocrinol (Paris)*, 69, 164–165

Wolf R, Frederich R, Fiedorek FT, Donovan M, Xu Z, Harris S, Chen R (2009). Evaluation of CV risk in the saxagliptin clinical trials. *Diabetes*, 59(Suppl 1), 8

Yoo BK, Triller DM, Yoo DJ (2006). Exenatide: a new option for the treatment of type 2 diabetes. *Ann Pharmacother*, 40, 1777–1784

Zander M, Madsbad S, Madsen JL, Holst JJ (2002). Effect of 6-week course of glucagon-like peptide 1 on glycaemic control, insulin sensitivity, and beta-cell function in type 2 diabetes: a parallel-group study. *Lancet,* 359, 824–830

Zinman B, Gerich J, Buse JB, Lewin A, Schwartz S, Raskin P, Hale PM, Zdravkovic M, Blonde L (2009). Efficacy and safety of the human glucagon-like peptide-1 analog liraglutide in combination with metformin and thiazolidinedione in patients with type 2 diabetes (LEAD-4 Met+TZD). *Diabetes Care,* 32,1224–1230

Zunz E, La Barre J (1929). Contributions a l'étude des variations physiologiques de la sécrétion interne du pancréas: relations entre les sécrétions externe et interne du pancréas. *Arch Int Physiol Biochim,* 31, 20–44

16

Zinc Translocation Causes Hypoglycemia-Induced Neuron Death

Sang Won Suh
Department of Physiology, Hallym University, College of Medicine, Chuncheon, Korea

1. Introduction

Hypoglycemia is a common but serious problem among type1 and type 2 diabetic patients receiving intensive treatment with glucose-lowering drugs such as insulin or sulfonylurea. Moderate hypoglycemia is occurring 0.1-0.3 episode/patient per day and is usually corrected by patients themselves or just ignored. However, severe hypoglycemia causes unconsciousness and it may lead to neuronal injury in the cerebral cortex and hippocampus. Hypoglycemic neuronal death is resulted from a cascade of several events after prolonged period of lack of glucose since brain exclusively use glucose (Auer et al., 1984a; Auer and Siesjo, 1993; Auer et al., 1984b). Sustained release of glutamate from presynaptic terminals into the extracellular space and activation of glutamate receptors has been suggested as a necessary upstream event in this neuron death cascade (Auer and Siesjo, 1993; Wieloch, 1985). Also mitochondrial membrane permeability (Friberg et al., 1998), calpain activation (Ferrand-Drake et al., 2003), PARP-1 activation (Suh et al., 2003) and NADPH oxidase activation-induced ROS production (Suh et al., 2007; Suh et al., 2008) have been shown to be possible downstream events. Our lab has undertaken studies to establish whether vesicular zinc release and subsequent zinc translocation into postsynaptic neurons is an important upstream step in this hypoglycemia-induced neuron death process. Using an animal model of insulin-induced hypoglycemia we have shown that: (I) vesicular zinc is released from hippocampal mossy fiber terminals; (II) intracellular zinc accumulation is induced in the hippocampal neurons; (III) neuronal death is reduced by zinc chelation or zinc transporter gene deletion; (IV) PARP-1 activation is reduced by zinc chelation; (V) ROS production is reduced by zinc chelation after hypoglycemia and glucose reperfusion (HG/GR); and (VI) hypothermia prevented hypoglycemia-induced zinc release and neuron death. Together, these results suggest that zinc translocation is an upstream step linking HG/GR to PARP-1 activation, to NADPH oxidase activation and neuronal death in brain regions containing high concentrations of vesicular zinc. Zinc translocation into postsynaptic neurons was also demonstrated in the hippocampal slice model with combined oxygen and glucose deprivation (OGD) where neuronal zinc accumulation into the hippocampal CA1 neurons is blocked by extracellular zinc chelator, CaEDTA (Yin et al., 2002). In addition, hippocampal slices prepared from zinc transporter 3 (ZnT3) knockout mouse, which have little or no vesicular zinc in neuronal terminals, showed no zinc accumulation in post-synaptic neurons following OGD and hypoglycemia (Suh et al., 2008). These hippocampal slice experiments with zinc chelator or with ZnT3 KO mice suggest that the zinc signal observed in post-synaptic hippocampal neurons as shown in our previous study (Suh et al., 2003) was a result of zinc translocation from the presynaptic terminals.

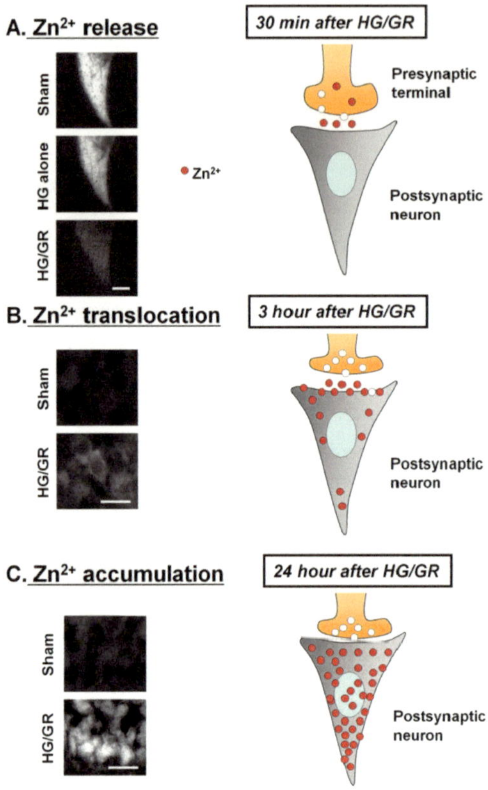

Fig. 1. Vesicular zinc release and translocation after hypoglycemia.
A) TSQ fluorescent images show vesicular zinc release from presynaptic terminals of hippocampal mossy fibers after hypoglycemia/ glucose reperfusion (HG/GR). Intense TSQ fluorescent signal (white color in the figure) in the mossy fiber of sham operated rats indicates high vesicular zinc contents in the vesicle. However, the diminished TSQ fluorescent intensity in the HG/GR rats indicates that bulk of vesicular zinc has been released and therefore presynaptic vesicular zinc contents are reduced at the time when the brain section was evaluated. TSQ fluorescent intensity in mossy fiber is decreased after 60 minutes of hypoglycemia (HG alone). TSQ fluorescent intensity is further decreased after 30 minutes hypoglycemia and 30 minutes glucose reperfusion (HG/GR), which represents mossy fiber vesicular zinc release from presynaptic terminals. A schematic drawing represents vesicular zinc release from presynaptic terminals after HG/GR. B) TSQ fluorescent images show zinc translocation into postsynaptic neurons of hippocampal CA1 pyramidal neurons 3 hours after hypoglycemia. Zinc accumulation in the intracellular space can be detected in this early time point. A schematic drawing represents intracellular zinc accumulation 3 hours after HG/GR. C) TSQ fluorescent images show zinc accumulation into postsynaptic neurons 24 hours after HG/GR. Intense zinc accumulation in the intracellular space is detected in this time point. A schematic drawing represents intracellular zinc accumulation 24 hours after HG/GR. Scale bar in (A) is 200 µm and in (B) and (C) are 20 µm.

2. Role of zinc in hypoglycemic neuronal death

Chelatable zinc (free or weakly bound to proteins) is present in a subset of glutamatergic axon terminals throughout the mammalian forebrain, especially in the hippocampus and in the cerebral cortex (Danscher et al., 1985) (Frederickson, 1989). The chelatable zinc is mainly localized in synaptic vesicles of excitatory presynaptic neuron terminals (Perez-Clausell and Danscher, 1985) and is released into the extracellular space during paroxysmal neuronal activity or membrane depolarization (Assaf and Chung, 1984; Howell et al., 1984). This zinc release has been suggested to contribute to neuronal death in several disease conditions, such as seizure (Frederickson et al., 1988; Suh et al., 2001), ischemia (Koh et al., 1996; Tonder et al., 1990) and traumatic brain injury (Suh et al., 2000). Zinc can induce the production of reactive oxygen species (ROS) and PARP-1 activation in cell cultures (Kim et al., 1999; Sensi et al., 1999a; Sheline et al., 2000), suggesting a possible role of zinc in hypoglycemia-induced neuronal death. Our previous study showed that hypoglycemia induces vesicular zinc release from the synaptic terminals. We also found that hypoglycemia increases neuronal zinc accumulation in postsynaptic neurons, which is prevented by intracerebroventricular injection of the Zn^{2+} chelator CaEDTA (Suh et al., 2004; Suh et al., 2008) or intraperitoneal injection of clioquinol (CQ) (Shin et al., 2010).

2.1 Vesicular zinc release and translocation after hypoglycemia

Oxidative stress and zinc release are both known to contribute to neuronal death after hypoglycemia; however, the temporal relationships between these events are not well established. Our study demonstrated that the vesicular zinc release from hippocampal mossy fiber and subsequent translocation into postsynaptic neurons occurs immediately after HG/GR. We used the fluorescent dye TSQ, which binds free zinc (Frederickson et al., 1987). The vesicular zinc signal detected by TSQ showed a partial decrease (release from mossy fiber terminal) after 60 minutes of hypoglycemia alone (HG alone), but was almost completely absent after 30 minutes of hypoglycemia followed by 30 minutes of glucose reperfusion (HG/GR) (Figure 1A) (Suh et al., 2004; Suh et al., 2007). This result suggests that vesicular zinc release from hippocampal mossy fiber is not caused by hypoglycemia itself but caused by a combination of hypoglycemia and subsequent glucose reperfusion. Conversely, TSQ staining in the postsynaptic pyramidal neuron bodies was absent under sham operated conditions or hypoglycemia alone, but TSQ intensity in the cytoplasm of CA1 neurons was increased 3 hours after 30 minutes of hypoglycemia and 30 minutes glucose reperfusion (HG/GR) (Figure 1B). This represents translocation of presynaptic zinc to postsynaptic neuron of CA1 pyramidal neurons. This initial cytoplasmic zinc increase was prevented by intracerebroventricular (i.c.v) injection of the zinc chelator, CaEDTA. Without zinc chelation, this intraneuronal zinc accumulation continued to increase until 24 hours after hypoglycemia and glucose reperfusion (Suh et al., 2008). However, CaEDTA treatment also prevented this continuous intracellular zinc accumulation when evaluated at 24 hours later, suggesting that released zinc from the synaptic vesicles translocated into the post-synaptic neurons during several hours after hypoglycemia and glucose reperfusion conditions (Figure 1C). From these findings, we speculate that zinc release/translocation is a key upstream step in the sequence of events leading to neuronal death after HG/GR (Suh et al., 2004; Suh et al., 2007). However, the identity of the factor(s) involved in the intermediating step(s) for HG/GR-induced vesicular zinc release and translocation process is unknown. In our prior study, nitrotyrosine formation was detected shortly after glucose reperfusion, but not during hypoglycemia per se (Suh et al., 2003). Subsequently we found that a neuron specific NOS inhibitor, 7-NI, significantly inhibited hypoglycemia-induced vesicular zinc release from hippocampal mossy fiber (Fig 2A). 7-NI also prevented intracellular zinc accumulation and neuronal death at 24 hour post-HG/GR time point (Fig. 2B) (Suh et al., 2003). These findings suggest that nitric oxide production is an event upstream of vesicular zinc release and postsynaptic zinc accumulation. This observation is consistent with previous studies in which intra-hippocampal injection of nitric oxide donor (Spermino-NONOate) induced vesicular zinc release and intracellular zinc accumulation (Cuajungco and Lees, 1998; Frederickson et al., 2002).

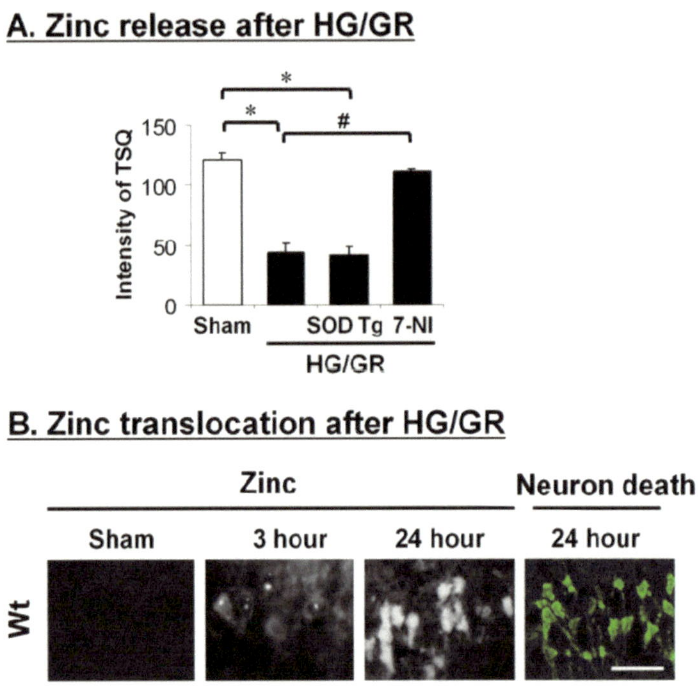

Fig. 2. A) Vesicular zinc release after hypoglycemia/glucose reperfusion is prevented by NOS inhibitor. Vesicular zinc release was evaluated at hippocampal hilus by TSQ fluorescence. The TSQ signal loss is apparent after 30 minutes of HG and 30 minutes of GR. SOD-1 over-expressing rats (SOD-1 Tg) show similar zinc release after HG/GR (HG+GR+SOD), whereas the NOS inhibitor 7-NI almost completely prevented vesicular zinc release from the hilus mossy fiber area. Graph shows TSQ fluorescence intensity. Data are mean + s.e.m; n = 10; * $P < 0.05$. # $P < 0.05$. B) Intracellular zinc accumulation and neuronal death after hypoglycemia/ glucose reperfusion (HG/GR). Images show neuronal zinc accumulation at 3 or 24 hours after HG/GR and neuronal death at 24 hours after HG/GR. TSQ intensity in CA1 pyramidal neurons is increased compared to sham operated rats by 3 hours after HG, and further increased at 24 hours. CA1 pyramidal neurons show Fluoro-Jade B staining (green) at 24 hours after HG/GR. Scale bar = 50 µm. n = 3-4. This figure is modified from our previous published paper (Suh et al., JCBFM, 2008).

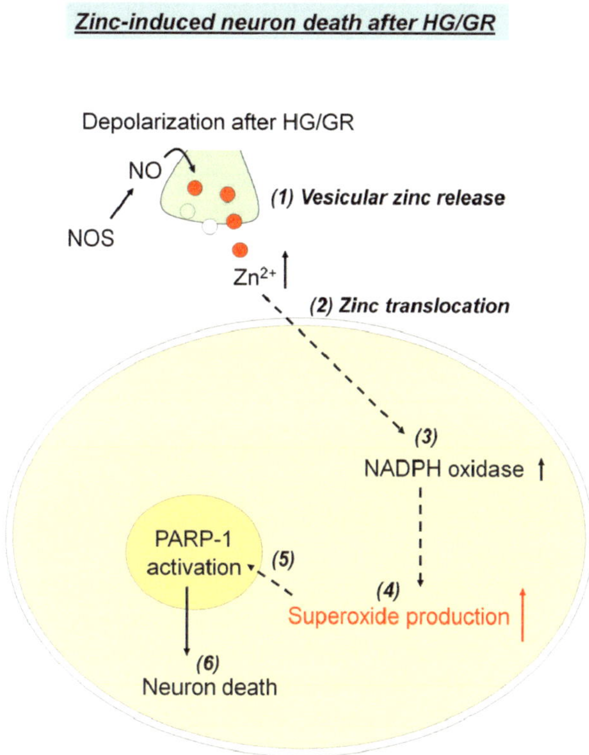

Fig. 3. Key aspects of hypoglycemia-induced neuronal death by zinc.
1) Nitric oxide (NO) production after hypoglycemia/ glucose reperfusion leads to release of zinc together with glutamate from presynaptic terminals. 2) Zinc translocates into intracellular space. 3) Translocated zinc activates NADPH oxidase. 4) NADPH oxidase activation induces ROS production. 5) Production of superoxide from NADPH oxidase induces DNA damage and activation of poly(ADP-ribose) polymerase-1 (PARP-1) in the nucleus. 6) Neuron death.

Since peroxynitrite (highly neurotoxic) is formed by reaction of nitric oxide (NO) with superoxide (Beckman and Koppenol, 1996), our previous study also sought to clarify the role of superoxide formation on presynaptic zinc release from hippocampal mossy fiber and postsynaptic zinc accumulation in the hippocampal CA1 neurons after hypoglycemic insult. This study showed that over-expression of SOD-1 significantly reduced hypoglycemia-induced neuronal death (Suh et al., 2007). To determine whether the neuroprotective role of SOD-1 over-expression was due to reduced release of vesicular zinc, SOD-1 transgenic rats were subjected to hypoglycemia. From this study, we concluded that SOD-1 overexpression had no effect on hypoglycemia-induced vesicular zinc release or on the initial zinc translocation into hippocampal postsynaptic neurons when evaluated at 3 hours after hypoglycemia, but that SOD-1 overexpression did reduce neuronal death and neuronal zinc accumulation when evaluated at 24 hours after hypoglycemia. These results suggest that vesicular zinc release occurs upstream of ROS production, but that ROS production continues to promote to zinc accumulation in post-synaptic neurons at later time points

(Figure 2, 3). This suggests that protein-bound zinc can be liberated by reactive oxygen species (ROS) such as superoxide. Thus, if neuronal SOD concentrations are adequate for clearance of superoxide, further intracellular free zinc release can be prevented even though initial zinc translocation event has occurred. Conversely, if superoxide production is not cleared or stabilized, intracellular free zinc will continue to increase to the point of neuronal demise. This result suggests that in addition to presynaptically-released Zn^{2+} , hippocampal neurons also have a pool of intracellularly releasable Zn^{2+}. Intracellularly derived zinc may arise from metallothionein (MTs) or other zinc binding proteins. MTs play a major role in modulating neuron death after seizure or ischemia as these proteins release a substantial amount of Zn^{2+} under conditions of oxidative stress. This notion is supported by prior studies suggesting that non-vesicular zinc may be also important in promoting brain injury (Lee et al., 2000).

2.2 The role of zinc on hypoglycemia-induced ROS production

The mechanism by which ROS production is aggravated by intracellular zinc influx has not been firmly established. Several lines of evidence suggest that zinc induces increased mitochondrial ROS production (Sensi et al., 1999b). However, in cell culture models, zinc has been identified as an activator of NADPH oxidase, an enzyme that produces superoxide. NADPH oxidase is present in many cell types including neurons (Kim and Koh, 2002; Noh and Koh, 2000). NADPH oxidase is a multi-component enzyme comprising a plasma membrane-bound subunit, gp91; a membrane-associated flavocytochrome, cytochrome b558; and at least three cytosolic subunits, $p47^{phox}$, $p67^{phox}$ and the small G protein Rac2 (Groemping and Rittinger, 2005). During activation, the $p47^{phox}$ component is phosphorylated and translocates to the plasma membrane, where it associates with the other subunits to form the active enzyme complex. The methoxy-substituted catechol, apocynin, blocks this assembly but does not inhibit mitochondrial dehydrogenases (Dodd and Pearse, 2000; Stolk et al., 1994). Interestingly, our previous studies examining the production of ROS in the brain during hypoglycemic insult suggest that superoxide is formed primarily during the glucose reperfusion period. The mechanism by which NADPH oxidase is activated in non-phagocytic cells is not well understood, but zinc has been identified as both an inducer of neuronal NADPH oxidase activity (Kim and Koh, 2002; Noh and Koh, 2000) and a contributor to hypoglycemic neuronal death (Suh et al., 2008). High concentrations of presynaptic zinc are present in the brain regions most vulnerable to hypoglycemic injury (Frederickson et al., 2005; Suh et al., 2004). Recently, we published that vesicular zinc release is required for NADPH oxidase activation in HG/GR (Suh et al., 2007). Rats pre-treated with an intracerebroventricular injection of the zinc chelator CaEDTA showed reduced neuronal ROS formation, suggesting that vesicular zinc release is an upstream event of NADPH oxidase activation. ZnEDTA, used as a control, showed no effect on ROS production. The translocation of NADPH oxidase subunits, $p47^{phox}$ or $p61^{phox}$, to the plasma membrane in cortical neuronal cultures subjected to glucose deprivation followed by glucose reperfusion was blocked by CaEDTA, but not by ZnEDTA (Figure 4). Moreover we demonstrated that zinc-induced ROS production in neuron cultures was almost completely absent in cultures from mice deficient in the $p47^{phox}$ subunit of NADPH oxidase and in wt neurons treated with the NADPH oxidase assembly inhibitor apocynin (Stolk et al., 1994; Suh et al., 2008). These results suggest that NADPH oxidase subunit assembly is triggered by glucose reperfusion through a process requiring extracellular zinc signaling. To further confirm that vesicular zinc release is involved in HG/GR-induced ROS production and neuron death, we used the ZnT3-/- mouse, which has no vesicular zinc in the presynaptic terminals (Suh et al., 2007). The ZnT3-/- mice showed diminished ROS production at 3 hours after HG/GR and reduced neuronal death 7 days after HG/GR (Figure 5). This result confirms prior reports that zinc chelation prevents ROS production and neuron death after HG/GR (Suh et al., 2004; Suh et al., 2007) and strongly suggests that it is the vesicular zinc pool that contributes to neuronal demise in this setting.

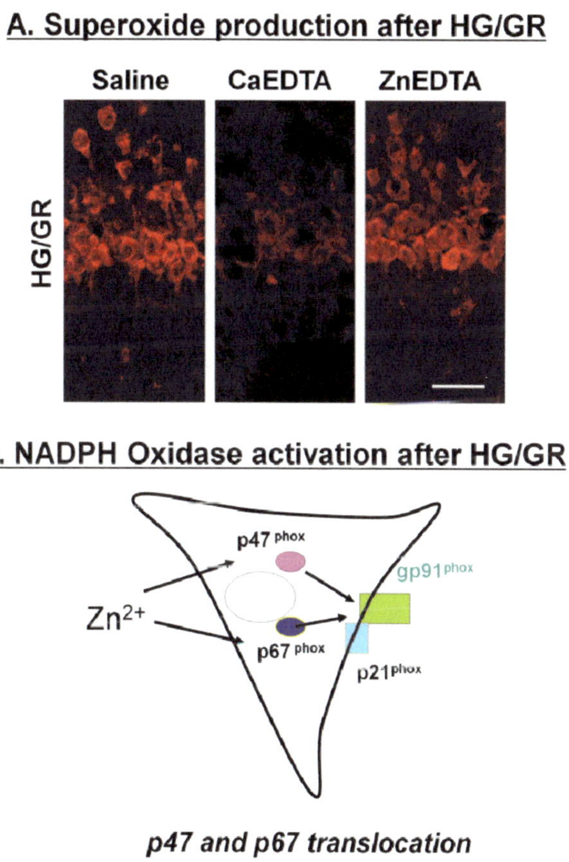

Fig. 4. Hypoglycemia/ glucose reperfusion-induced ROS production is mediated by zinc-induced NADPH oxidase activation. ROS production in neurons detected by ethidium (Et) fluorescence.
A) The zinc chelator, CaEDTA, reduces HG/GR-induced Et production in the CA1 neurons. ZnEDTA is the control. Rats were treated with saline, 100 mM CaEDTA, or 100 mM ZnEDTA. Scale bar is 50 μm. B) Schematic drawing of p47phox and p67phox translocation to plasma membrane by zinc translocation into neuron.

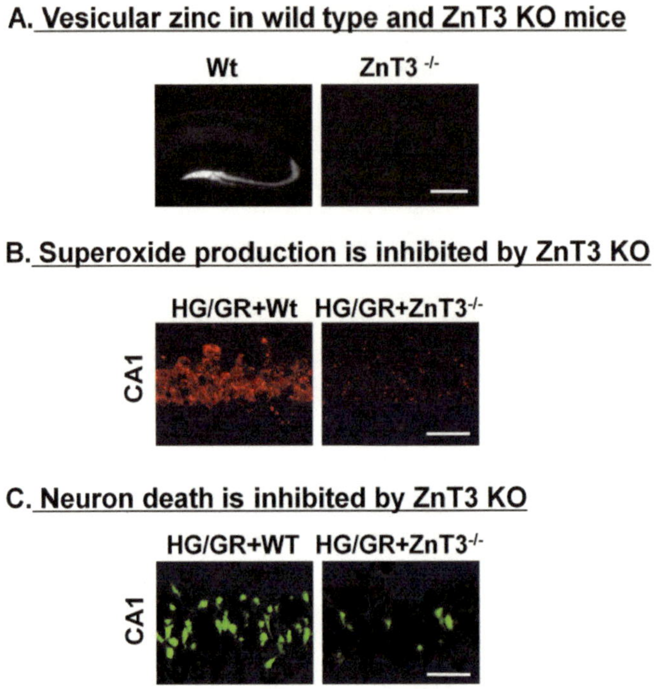

Fig. 5. Hypoglycemia/ glucose reperfusion-induced ROS production and neuronal injury is prevented by ZnT3 gene deletion in mice.
A) Vesicular zinc in the mouse hippocampus imaged with TSQ fluorescence (white) from wild-type mice and from ZnT3-/- mice. Scale bar is 500 µm. B) To characterize the source of ROS production in hypoglycemic neuronal injury, we used a rat model of insulin-induced hypoglycemia and evaluated the production of reactive oxygen species with dihydroethidium. Dihydroethidium is oxidized by superoxide and superoxide reaction products to form fluorescent ethidium (Et) species, which are then trapped within cells by DNA binding. In the ZnT3-/- mice, hypoglycemia-induced ROS production is almost completely prevented. Scale bar is 50 µm. C) Neuronal death (FJB (+) neurons) in ZnT3-/- mice was significantly less than wild type mice. Scale bar is 100 µm. Part of this figure is modified from our previous published paper (Suh et al., JCBFM, 2008).

2.3 The role of zinc on hypoglycemia-induced PARP-1 activation

PARP-1 activation has been shown to mediate neuronal death in a variety of disorders including ischemia, trauma, and inflammation (Virag and Szabo, 2002). PARP-1 uses the ADP-ribose group of NAD+ to form branched ADP-ribose polymers on specific acceptor proteins in the vicinity of DNA strand breaks or kinks (Burzio et al., 1979; D'Amours et al., 1999). Formation of these polymers facilitates DNA repair and prevents chromatid exchange, but extensive PARP-1 activation can promote cell death through a processes involving mitochondrial permeability transition and release of apoptosis inducing factor (Alano et al., 2004; Ha and Snyder, 1999; Yu et al., 2002). Our previous study showed that PARP-1 activation was substantially increased in hippocampal neurons after HG/GR. Rats treated with PARP-1 inhibitors after HG/GR showed a striking reduction in neuronal death, coupled with improved performance on the Morris water maze, a test of spatial learning and memory (Suh et al., 2003). Administration of PARP-1 inhibitors at time points up to 3 hours after HG/GR was effective in reducing neuronal death, suggesting both that PARP-1 is a downstream event in the HG/GR cell death pathway and that PARP-1 inhibitors might be useful in the clinical treatment of hypoglycemic brain injury (Figure 6).

A link between zinc release and PARP-1 activation has been suggested by studies showing PARP-1 activation and PARP-1 mediated neuronal death after neuronal exposure to zinc in cell culture, and the ability of PARP-1 inhibitors to abrogate zinc-induced cell death (Kim and Koh, 2002; Sheline et al., 2000; Sheline et al., 2003; Virag and Szabo, 2002). How zinc leads to PARP-1 activation has not been firmly established, but zinc has been shown to induce formation of reactive oxygen species through actions on mitochondria (Ichord et al., 1999) and through up-regulation of NADPH oxidase and neuronal nitric oxide synthase (Kim et al., 2002). Our previous study showed that the zinc chelator CaEDTA attenuated poly(ADP-ribose) formation in the post-synaptic pyramidal cells after HG/GR, suggesting that zinc translocation may be an upstream event in hypoglycemia-induced PARP-1 activation. This result, coupled with the marked reduction in neuronal death observed with CaEDTA, and the prior observation that PARP-1 inhibitors reduce hypoglycemic neuronal death (Frederickson et al., 2002), suggests a sequential process of zinc entry, PARP-1 activation, and cell death triggered by HG/GR. These results do not, however, exclude other mechanisms by which vesicular zinc release could contribute to hypoglycemic neuronal death.

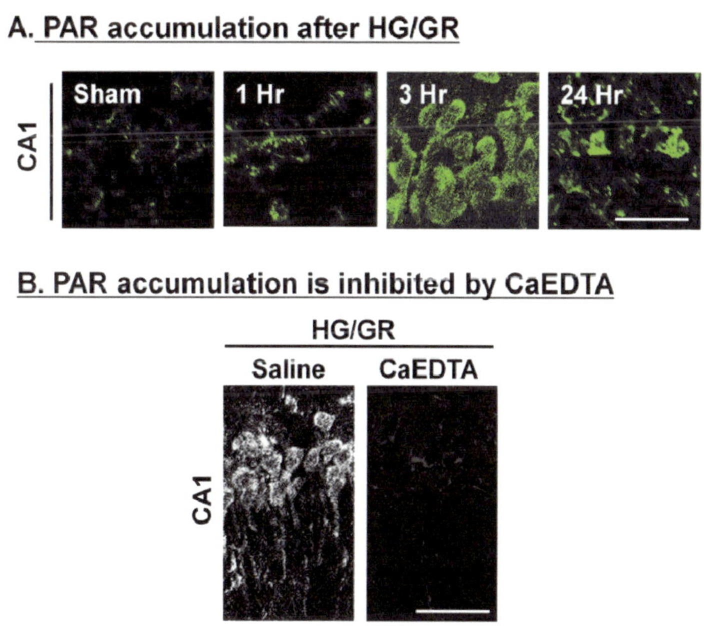

Fig. 6. Hypoglycemia/ glucose reperfusion-induced poly(ADP-ribose) formation in CA1 hippocampus in rats.
A) Poly(ADP-ribose) immunoreactivity was only modestly increased at termination of immediately after HG/GR (0 hr), but was markedly increased at 3 hr after insult, and then slowly declined after that point in the hippocampal CA1 and DG area. Scale bar is 50 µm.
B) Poly(ADP-ribose) formation was reduced by administration of zinc chelator, CaEDTA, at the time of glucose correction. Scale bar is 50 µm.

2.4 The role of zinc on hypoglycemia-induced microglia activation

Microglia is thought to be the resident immune cells of the central nervous system (CNS). Under physical conditions, resting microglia adopts the characteristic ramified morphological appearance and scatter throughout mature CNS to play role in the immune surveillance and host defense. The resting microglia transform into an activated states including amoeboid morphology, up-regulation of proliferation and release of proinflammatory mediators, when the cells bind to pathogen-derived molecules or other microglial activating agents. The pro-inflammatory cytokines such as interleukin-1 and tumor necrosis factor alpha, released from activated microglia following ischemia, brain trauma and the other brain damages (Clausen et al., 2005; Sairanen et al., 1997; Saito et al., 1996; Taupin et al., 1993), are thought to be associated with neuronal death (Loddick and Rothwell, 1996; Lu et al., 2005; Yamasaki et al., 1995). On the other hand, these cytokines have been reported to induce nerve growth factor expression or cell survival signaling (DeKosky et al., 1994), (Fontaine et al., 2002) (Herx et al., 2000). Moreover activated microglia have been reported to release neurotrophic factors such as brain-derived neurotrophic factor (Lee et al., 2002b). These reports are implying that microglia activation is not only neurotoxic but neurotrophic. However, the factors that trigger microglial activation have not been completely understood. Recently, poly (ADP-ribose) polymerase (PARP)-1 has been known to act as a coactivator of nuclear factor kappa B (NF-kB), which leads to microglial migration on excitotoxically damaged organotypic hippocampal slice culture, and neuronal cell death (Chiarugi and Moskowitz, 2003) and (Ullrich et al., 2001). Furthermore, in zinc-induced cell death of neuron cultures, PARP-1 has been reported to be activated by zinc through NADPH oxidase pathway (Sheline et al., 2003), (Kim and Koh, 2002). In our previous study, we sought to examine whether zinc induces microglial activation and how microglia is activated by zinc. We found that zinc can induce microglial activation which mediated by PARP-1 activation though NADPH oxidase pathway and that microglial activation in mice ischemic brain are blocked by zinc chelator (Kauppinen et al., 2008). During severe hypoglycemia, glucose reperfusion and its neurotoxic cascade may not only damage neurons directly, but may also promote neuronal injury indirectly via microglia activation. Microglia activation is a gradual process including change of morphology from highly ramified into an amoeboid shape, proliferation, migration to injury site, increased expression of surface molecules, increased secretion of cytokines, chemokines, free radicals and proteases, and assumption of phagocytotic activity (Kreutzberg, 1996). We tested whether zinc chelation prevents microglia activation after hypoglycemia. Both CaEDTA and CQ substantially decreased hypoglycemia-induced microglia activation in the hippocampal CA1 pyramidal area (Figure 7).

2.5 Prevention of hypoglycemia-induced neuronal death by hypothermia

Our previous study presented that mild hypothermia reduces hypoglycemia-induced neuronal death in the hippocampus, whereas hyperthermia aggravates those brain injuries. We suggested that hypothermia (lowering brain temperature) prevents hypoglycemia-induced neuronal death by reduction of vesicular zinc release, superoxide production and microglia activation, where temperature dependent vesicular zinc release was a key event upstream of hypoglycemia-induced superoxide production and microglia activation.

Mild hypothermia has been known as the most effective approach to prevent neuronal death after cerebral ischemia (Busto et al., 1987; Maier et al., 2002), traumatic brain injury (Clifton et al., 1991; Suh et al., 2006) and prolonged seizure (Liu et al., 1993). We found that

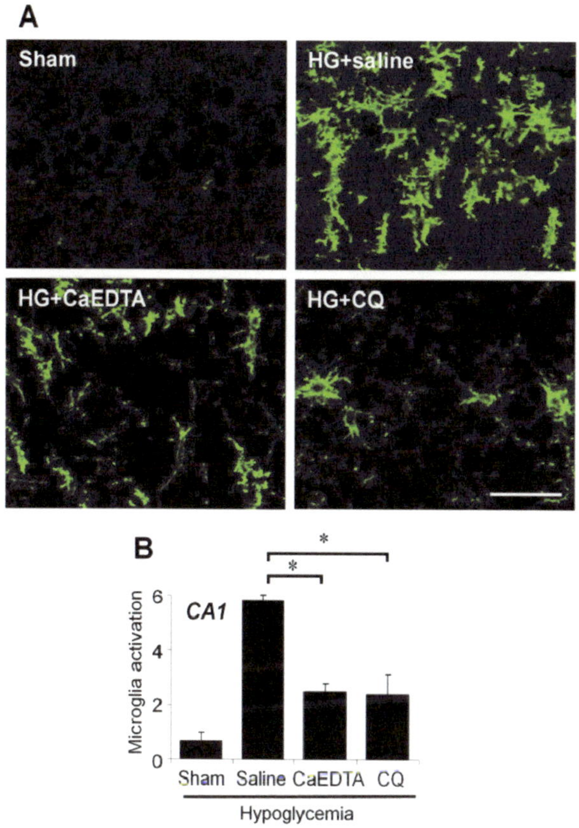

Fig. 7. Hypoglycemia-induced microglia activation is prevented by zinc chelation. (A) Morphological change and intensity of immunostaining of microglia after hypoglycemia is affected by zinc chelation. Hypoglycemia (HG+saline) substantially increased microglia activation in the hippocampal CA1 region. However, zinc chelation by CaEDTA (HG+CaEDTA) or clioquinol (HG+CQ) significantly reduced microglia activation in the above areas. Scale bar=100 μm. (B) Quantification of microglia activation was performed in the hippocampal CA1 area. As shown in the images, microglia activation is strongly prevented by zinc chelation. Data are mean±s.e.m. (n=3 to 6); $^*P<0.05$ compared with the saline treated group.

mild hypothermia also can prevent hypoglycemia-induced neuronal death. Neuronal death evaluated in hippocampal area shows that hypothermia significantly reduced neuronal death while hyperthermia applied after hypoglycemic events aggravated the neuronal death (Shin et al., 2010). The neuroprotective effects of hypothermia after hypoglycemia in our previous study, however, differ from those reported in previous studies (Agardh et al., 1992). Agardh et al. reported that mild hypothermia applied before and during of hypoglycemia (before and entire period of iso-EEG period) produced a similar degree of neuronal death compared to normothermic animals. No neuroprotective effect of hypothermia was seen in the hypoglycemic animals. The differences between our study and Agardh et al.'s may be explained by the onset of hypothermia application. Agardh et al. applied hypothermia before and during the iso-EEG period. However, in our study, hypothermia applied after the iso-EEG period was terminated, i.e. brain temperature was decreased during the glucose reperfusion period after hypoglycemia. Since we have previously shown that hypoglycemia-induced neuronal death is not initiated during the period of glucose deprivation but instead during glucose reperfusion period, it may be that the hypothermic application before and during the isoelectric period was not sufficient to prevent neuronal death after hypoglycemic events. In our experimental setting we also found that hypothermia application before and during the iso-EEG period had no statistically significant neuroprotective effects as seen in the previous study (Agardh et al., 1992), strengthening our hypothesis that brain temperature is a critical factor during glucose reperfusion period after hypoglycemia.

Suggested neuroprotective mechanisms of mild hypothermia on several brain injuries are based on decreases in cerebral metabolic requirement (Erecinska et al., 2003), intracranial pressure (Soukup et al., 2002), glutamate release from presynaptic vesicles (Arai et al., 1993; Ichord et al., 1999), free radical generation (Globus et al., 1995; Horiguchi et al., 2003) and inflammatory reaction (Kumar and Evans, 1997; Wang et al., 2002). Previously, we have shown that hypothermia reduced vesicular zinc release and subsequent neuronal death after traumatic brain injury (Suh et al., 2006). We also have shown that hypoglycemia-induced neuronal death is mediated by vesicular zinc release and translocation (Suh et al., 2004; Suh et al., 2008). Therefore, we hypothesized that mild hypothermia has neuroprotective effects by reduction of the vesicular zinc release after hypoglycemia. Although zinc is released from presynaptic terminals as a component of normal physiologic signaling at zinc-modulated synapses (Li et al., 2001), a large amount of vesicular zinc released together with glutamate may enter postsynaptic neurons through glutamate receptors (Weiss and Sensi, 2000; Weiss et al., 2000) or voltage-sensitive calcium channels (Sensi et al., 1999b). Zinc translocation into post-synaptic neurons after hypoglycemia has been demonstrated by our lab (Suh et al., 2004; Suh et al., 2007; Suh et al., 2008). Many brain areas with high vesicular zinc level exhibit high vulnerability to hypoglycemia, but this correlation is not always true. Some brain areas with high vesicular zinc concentration are not correspondingly sensitive to hypoglycemia, and conversely some brain areas that are highly sensitive to hypoglycemia are not rich in vesicular zinc (Frederickson et al., 2000). Thus vesicular zinc is not the sole determinant of neuronal vulnerability to hypoglycemia, but may be a contributory factor in areas where vesicular concentrations are high. The zinc chelator CaEDTA was used to evaluate a causal role for extracellular zinc elevations in subsequent post-synaptic neuronal zinc accumulation and death after hypoglycemia. The utility of CaEDTA as a zinc chelator has been established in ischemia, brain trauma and epilepsy studies (Frederickson et al., 2002; Koh et al., 1996; Lee et al., 2002a). Interestingly, Aizenmann et al. suggested that the large fraction of zinc existing in the form of thiol-zinc-metalloproteins can be released from oxidation of intracellular zinc binding proteins (e.g. metallothionein) by oxidative stress. Zinc liberated in such a manner may then become cytotoxic (Aizenman et al., 2000). Our study showed that application of mild hypothermia significantly reduced hypoglycemia-induce neuronal death by reducing presynaptic zinc release and translocation into postsynaptic neurons (Figure 8) (Shin et al., 2010). Hyperthermia applied after hypoglycemia aggravates this zinc release and translocation compared to normothermia applied animals. From these results, we conclude that neuroprotective effects of mild hypothermia after hypoglycemia can be achieved by reduction of synaptic zinc release and subsequent zinc translocation. However, our study also found that zinc dependent DG neuron degeneration was prevented by the cell permeable zinc chelator, CQ. We therefore

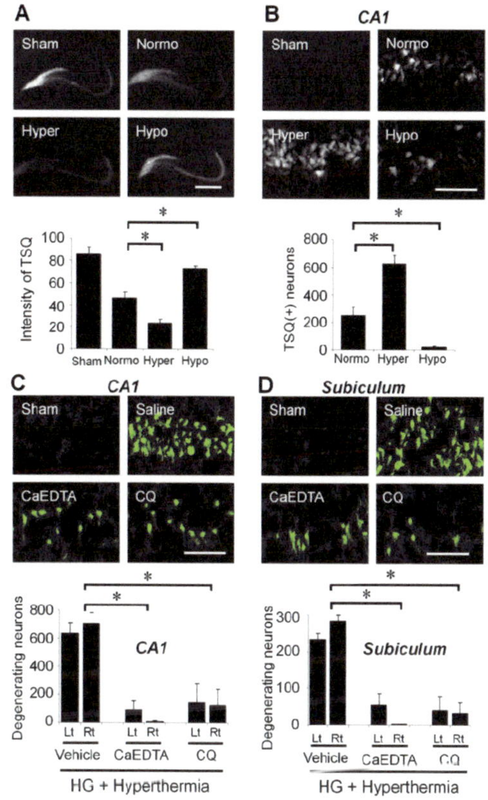

Fig. 8. Temperature dependent hypoglycemic neuronal death is mediated by zinc release and translocation.
(A-D) Vesicular zinc release and translocation is aggravated by hyperthermia but is prevented by hypothermia. (A) represents TSQ fluorescence images of hippocampus from sham operated (Sham) and hypoglycemia (HG) experienced rats. Hypothermia group (Hypo) almost completely prevented synaptic zinc release. Scale bar = 500 μm. (B) Bar graph shows quantitated TSQ fluorescence intensity from hilus area. Data are mean + s.e.m. (n=7-12). * $P < 0.05$ compared with normothermic reperfusion group. (C) Photomicrographs of TSQ fluorescence staining shows zinc accumulation in the hippocampal CA1 neurons after hypoglycemia. Scale bar = 100 μm. (D) Bar graph shows quantitated TSQ (+) neurons in the CA1 area. Data are mean ± s.e.m. (n = 5-7). *$p < 0.05$ compared with normothermic glucose reperfusion group. (E-H) Zinc chelators, CaEDTA or clioquinol (CQ), prevents hypoglycemia-induced neuronal death. (E and G). FJB (+) neurons were reduced by CaEDTA or CQ injection even after hyperthermic reperfusion. Scale bar = 100 μm. (F and G) graphs represent quantitated neuronal death in the hippocampal CA1 and subiculum area after hypoglycemia. Data are the mean ± s.e.m (n=5-7) *$p < 0.05$ compared with saline treated rats. Part of this figure is modified from our previous published paper (Suh et al., JCBFM, 2010).

cannot exclude the possibility that intracellularly originated free zinc also contributes to hippocampal neuron cell death after hypoglycemia as previously suggested (Aizenman et al., 2000). Anatomical and physiological studies have shown that DG neurons contain a high concentration of vesicular zinc in their synaptic terminals which is released with neuronal activity. Intraneuronal accumulation of zinc may arise from cytoplasmic organelles or proteins rather than from presynaptic terminals of stratum moleculare. However, the source of intraneuronal accumulation of zinc in DG neurons still requires further study. An additional unsolved question arises regarding how the extracellular zinc chelator, CaEDTA also prevented DG neuron death if intraneuronal zinc accumulation originates from cytoplasmic sources.

Taken together, the present study shows that post-hypoglycemic (glucose reperfusion period) brain temperature can modulate the outcome of brain injury, i.e. hypothermia significantly reduces, while hyperthermia aggravates, neuronal death after hypoglycemia through inhibition of vesicular zinc release, reduction of ROS production and prevention of microglia activation. Therefore, cautious brain temperature monitoring and maintaining lower brain temperature during glucose reperfusion period may predict a better clinical outcome after a severe hypoglycemic episode.

3. Proposed intervention strategies for hypoglycemia-induced neuron death

Taken together the present book chapter suggests a sequence of events that lead to neuronal death after HG/GR. Glucose reperfusion initiates nitric oxide production, which leads to vesicular zinc release, which in turn activates neuronal NADPH oxidase. ROS produced by NADPH oxidase leads to increased zinc accumulation, PARP-1 activation, and resultant cell death. Therefore, based on these studies, the present review suggests that following intervention strategies for preventing hypoglycemia-induced neuron death. As we described in schematic drawing (Figure 9), there are at least 6 different possible approaches.

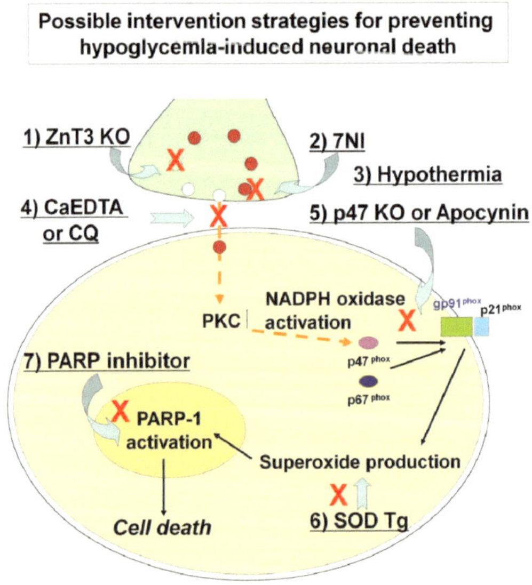

Fig. 9. Proposed intervention strategies for preventing hypoglycemia/ glucose reperfusion-induced neuron death. This schematic drawing indicates that hypoglycemia/ glucose reperfusion-induced neuron death can be prevented by several intervention methods. 1) Vesicular zinc content modulation by gene or chemical manipulation. 2) Vesicular zinc release inhibition by NO inhibitor. 3) Vesicular zinc release inhibition by hypothermia. 4) Zinc chelation in the extracellular space. 5) Inhibition of NADPH oxidase activation. 6) Scavenging or dismutating of reactive oxygen species. 7) Inhibition of PARP-1 activation. Round red colored dot represents ionic zinc. Symbol X represents intervention.

1) Modulation of vesicular zinc release by gene manipulation; 2) Prevention of vesicular zinc release by NOS inhibition; 3) hypothermia; 4) Chelation of extracellular zinc by zinc chelators; 5) Inhibition of NADPH oxidase activation; 6) Increase of SOD function; 7) PARP-1 inhibition. Among them, we speculate that prevention of vesicular zinc release and translocation would be the most promising intervention strategies. However, this intervention strategy requires a highly zinc specific chelator, which also can permeate blood brain barrier and has no side effects. No such agent is currently available and further investigation will be necessary to identify and develop candidate drugs for this purpose.

4. Conclusion

Vesicular zinc release and subsequent translocation of this ion into postsynaptic neurons has been known as a key upstream event of hypoglycemia-induced neuron death. Thus, zinc chelation is a promising target for the treatment of severe hypoglycemia-induced neuron death. However, still further studies will be needed to apply this concept to human.

5. Acknowledgement

This study was supported by a grant of the Korea Healthcare technology R&D Project, Ministry of Health & Welfare, Republic of Korea (A100687) and Korea Science and Engineering Foundation (KOSEF- 2009-0078399).

6. References

Agardh, C.D., Smith, M.L., and Siesjo, B.K. (1992). The influence of hypothermia on hypoglycemia-induced brain damage in the rat. Acta Neuropathol *83*, 379-385.

Aizenman, E., Stout, A.K., Hartnett, K.A., Dineley, K.E., McLaughlin, B., and Reynolds, I.J. (2000). Induction of neuronal apoptosis by thiol oxidation: putative role of intracellular zinc release. J Neurochem *75*, 1878-1888.

Alano, C.C., Ying, W., and Swanson, R.A. (2004). Poly(ADP ribose) polymerase-1-mediated cell death in astrocytes requires NAD+ depletion and mitochondrial permeability transition. J Biol Chem *279*, 18895-18902.

Arai, H., Uto, A., Ogawa, Y., and Sato, K. (1993). Effect of low temperature on glutamate-induced intracellular calcium accumulation and cell death in cultured hippocampal neurons. Neurosci Lett *163*, 132-134.

Assaf, S.Y., and Chung, S.H. (1984). Release of endogenous Zn2+ from brain tissue during activity. Nature *308*, 734-736.

Auer, R.N., Olsson, Y., and Siesjo, B.K. (1984a). Hypoglycemic brain injury in the rat. Correlation of density of brain damage with the EEG isoelectric time: a quantitative study. Diabetes 33, 1090-1098.

Auer, R.N., and Siesjo, B.K. (1993). Hypoglycaemia: brain neurochemistry and neuropathology. Baillieres Clin Endocrinol Metab *7*, 611-625.

Auer, R.N., Wieloch, T., Olsson, Y., and Siesjo, B.K. (1984b). The distribution of hypoglycemic brain damage. Acta Neuropathol *64*, 177-191.

Beckman, J.S., and Koppenol, W.H. (1996). Nitric oxide, superoxide, and peroxynitrite: the good, the bad, and ugly. Am J Physiol *271*, C1424-1437.

Burzio, L.O., Riquelme, P.T., and Koide, S.S. (1979). ADP ribosylation of rat liver nucleosomal core histones. J Biol Chem *254*, 3029-3037.

Busto, R., Dietrich, W.D., Globus, M.Y., Valdes, I., Scheinberg, P., and Ginsberg, M.D. (1987). Small differences in intraischemic brain temperature critically determine the extent of ischemic neuronal injury. J Cereb Blood Flow Metab *7*, 729-738.

Chiarugi, A., and Moskowitz, M.A. (2003). Poly(ADP-ribose) polymerase-1 activity promotes NF-kappaB-driven transcription and microglial activation: implication for neurodegenerative disorders. J Neurochem *85*, 306-317.

Clausen, B.H., Lambertsen, K.L., Meldgaard, M., and Finsen, B. (2005). A quantitative in situ hybridization and polymerase chain reaction study of microglial-macrophage expression of interleukin-1beta mRNA following permanent middle cerebral artery occlusion in mice. Neuroscience *132*, 879-892.

Clifton, G.L., Jiang, J.Y., Lyeth, B.G., Jenkins, L.W., Hamm, R.J., and Hayes, R.L. (1991). Marked protection by moderate hypothermia after experimental traumatic brain injury. J Cereb Blood Flow Metab *11*, 114-121.

Cuajungco, M.P., and Lees, G.J. (1998). Nitric oxide generators produce accumulation of chelatable zinc in hippocampal neuronal perikarya. Brain Res *799*, 118-129.

D'Amours, D., Desnoyers, S., D'Silva, I., and Poirier, G.G. (1999). Poly(ADP-ribosyl)ation reactions in the regulation of nuclear functions. Biochem J *342*, 249-268.

Danscher, G., Howell, G., Perez-Clausell, J., and Hertel, N. (1985). The dithizone, Timm's sulphide silver and the selenium methods demonstrate a chelatable pool of zinc in CNS. A proton activation (PIXE) analysis of carbon tetrachloride extracts from rat brains and spinal cords intravitally treated with dithizone. Histochemistry *83*, 419-422.

DeKosky, S.T., Goss, J.R., Miller, P.D., Styren, S.D., Kochanek, P.M., and Marion, D. (1994). Upregulation of nerve growth factor following cortical trauma. Exp Neurol *130*, 173-177.

Dodd, O.J., and Pearse, D.B. (2000). Effect of the NADPH oxidase inhibitor apocynin on ischemia-reperfusion lung injury. Am J Physiol Heart Circ Physiol *279*, H303-312.

Erecinska, M., Thoresen, M., and Silver, I.A. (2003). Effects of hypothermia on energy metabolism in Mammalian central nervous system. J Cereb Blood Flow Metab *23*, 513-530.

Ferrand-Drake, M., Zhu, C., Gido, G., Hansen, A.J., Karlsson, J.O., Bahr, B.A., Zamzami, N., Kroemer, G., Chan, P.H., Wieloch, T., and Blomgren, K. (2003). Cyclosporin A prevents calpain activation despite increased intracellular calcium concentrations, as well as translocation of apoptosis-inducing factor, cytochrome c and caspase-3 activation in neurons exposed to transient hypoglycemia. J Neurochem *85*, 1431-1442.

Fontaine, V., Mohand-Said, S., Hanoteau, N., Fuchs, C., Pfizenmaier, K., and Eisel, U. (2002). Neurodegenerative and neuroprotective effects of tumor Necrosis factor (TNF) in retinal ischemia: opposite roles of TNF receptor 1 and TNF receptor 2. J Neurosci *22*, RC216.

Frederickson, C.J. (1989). Neurobiology of zinc and zinc-containing neurons. Int Rev Neurobiol *31*, 145-238.

Frederickson, C.J., Cuajungco, M.P., LaBuda, C.J., and Suh, S.W. (2002). Nitric oxide causes apparent release of zinc from presynaptic boutons. Neuroscience *115*, 471-474.

Frederickson, C.J., Hernandez, M.D., Goik, S.A., Morton, J.D., and McGinty, J.F. (1988). Loss of zinc staining from hippocampal mossy fibers during kainic acid induced seizures: a histofluorescence study. Brain Res *446*, 383-386.

Frederickson, C.J., Kasarskis, E.J., Ringo, D., and Frederickson, R.E. (1987). A quinoline fluorescence method for visualizing and assaying the histochemically reactive zinc (bouton zinc) in the brain. J Neurosci Methods *20*, 91-103.

Frederickson, C.J., Koh, J.Y., and Bush, A.I. (2005). The neurobiology of zinc in health and disease. Nat Rev Neurosci *6*, 449-462.

Frederickson, C.J., Suh, S.W., Silva, D., and Thompson, R.B. (2000). Importance of zinc in the central nervous system: the zinc-containing neuron. J Nutr *130*, 1471S-1483S.

Friberg, H., Ferrand-Drake, M., Bengtsson, F., Halestrap, A.P., and Wieloch, T. (1998). Cyclosporin A, but not FK 506, protects mitochondria and neurons against hypoglycemic damage and implicates the mitochondrial permeability transition in cell death. J Neurosci *18*, 5151-5159.

Globus, M.Y., Busto, R., Lin, B., Schnippering, H., and Ginsberg, M.D. (1995). Detection of free radical activity during transient global ischemia and recirculation: effects of intraischemic brain temperature modulation. J Neurochem *65*, 1250-1256.

Groemping, Y., and Rittinger, K. (2005). Activation and assembly of the NADPH oxidase: a structural perspective. Biochem J *386*, 401-416.

Ha, H.C., and Snyder, S.H. (1999). Poly(ADP-ribose) polymerase is a mediator of necrotic cell death by ATP depletion. Proc Natl Acad Sci U S A *96*, 13978-13982.

Herx, L.M., Rivest, S., and Yong, V.W. (2000). Central nervous system-initiated inflammation and neurotrophism in trauma: IL-1 beta is required for the production of ciliary neurotrophic factor. J Immunol *165*, 2232-2239.

Horiguchi, T., Shimizu, K., Ogino, M., Suga, S., Inamasu, J., and Kawase, T. (2003). Postischemic hypothermia inhibits the generation of hydroxyl radical following transient forebrain ischemia in rats. J Neurotrauma *20*, 511-520.

Howell, G.A., Welch, M.G., and Frederickson, C.J. (1984). Stimulation-induced uptake and release of zinc in hippocampal slices. Nature *308*, 736-738.

Ichord, R.N., Northington, F.J., van Wylen, D., Johnston, M.V., Kwon, C., and Traystman, R.J. (1999). Brain O2 consumption and glutamate release during hypoglycemic coma in piglets are temperature sensitive. Am J Physiol *276*, H2053-2062.

Kauppinen, T.M., Higashi, Y., Suh, S.W., Escartin, C., Nagasawa, K., and Swanson, R.A. (2008). Zinc triggers microglial activation. J Neurosci *28*, 5827-5835.

Kim, T.Y., Hwang, J.J., Yun, S.H., Jung, M.W., and Koh, J.Y. (2002). Augmentation by zinc of NMDA receptor-mediated synaptic responses in CA1 of rat hippocampal slices: mediation by Src family tyrosine kinases. Synapse *46*, 49-56.

Kim, Y.H., Kim, E.Y., Gwag, B.J., Sohn, S., and Koh, J.Y. (1999). Zinc-induced cortical neuronal death with features of apoptosis and necrosis: mediation by free radicals. Neuroscience *89*, 175-182.

Kim, Y.H., and Koh, J.Y. (2002). The role of NADPH oxidase and neuronal nitric oxide synthase in zinc-induced poly(ADP-ribose) polymerase activation and cell death in cortical culture. Exp Neurol *177*, 407-418.

Koh, J.Y., Suh, S.W., Gwag, B.J., He, Y.Y., Hsu, C.Y., and Choi, D.W. (1996). The role of zinc in selective neuronal death after transient global cerebral ischemia. Science *272*, 1013-1016.

Kreutzberg, G.W. (1996). Microglia: a sensor for pathological events in the CNS. Trends Neurosci *19*, 312-318.

Kumar, K., and Evans, A.T. (1997). Effect of hypothermia on microglial reaction in ischemic brain. Neuroreport *8*, 947-950.

Lee, J.Y., Cole, T.B., Palmiter, R.D., and Koh, J.Y. (2000). Accumulation of zinc in degenerating hippocampal neurons of ZnT3-null mice after seizures: evidence against synaptic vesicle origin. J Neurosci *20*, RC79.

Lee, J.Y., Cole, T.B., Palmiter, R.D., Suh, S.W., and Koh, J.Y. (2002a). Contribution by synaptic zinc to the gender-disparate plaque formation in human Swedish mutant APP transgenic mice. Proc Natl Acad Sci U S A *99*, 7705-7710.

Lee, T.H., Kato, H., Chen, S.T., Kogure, K., and Itoyama, Y. (2002b). Expression disparity of brain-derived neurotrophic factor immunoreactivity and mRNA in ischemic hippocampal neurons. Neuroreport *13*, 2271-2275.

Li, Y., Hough, C.J., Suh, S.W., Sarvey, J.M., and Frederickson, C.J. (2001). Rapid translocation of Zn(2+) from presynaptic terminals into postsynaptic hippocampal neurons after physiological stimulation. J Neurophysiol *86*, 2597-2604.

Liu, Z., Gatt, A., Mikati, M., and Holmes, G.L. (1993). Effect of temperature on kainic acid-induced seizures. Brain Res *631*, 51-58.

Loddick, S.A., and Rothwell, N.J. (1996). Neuroprotective effects of human recombinant interleukin-1 receptor antagonist in focal cerebral ischaemia in the rat. J Cereb Blood Flow Metab *16*, 932-940.

Lu, K.T., Wang, Y.W., Yang, J.T., Yang, Y.L., and Chen, H.I. (2005). Effect of interleukin-1 on traumatic brain injury-induced damage to hippocampal neurons. J Neurotrauma *22*, 885-895.

Maier, C.M., Sun, G.H., Cheng, D., Yenari, M.A., Chan, P.H., and Steinberg, G.K. (2002). Effects of mild hypothermia on superoxide anion production, superoxide dismutase expression, and activity following transient focal cerebral ischemia. Neurobiol Dis *11*, 28-42.

Noh, K.M., and Koh, J.Y. (2000). Induction and activation by zinc of NADPH oxidase in cultured cortical neurons and astrocytes. J Neurosci *20*, RC111.

Perez-Clausell, J., and Danscher, G. (1985). Intravesicular localization of zinc in rat telencephalic boutons. A histochemical study. Brain Res *337*, 91-98.

Sairanen, T.R., Lindsberg, P.J., Brenner, M., and Siren, A.L. (1997). Global forebrain ischemia results in differential cellular expression of interleukin-1beta (IL-1beta) and its receptor at mRNA and protein level. J Cereb Blood Flow Metab *17*, 1107-1120.

Saito, K., Suyama, K., Nishida, K., Sei, Y., and Basile, A.S. (1996). Early increases in TNF-alpha, IL-6 and IL-1 beta levels following transient cerebral ischemia in gerbil brain. Neurosci Lett *206*, 149-152.

Sensi, S.L., Yin, H.Z., Carriedo, S.G., Rao, S.S., and Weiss, J.H. (1999a). Preferential Zn2+ influx through Ca2+-permeable AMPA/kainate channels triggers prolonged mitochondrial superoxide production. Proc Natl Acad Sci U S A *96*, 2414-2419.

Sensi, S.L., Yin, H.Z., and Weiss, J.H. (1999b). Glutamate triggers preferential Zn2+ flux through Ca2+ permeable AMPA channels and consequent ROS production. Neuroreport *10*, 1723-1727.

Sheline, C.T., Behrens, M.M., and Choi, D.W. (2000). Zinc-induced cortical neuronal death: contribution of energy failure attributable to loss of NAD(+) and inhibition of glycolysis. J Neurosci *20*, 3139-3146.

Sheline, C.T., Wang, H., Cai, A.L., Dawson, V.L., and Choi, D.W. (2003). Involvement of poly ADP ribosyl polymerase-1 in acute but not chronic zinc toxicity. Eur J Neurosci *18*, 1402-1409.

Shin, B.S., Won, S.J., Yoo, B.H., Kauppinen, T.M., and Suh, S.W. (2010). Prevention of hypoglycemia-induced neuronal death by hypothermia. J Cereb Blood Flow Metab *30*, 390-402.

Soukup, J., Zauner, A., Doppenberg, E.M., Menzel, M., Gilman, C., Young, H.F., and Bullock, R. (2002). The importance of brain temperature in patients after severe head injury: relationship to intracranial pressure, cerebral perfusion pressure, cerebral blood flow, and outcome. J Neurotrauma *19*, 559-571.

Stolk, J., Hiltermann, T.J., Dijkman, J.H., and Verhoeven, A.J. (1994). Characteristics of the inhibition of NADPH oxidase activation in neutrophils by apocynin, a methoxy-substituted catechol. Am J Respir Cell Mol Biol *11*, 95-102.

Suh, S.W., Aoyama, K., Chen, Y., Garnier, P., Matsumori, Y., Gum, E., Liu, J., and Swanson, R.A. (2003). Hypoglycemic neuronal death and cognitive impairment are prevented by poly(ADP-ribose) polymerase inhibitors administered after hypoglycemia. J Neurosci *23*, 10681-10690.

Suh, S.W., Chen, J.W., Motamedi, M., Bell, B., Listiak, K., Pons, N.F., Danscher, G., and Frederickson, C.J. (2000). Evidence that synaptically-released zinc contributes to neuronal injury after traumatic brain injury. Brain Res *852*, 268-273.

Suh, S.W., Frederickson, C.J., and Danscher, G. (2006). Neurotoxic zinc translocation into hippocampal neurons is inhibited by hypothermia and is aggravated by hyperthermia after traumatic brain injury in rats. J Cereb Blood Flow Metab *26*, 161-169.

Suh, S.W., Garnier, P., Aoyama, K., Chen, Y., and Swanson, R.A. (2004). Zinc release contributes to hypoglycemia-induced neuronal death. Neurobiol Dis *16*, 538-545.

Suh, S.W., Gum, E.T., Hamby, A.M., Chan, P.H., and Swanson, R.A. (2007). Hypoglycemic neuronal death is triggered by glucose reperfusion and activation of neuronal NADPH oxidase. J Clin Invest *117*, 910-918.

Suh, S.W., Hamby, A.M., Gum, E.T., Shin, B.S., Won, S.J., Sheline, C.T., Chan, P.H., and Swanson, R.A. (2008). Sequential release of nitric oxide, zinc, and superoxide in hypoglycemic neuronal death. J Cereb Blood Flow Metab *28*, 1697-1706.

Suh, S.W., Thompson, R.B., and Frederickson, C.J. (2001). Loss of vesicular zinc and appearance of perikaryal zinc after seizures induced by pilocarpine. Neuroreport *12*, 1523-1525.

Taupin, V., Toulmond, S., Serrano, A., Benavides, J., and Zavala, F. (1993). Increase in IL-6, IL-1 and TNF levels in rat brain following traumatic lesion. Influence of pre- and post-traumatic treatment with Ro5 4864, a peripheral-type (p site) benzodiazepine ligand. J Neuroimmunol *42*, 177-185.

Tonder, N., Johansen, F.F., Frederickson, C.J., Zimmer, J., and Diemer, N.H. (1990). Possible role of zinc in the selective degeneration of dentate hilar neurons after cerebral ischemia in the adult rat. Neurosci Lett *109*, 247-252.

Ullrich, O., Diestel, A., Eyupoglu, I.Y., and Nitsch, R. (2001). Regulation of microglial expression of integrins by poly(ADP-ribose) polymerase-1. Nat Cell Biol *3*, 1035-1042.

Virag, L., and Szabo, C. (2002). The therapeutic potential of poly(ADP-ribose) polymerase inhibitors. Pharmacol Rev *54*, 375-429.

Wang, G.J., Deng, H.Y., Maier, C.M., Sun, G.H., and Yenari, M.A. (2002). Mild hypothermia reduces ICAM-1 expression, neutrophil infiltration and microglia/monocyte accumulation following experimental stroke. Neuroscience *114*, 1081-1090.

Weiss, J.H., and Sensi, S.L. (2000). Ca2+-Zn2+ permeable AMPA or kainate receptors: possible key factors in selective neurodegeneration. Trends Neurosci *23*, 365-371.

Weiss, J.H., Sensi, S.L., and Koh, J.Y. (2000). Zn(2+): a novel ionic mediator of neural injury in brain disease. Trends Pharmacol Sci *21*, 395-401.

Wieloch, T. (1985). Hypoglycemia-induced neuronal damage prevented by an N-methyl-D-aspartate antagonist. Science *230*, 681-683.

Yamasaki, Y., Matsuura, N., Shozuhara, H., Onodera, H., Itoyama, Y., and Kogure, K. (1995). Interleukin-1 as a pathogenetic mediator of ischemic brain damage in rats. Stroke *26*, 676-680; discussion 681.

Yin, H.Z., Sensi, S.L., Ogoshi, F., and Weiss, J.H. (2002). Blockade of Ca2+-permeable AMPA/kainate channels decreases oxygen-glucose deprivation-induced Zn2+ accumulation and neuronal loss in hippocampal pyramidal neurons. J Neurosci *22*, 1273-1279.

Yu, S.W., Wang, H., Poitras, M.F., Coombs, C., Bowers, W.J., Federoff, H.J., Poirier, G.G., Dawson, T.M., and Dawson, V.L. (2002). Mediation of poly(ADP-ribose) polymerase-1-dependent cell death by apoptosis-inducing factor. Science *297*, 259-263.

17

Congenital Hyperinsulinism

Xinhua Xiao and Si Chen
Key Laboratory of Endocrinology, the Ministry of Health,
Department of Endocrinology, Peking Union Medical College Hospital,
Chinese Academy of Medical Sciences & Peking Union Medical College,
1 Shuaifuyuan, Wangfujing ST, Beijing ,
Diabetes Institute, Shanghai Sixth Hospital Affiliated to
Shanghai Jiaotong University, Shanghai,
China

1. Introduction

Congenital hyperinsulinism (CHI) is the most common cause of persistent and recurrent hypoglycaemia in neonates and infants during their first year of livies. CHI may lead to severe mental retardation and epilepsy if not treated properly. Both sporadic and familial variants of CHI are recognized, and of which sporadic forms is relatively uncommon (incidence 1 per 35,000 live births), comparing with the highly consanguinious familial forms high rates of consanguinity; with incidence may be as high as 1 in 2,500 live births in the corresponding communities. The clinical severity of CHI varies mainly with age of onset of hypoglycaemia (severe hypoglycaemia in neonates) and is remarkedly predictive in terms of therapeutic outcome and genetic counseling.

2. Physiopathology of hypoglycemia

Hypoglycemia in children is defined by a glucose plasma level below 2.8 or 3 mmol/l, It is a life-threatening condition that requires being diagnosed and treated promptly and appropriately to avoid brain damage and general distress. Congenital hyperinsulinism is due to an inappropriate insulin over-secretion by the β-cells. Insulin is known to be the only hormone to decrease plasma glucose level, and the function of which is realized by inhibiting hepatic glycogenolysis and boosting muscle uptake as well as reducing lipolysis and ketogenesis. Mechanisms above might explain the major characteristic clinical findings of neonatal hyperinsulinism (HI): the increased glucose requirement to correct hypoglycemia, the responsiveness to exogenous glucagon , and the absence of ketone bodies detected.
Several pathways are involved in the regulation of insulin secretion by the pancreatic β-cell, helping explaining the effectiveness of diazoxide, somatostatin, calcium channel inhibitors and protein restricted diet treatments(Fig. 1). Glucose and other substrates, such as amino acids, stimulate insulin secretion , by raising the intracytosolic ATP/ADP ratio. Glucokinase enzyme initiates the β-cell glucose metabolism. It has a high Km for glucose so that the blood concentration of glucose directly determines the rate in glucose oxidation of β-cell and

subsequently controls the insulin release. The increase in the cytosolic ATP/ADP ratio activates the plasma membrane sulfonylurea receptor 1 (SUR1), leading to the closure of the potassium channel (K_{ATP} channel) which depolarizes the plasma membrane and opens a voltage dependant calcium channel. The calcium cellular concentration consequently increases, which triggers the release of insulin from storage granules. Leucine, one of the most potent amino acids in stimulating insulin secretion, acts indirectly as a positive allosteric affector of glutamate dehydrogenase (GDH) which catalyses the oxidative deamination of glutamate to alpha-ketoglutarate and ammonia, using NAD or NADP as co-factor. Hyperactivation of GDH is responsible for an increased alpha of the β-cell ATP/ADP ratio. Diazoxide blocks insulin secretion by activating (opening) the SUR1. Somatostatin analogues act by inhibiting the insulin release through different mechanisms involving adenylyl cyclase and protein kinase A, and dietary protein restriction decreases the stimulation of GDH by leucine

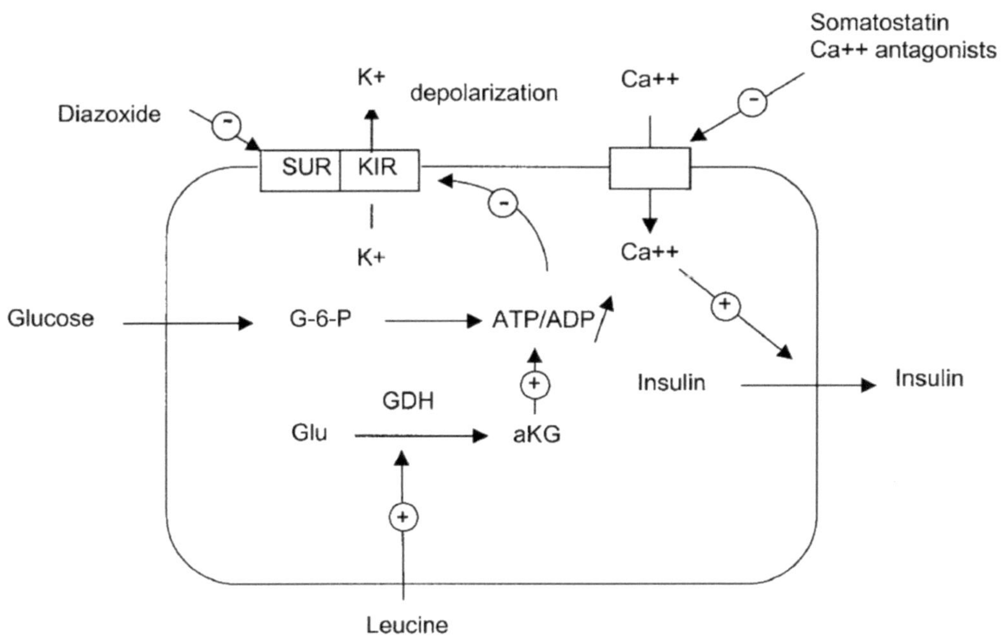

Fig. 1. Mechanisms of insulin secretion by the pancreatic beta cell. +: stimulation; -: inhibition; ADP: adenosine diphosphate; ATP: adenosine triphosphate; α-KG: α-ketoglutarate; G-6-P: glucose-6-phosphate; GDH: glutamate dehydrogenase.

3. Genetics

Insulin secretion from β-cells is precisely regulated to maintain plasma glucose levels within a normal range (3.5–5.5 mmol/l). The genetic basis of CHI involves defects in key genes which regulate insulin secretion from β-cells. The most common cause of CHI are recessive inactivating mutations in ABCC8 and KCNJ11 which encode the two subunits of the adenosine triphosphate sensitive potassium channels (ATP sensitive K_{ATP} channels) in the pancreatic β-cell. These β-cell K_{ATP} channels play a key role in transducing signals derived from glucose metabolism to β-cell membrane depolarisation and regulated insulin secretion. Another recessive form of CHI is due to mutations in HADH (encoding for-3-hydroxyacyl-coenzyme A dehydrogenase). Dominant forms of CHI are due to inactivating mutations in ABCC8 and KCNJ11 and activating mutations in GLUD1 (encoding glutamate dehydrogenase), GCK (encoding glucokinase), HNF4A (encoding hepatocyte nuclear factor 4a) and SLC16A1 (encoding monocarboxylate transporter 1). Mutations in all these genes account for about 50% of the revealed causes of CHI, and in some populations mutations in these genes contributes to only about 20% of CHI cases, suggesting other novel genetic aetiologies. Table 1 summarises the known genetic causes of CHI.

Gene	locus	OMIM	Protein	Mechanism
ABCC8	11p15.1	600509	Sulfonylurea receptor1 (SUR1)	Defects in KATP biogenesis and turnover, trafficking and nucleotide regulation
KCNJ11	11p15.1	600937	Inward rectifying potassium channel (Kir6.2)	Defects in KATP biogenesis and turnover, trafficking and nucleotide regulation
GLUD1	10q23.3	138130	Glutamate dehydrogenase (GDH)	Loss of inhibition of GDH by GTP and increased basal GDH activity
GCK	7p15–13	138079	Glucokinase	Increased affinity of GCK for glucose
HADH	4q22–26	601609	3-hydroxyacyl-CoA dehydrogenase	Unknown
SLC16A1	1p13.2–p12	600682	Monocarboxylate transporter 1 (MCT1)	Increased expression of MCT1
HNF4A	20q12–13.1	600281	Hepatocyte nuclear factor 4 alpha	Unknown

Table 1. The genes implicated in congenital hyperinsulinism with the gene loci and proteins affected

3.1 Role of pancreatic β-cell K_{ATP} channels in glucose-induced insulin secretion

K_{ATP} channels have a key role in the physiology of many cells, and defects in either structure or regulation is pathogenic. Functionally K_{ATP} channels provide a means of linking the electrical activity of a cell to its metabolic state by sensing changes in the concentration of intracellular nucleotides, and in some cases they mediate the actions of hormones and transmitters. The pancreatic K_{ATP} channel is a functional complex of the sulfonylurea receptor 1(SUR1) and an inward rectifier potassium channel subunit (Kir6.2) and acts pivotally in regulating insulin secretion from the β-cell. The Kir6.2 forms the pore of the channel and the SUR1 (an ATP binding cassette transporter) acts as a regulatory subunit.

K_{ATP} channels are regulated by adenine nucleotides to convert changes in cellular metabolic levels into membrane excitability. Each subunit of the K_{ATP} channel is known to be regulated differentially. The Kir6.2 subunit determines the biophysical properties of the channel complex including K+ selectivity, rectification, inhibition by ATP and activation by acyl-CoAs. The sulfonylurea receptors endow K_{ATP} channels with sensitivity to the stimulatory actions of Mg-nucleotides and K_{ATP} channel openers (for example, diazoxide, nicorandil) and the inhibitory effects of sulfonylureas and glinides and endosulfins.
K_{ATP} channels can only function if they are assembled and correctly transported to the cell membrane surface (trafficking). The assembly and trafficking of K_{ATP} channels are intricately linked processes. Only octameric K_{ATP} channel complexes are capable of expressing on the cell membrane surface. For example both Kir6.2 and SUR1 possess an endoplasmic reticulum (ER) retention signal (RKR) that prevents the trafficking of each subunit to the plasma membrane in the absence of the other subunit. Correct assembly of the two subunits masks these retention signals, allowing them to traffic to the plasma membrane. The retention signal is present in the C-terminal region of Kir6.2 and in an intracellular loop between TM11 and NBF-1 in SUR1. Truncation of the C-terminus of Kir6.2 deletes its retention signal, allowing functional expression of Kir6.2 in the absence of SUR1 subunit. In addition to these retrograde signals, the C-terminus of SUR1 has an anterograde signal, composed in part of a dileucine motif and downstream phenylalanine, which is required for K_{ATP} channels to exit the ER/cis-Golgi compartments and transit to the cell surface. Deletion of as few as seven amino acids, including the phenylalanine, from SUR1 markedly reduces surface expression of K_{ATP} channels. Thus,one function of SUR is as a chaperone protein, to facilitate the surface expression of Kir6.2. There is also some evidence that Kir6.2 provides a reciprocal service for SUR.

3.2 Mutations that affect K_{ATP} channels in pancreatic β-cells

The commonest genetic causes of CHI are autosomal recessive mutations in ABCC8 and KCNJ11 genes encoding the two subunits of the pancreatic β-cell K_{ATP} channels. Autosomal dominant mutations have also been described. These mutations result in differing abnormalities of recombinant K_{ATP} channels including protein folding, protein synthesis defects, assembly and trafficking defects, and alterations in both nucleotide regulation and open-state frequency.
The SUR1 and Kir6.2 proteins are encoded by adjacent genes (ABCC8 and KCNJ11, respectively) located on chromosome 11p15.1. Recessive inactivating mutations in ABCC8 and KCNJ11 cause the most common and most severe forms of CHI. Patients with mutations in these genes are usually unresponsive to medical therapy and may require pancreatectomy. Autosomal-dominant mutations in ABCC8 and KCNJ11 cause mild, medically responsive HH. In general, mutations in ABCC8 and KCNJ11 account for approximately 50% of the cases of CHI.
Recessive inactivating mutations in ABCC8 and KCNJ11 are typically associated with the diffuse type of CHI. Typical diffuse disease is characterized by enlarged nuclei of pancreatic β-cells, although the degree of nuclear enlargement might show variation from one islet to another. Other changes in the β-cells include an increase in quantity of proinsulin in the Golgi area and an increased amount of cytoplasm.By contrast, the focal form of the disease is characterized by the presence of adenomatous hyperplasia confined to a single region of the pancreas. In the majority of cases this hyperplasia is macroscopically invisible; loci can be 2–10 mm in diameter.

The genetic basis of focal disease involves the paternal inheritance of a recessive ABCC8 or KCNJ11 mutation and the somatic loss of heterozygosity in the distal portion of the short arm of the maternal chromosome 11. Somatic loss of heterozygosity represents the loss of normal function of one allele of a gene, the other allele of which was already inactivated in a cell (in this case, a pancreatic β-cell). Patients with focal, congenital HH might have more than one focal pancreatic lesion, which can be caused by a separate somatic maternal deletion of the 11p15.1 region. Focal lesions are different from insulinomas (which are also called adenomas) in terms of their histology and molecular mechanisms of insulin secretion.

3.3 Mutations that affect leucine and glucose metabolism in pancreatic β-cells

Metabolopathies cause CHI either by altering the concentration of intracellular signalling molecules (such as ATP/ADP) or by the accumulation of intermediary metabolites. Autosomal dominant mutations in the genes encoding glutamate dehydrogenase (GDH) (GLUD1) and glucokinase (GCK) lead to inappropriate insulin secretion by increasing the amount of ATP in the β-cells. More recently autosomal recessive mutations in short-chain L-3-hydroxyacyl- CoA dehydrogenase (HADHSC) have been linked to defects in fatty acid oxidation and hyperinsulinism.

3.3.1 Gain of function mutations in glutamate dehydrogenase

The GLUD1 gene is located on chromosome 10q23.3 and contains 13 exons coding for a 505 amino acid mature enzyme, glutamate dehydrogenase (GDH). This enzyme catalyses the oxidative deamination of glutamate to α-ketoglutarate and ammonia using NAD+ and/or NADP+ as co-factors.In the β-cells α-ketoglutarate enters the tricarboxylic acid cycle and leads to an increase in the cellular ATP concentration. This increases the ATP/ADP ratio which triggers closure of the K_{ATP} channels and depolarisation of the β-cell membrane. This, in turn, opens the voltage gated calcium channel, raises the cytosolic calcium, and triggers the release of insulin.

Activating mutations (heterozygous missense single amino acid substitutions) in the GLUD1 gene are the second most common cause of CHI. GLUD1 gene mutations cause a form of CHI in which affected children have recurrent symptomatic HH together with a persistently elevated plasma ammonia value, the hyperinsulinism/hyperammonaemia (HI/HA) syndrome. The mutations causing HI/HA reduce the sensitivity of the enzyme to allosteric inhibition by the high energy phosphate GTP and in rare cases increase basal GDH activity. The loss of inhibition by GTP increases the rate of oxidation of glutamate in the presence of leucine, thereby increasing insulin secretion. The clinical picture is hence characterised by postprandial hypoglycaemia following a protein meal (fasting hypoglycaemia may also occur). The hypoglycaemia in patients with HI/HA syndrome is usually responsive to medical treatment with diazoxide. The hyperammonaemia is considered to be asymptomatic and hence efforts to reduce plasma ammonia values with sodium benzoate or N-carbamylglutamate do not seem to be beneficial.

3.3.2 Congenital hyperinsulinism due to gain of function mutations in glucokinase

Heterozygous inactivating mutations in GCK cause maturity onset diabetes of the young (MODY), homozygous inactivating in GCK mutations result in permanent neonatal diabetes, whereas heterozygous activating GCK mutations cause CHI. So far seven activating GCK mutations (V455M, A456V, Y214C, T65I, W99R, G68V, S64Y) have been

described that lead to CHI. Activating GCK mutations increase the affinity of GCK for glucose and alter (reset) the threshold for glucose stimulated insulin secretion. All reported activating mutations cluster in a region of the enzyme, which has been termed the allosteric activator site and is remote to the substrate binding site. The allosteric site of GCK is where small molecule activators bind, suggesting a critical role of the allosteric site in the regulation of GCK activities. There is no evidence to suggest that over-expression of GCK (increased gene dosage effect) is a likely cause of CHI.
The clinical symptoms and course of patients with GCK mutations cover a broad spectrum from asymptomatic hypoglycaemia to unconsciousness and seizures, even within the same family with the same mutation, implicating a complex mechanism for GCK regulation. Patients with activating GCK mutations may present with postprandial hyperinsulinaemic hypoglycaemia. Most of the GCK mutations reported to date cause mild diazoxide responsive CHI.

3.4 Mutations in the HNF4A gene

Heterozygote mutations in the human HNF4A gene classically lead to maturity onset diabetes of the young subtype 1 (MODY1), which is characterised by autosomal dominant inheritance and impaired glucose stimulated insulin secretion from pancreatic β-cell. These mutations in the HNF4A gene cause multiple defects in glucose stimulated insulin secretion and in expression of HNF4A dependent genes.Recently mutations in the HNF4A gene were reported to cause macrosomia and both transient and persistent HH.In one retrospective study the birth weight of the HNF4A mutation carriers compared to non-mutation family members was increased by a median of 790 g.Transient hypoglycaemia was reported in 8/54 infants with heterozygous HNF4A mutations and documented HH in three cases.

3.5 Mutations that cause defective fatty-acid metabolism in pancreatic β-cells

Loss-of-function mutations in the HADH gene are associated with CHI. The clinical presentation of all patients reported is heterogeneous, with either mild late onset intermittent HH or severe neonatal hypoglycaemia. All reported cases have presented with increased 3-hydroxyglutarate in urine and hydroxybutyrylcarnitine in blood which may be diagnostically useful markers for HADH deficiency. In the first patient reported sequencing of the HADH genomic DNA from the fibroblasts showed a homozygous mutation (C773T) changing proline to leucine at amino acid 258.Analysis of blood from the parents showed they were heterozygous for this mutation. Western blot studies showed undetectable levels of immunoreactive HADH protein in the patient's fibroblasts.
The molecular mechanism of how loss of function in the HADH gene leads to unregulated insulin secretion is still unclear. Several recent studies in rodents have begun to give some insights into how HADH regulates insulin secretion and its interaction with other genes involved in β-cell development and function. The normal β-cell phenotype is characterised by a high expression of HADH and a low expression of other b-oxidation enzymes. Downregulation of HADH causes an elevated secretory activity suggesting that this enzyme protects against inappropriately high insulin values and hypoglycaemia. Hence, HADH seems to be a negative regulator of insulin secretion in β-cells. Further studies will be required to understand fully the biochemical pathways by which defects in HADH lead to dysregulated insulin secretion.

4. Histology

Two major histological forms of CHI have been described (diffuse and focal), there are still some cases which represent a diagnostic challenge, as they cannot be easily classified into focal or diffuse. Both the diffuse and focal forms share a similar clinical presentation, but result from different pathphysiological and molecular mechanisms. The histological form of CHI can be a guide as to the mode of inheritance,diffuse CHI usually presents as an autosomal recessive disorder, whereas focal CHI is sporadic.

The typical diffuse form affects all the β-cells within the islets of Langerhans and is most commonly due to recessive mutations in the genes encoding the two subunits of the K_{ATP} channel. Typical diffuse disease is characterized by an increase in the size of the pancreatic β -cell nuclei throughout the pancreas.

The 'focal' form (focal adenomatous pancreatic hyperplasia) of CHI is found in about 40–50% of the children and appears to be localized to one region of the pancreas. Focal pancreatic lesions appear as small regions of islet adenomatosis measuring 2–10 mm, which are characterized by β-cells with enlarged nuclei surrounded by normal tissue.Focal disease results from paternal uniparental disomy (UPD) encompassing chromosome 11p15.5-11p15.1 within a single pancreatic β-cell which unmasks a paternally inherited K_{ATP} channel mutation at 11p15.1. In addition, the lesion exhibits a somatic loss of a part of the maternally inherited chromosome 11p which includes imprinted maternally expressed tumour suppressor genes (H19 and P57 KIP2) , paternally expressed insulin growth factor-2, as well as (non-imprinted) SUR1/Kir6. This results in a corresponding reduction to homozygosity of the paternal mutation, and the outcome is unregulated insulin secretion.β -cells within the focal lesion do not express p57 KIP2 , but insulin growth factor-2 is mildly increased. The somatic loss of heterozygosity is associated with increased proliferation. The focal lesion is different from the insulinoma (also called adenoma) in histology and molecular mechanisms of insulin secretion.

5. Clinical presentation

CHI typically presents in the first few days after birth in term and preterm infants with symptomatic hypoglycaemia. The patients may present with non-specific symptoms of hypoglycaemia such as poor feeding, lethargy, and irritability or symptoms such as seizures and coma. In CHI a blood sample taken at the time of hypoglycaemia will show an inappropriately raised serum insulin level with low serum fatty acid levels and ketone bodies. Most infants with hyperinsulinism present within the early neonatal period although infantile and childhood onset forms are also recognized. Transient hyperinsulinism is seen in association with maternal diabetes, birth asphyxia, polycythaemia,and rhesus incompatibility. Other syndromic associations which might be evident at birth include Beckwith syndrome, Sotos' syndrome, Perlman's syndrome, and the clinical phenotype characteristic of phosphomannose isomerase deficiency (carbohydrate-deficient glycoprotein syndrome type 1b).

Most neonates with HI are born at term and are either normal or large for gestational age, although HI is described in preterm infants. Many of these infants are overtly macrosomic and plethoric and may have characteristic facial appearances comprising high forehead, small nasal tip, and short columella giving the impression that the nose is large and bulbous, smooth philtrum, and thin upper lip. The key events in early neonatal management of

infants with HI involve avoidance of hypoglycaemia and careful definition of clinical and biochemical phenotype. Infants with severe HI will not uncommonly have glucose requirements of 15—20 mg/kg/min and as such will usually be dependent upon intravenous glucose infusions. Blood sugar concentrations are usually very labile and it is of paramount importance that venous access is secure in these cases—usually necessitating placement of a central venous catheter. Infants with persistent forms of HI should normally be assessed in a referral centre for HI which has the necessary resource for timely definition of clinical and biochemical phenotype, genotype, and, if appropriate, structural phenotype.
The main differential diagnosis of congenital HI remains the factitious hyperinsulinism secondary to Munchausen by proxy syndrome, one of the parents administering insulin or sulfonylurea surreptitiously to their own child. Another period of onset for HI occurs later in infancy, between 1 and 20 months of life and is revealed in half of the patients by seizures. Macrosomy at birth can be noted. The characteristics of hypoglycemia are similar, although lower rates of intravenous glucose are required.

6. The diagnostic criteria for HI

The diagnostic criteria for congenital HI include: i) fasting and post-prandial hypoglycemia (<2.5 - 3 mmol/l) with unsuppressed insulin secretion (plasma insulin concentrations >1 mU/l), ii) a positive response to the subcutaneous or intramuscular administration of glucagon (plasma glucose concentration increase by 2 to 3 mmol/l following a 0.5 mg glucagon subcutaneous injection), iii) negative ketone bodies in urine (and in plasma) and iv) prolonged dependence on treatment to prevent hypoglycemia throughout the first months/years of life. Nevertheless, in infancy and childhood, normal plasma insulin and C-peptide concentrations during hypoglycemia do not exclude the diagnosis of HI and measurements have to be repeated. In the absence of clearly abnormal insulin levels during hypoglycemic episodes, an 8 to 12 hours fasting test aiming at revealing inappropriately low levels of ketone bodies, free fatty acid and branched chain amino acids can be helpful.
In some patients with protein-sensitive congenital HH owing to GLUD1 mutations, a leucine provocation test might be required to demonstrate HH. Analyses of urinary organic acids and acylcarnitine should also be performed, as results could aid in the diagnosis of HADH deficiency. Serum glucagon levels are decreased in congenital HH. Patients with HH demonstrate a positive glycemic response (a rise in blood glucose level of >1.5 mmol/l) to intramuscularly or intravenously administered glucagon during times of hypoglycemia. Decreased serum levels of insulin-like growth-factor binding protein 1 (IGFBP-1) aid the diagnosis in some patients, because insulin suppresses transcription of the IGFBP1 gene. Patients with exercise-induced HH will require an exercise provocation test and/or a pyruvate load to induce hypoglycemia.
All new HI patients should be screened for hyperammonemia to diagnose the HI/HA syndrome (GLUD1 gene), for short chain hydroxyacyl-CoA dehydrogenase (SCHAD) deficiency (HADH gene) with urine organic acids and plasma acylcarnitines chromatographies, and for CDG syndromes, as these 3 diseases may present in the neonatal period as apparently isolated HI. Other genes can be suspected depending on the context. SLC16A1 gene will be analyzed in case of Exercise-induced hyperinsulinism (EIHI), HNF4A gene when the newborn is macrosomic with a family history of MODY diabetes. Finally, familial forms or consanguinity and syndromic forms have to be checked as these are associated with a diffuse HI.

7. Medical management

Rapid diagnosis, avoidance of recurrent episodes of hypoglycemia and prompt management of hypoglycemia are the cornerstones of management to prevent brain damage and mental retardation in patients with CHI. Blood glucose levels must be maintained within the normal neonatal range (above 3.5 mmol/l), by administering glucose orally, enterally or intravenously. Usually, in neonates, the first step is a continuous enteral feeding of milk enriched with malto-dextrine. However, the severity of the hypoglycemias may straightaway or rapidly require more intensive treatments to prevent irreversible brain damages. The glucose rate administered has to be sufficient to normalize glucose levels, at least with a glucose flow equal to the physiological hepatic production of glucose (8–10 mg/kg/min for a neonate or young infant and 5–7 mg/kg/min for children). If hypoglycemia persists or recurs, the perfusion rate has to be increased, often requiring high concentration glucose solutions infused through a central venous line. However, in severe HI this may be insufficient and continuous glucagon infusion (intravenous or subcutaneous, 0.5 to 2 mg/day) along with glucose should be administered.
At the same time, specific treatments of HI must be initiated,which include diazoxide, octreotide and nifedipine.

7.1 Diazoxide

The clinical effectiveness of diazoxide is variable .Mutations in the ABCC8/KCNJ11 gene are not predictive of the response to diazoxide, and there is no correlation between the histology and the clinical efficacy of diazoxide. Patients with transient and syndromic forms of HH will usually respond to diazoxide, whereas those with severe neonatal CHI will show no response. Oral diazoxide is first used at 15 mg/kg/day (neonates) or 10 mg/kg/day (infants) in oral doses. Diazoxide efficiency is defined as the normalization of glycemia >3 mmol/l measured before and after each meal in patients fed normally with a physiological overnight fast, after stopping intravenous glucose and any other medications for at least five consecutive days. The most frequent adverse effect is hypertrichosis, which can be marked and distressing in young children. Hematological side effects are very rare with usual administration doses. Two confirmed hypoglycemias (<3 mmol/l) in a 24-hour glucose measurement cycle defined the patient as diazoxide unresponsive. Dietary measures and glucose perfusion should be started again to maintain normoglycemia.

7.2 Octreotide

Octreotide is a long-acting analog of the natural hormone somatostatin and is used in the short- and long-term management of CHI. In the short term (with and without glucagon), it is used to stabilize patients pending further investigations. Octreotide has been successively used in the long-term management of some CHI patients in combination with frequent feeding. The long-term medical management of diffuse disease with octreotide and frequent feeding should not be taken lightly, as it may impose a huge burden and be stressful on the family. A gastrostomy is recommend in these patients, as this will allow the delivery of bolus and continuous overnight feeds.
At initiation of octreotide treatment, some patients may present vomiting and/or diarrhea and abdominal distension, which will resolve spontaneously within 7 - 10 days. Gallbladder sludge or stones are rare but can necessitate ursodesoxycholic acid treatment. It should be

screened by abdominal ultrasound twice a year. Glycemia levels can rise significantly immediately after octreotide initiation, however this positive response can be transient, so that a 48 hour observation period should be performed to conclude definitively on the responsiveness to octreotide at a given dose.

7.3 Nifedipine

Other drugs as calcium channels blockers (like nifedipine, 0.5 - 2 mg/kg/day in 2 oral doses) can be proposed.
Patients who are resistant to medical treatment and require surgical treatment, must be assessed for their putative histological form of HI.

8. Differentiating focal from diffuse CHI

The gold standard method to determine which infants have fo-HI is intraoperative frozen section histology. This requires considerable histopathological expertise and will be most reliably performed in supraregional referral centres. Focal lesions are frequently not visible at laparotomy, although laporoscopic visualisation of the pancreas probably has an enhanced detection rate because of the magnification. It has been necessary to devise a number of strategies to differentiate fo-HI from di-HI preoperatively, as conventional imaging methods including ultrasound, octreotide scintigraphy, and magnetic resonance imaging are usually nondiscriminatory.

8.1 Invasive methods

Pancreatic venous sampling (PVS) has proven a valuable and reliable utility in differentiating foand di-HI and in localising focal lesions. The method relies upon transhepatic catheterization of the highly variable pancreatic venous anatomy and demonstration of persistent insulin secretion in the face of a low blood glucose concentration from one or more areas of the pancreas. The method requires that the infants medications are stopped for at least 48 h before the procedure, a specific method of general anaesthesia is administered and that blood glucose concentrations are kept <3.0 mmol/l throughout the procedure. Results may show generalised dysregulation of insulin secretion (di-HI), one or more hot spots of secretion (fo-HI), generalised suppression of secretion (focal disease with failure of catheterization of the region of the pancreas containing the lesion or an extrapancreatic source of insulin), or be uninformative (uninterpretable).
Where PVS has suggested the presence of fo-HI but not localised the lesion, and intra-arterial calcium stimulation test can be performed in which calcium is injected selectively into the gastroduodenal, superior mesenteric, and splenic arteries to stimulate insulin secretion. This method is good at localising focal disease but poor at confirming diffuse disease.
Some investigators have adopted a policy of early laparoscopic pancreatic biopsy. If no lesion is identified with the laparoscope, two or more biopsies from different regions of the pancreas are necessary.

8.2 Noninvasive methods

A variety of relatively noninvasive investigations including the i.v. tolbutamide test and the acute insulin response to an intravenous glucose load have been proposed to screen for fo-HI. The rationale for the tests depends either on the notion that, in fo-HI, the relatively quiescent pancreas outside the lesion can be further stimulated to secrete insulin.

Now 18fluoro-L-Dopa PET has been successfully used to localize the focal domain. The principle of this test is based on the fact that islets take up L-3,4-dihydroxyphenylalanine (L-dopa) and convert it to dopamine by dopa decarboxylase, present in the islet cells . However the precise role of dopamine in the pancreatic β-cells is currently unclear. 18fluoro-L-Dopa PET can also accurately locate ectopic focal lesions. 18fluoro-L-Dopa PET is highly sensitive in detecting focal lesions compared with the previous highly invasive techniques.

9. Surgical treatment

When medical and dietary therapies are ineffective, surgical treatment is required. If a focal lesion is identified and accurately located, it should be surgically removed, as this will "cure" the patient.As diffuse CHI is a heterogeneous disorder with respect to clinical presentation and response to medical therapy, the role of surgery in those cases that are diazoxide unresponsive is not so clear. Studies of predominantly Ashkenazi Jewish children with CHI suggest that the natural history of the disease is one of progressive glucose intolerance and clinical diabetes, possibly due to a slow progressive loss of β-cell function, and this may be due to the increased β -cell apoptosis, and, therefore, surgery may not be indicated in all patients. Similarly, some patients with diazoxide-responsive CHI go on to develop diabetes mellitus in adulthood .

Near-total pancreatectomy is a major operation and is associated with a high incidence of diabetes mellitus later in life. Clearly, surgery is indicated in those patients with severe diffuse disease who fail to respond to octreotide with frequent feeding regimens, and identification of this subgroup is important. The management of postpancreatectomy diabetes mellitus is complicated by the fact that these children have pancreatic exocrine insufficiency, glucagon deficiency, and have residual unregulated insulin secretion, and some patients show resistance to hyperketonaemia and diabetic ketoacidosis.

Before surgery, some precautions are necessary: i) stop medications several days before surgery (5 days before for diazoxide and 2 days before for octreotide) as they may interfere with the peroperative pathological analysis, ii) screen for gallbladder stones with a abdominal ultrasound, and treat if necessary and iii) supplement systematically with iron to prevent anemia.

10. Conclusion

CHI is a major cause of hypoglycaemia in the childhood period. Recognition and appropriate management of this type of hypoglycaemia are important to avoidlong-term neurological consequences. The genetic mechanisms that lead to some forms of transient and CHI are beginning to be understood. Recent experience using 18 FL -dopa PET/CT scanning to distinguish diffuse from focal hyperinsulinism has completely changed the diagnostic and management approach to these patients. For the future, the management of medically unresponsive diffuse disease remains a challenge, and identifying the genetic mechanisms leading to both transient and persistent hyperinsulinism in the remaining 50% of the patients will provide novel insights into pancreatic β-cell physiology.

11. Acknowledgment

This work was supported by grants from the Beijing Natural Science Foundation (No. 7092085, PI: Xinhua Xiao). We wish to express our sincere gratitude to all of the study participants.

12. References

Dunne et al.(2004). Hyperinsulinismin infancy from basic science to clinical disease. Physiol Rev;84:239 - 75.

Pearson et al.(2007) Macrosomia and hyperinsulinaemic hypoglycemia in patients with heterozygous mutations in the HNF4A gene. PLoS Med;4:e118.

Delonlay et al.(2007).Neonatal hyperinsulinism: clinicopathologic correlation. Hum Pathol ;38:387 - 99.

Verkarre et al.(1998).Paternal mutation of the sulfonylurea receptor (SUR1) gene and maternal loss of11p15 imprinted genes lead to persistent hyperinsulinism in focal adenomatoushyperplasia. J Clin Invest;102:1286 - 91.

Huopio et al.(2003). A newsubtype of autosomal dominant diabetes attributable to a mutation in the gene for sulfonyllurea receptor 1. Lancet;361:301 - 7.

18

Diabetes Control and Hypoglycemia

Paul Norwood and Alex Fogel
Valley Endocrine Research, Fresno, CA
University of California, San Francisco
USA

1. Introduction

Diabetes management has traditionally focused solely on lowering blood glucose levels to avoid the long term complications of diabetes. This approach sometimes neglects the detrimental effects of hypoglycemia on the diabetic patient. This is problematic, as hypoglycemia often places patients at risk of poor quality of life, increased medical costs and significant complications. As many instances of hypoglycemia are preventable by smarter treatment strategies, it is expected that accounting for the possibility of hypoglycemia may not only reduce a patient's health care costs, but will allow him or her a better quality of life, decrease the potential for disability and even increase life-expectancy. This article provides an overview of hypoglycemia and establishes guidelines for the management and prevention of hypoglycemia based on the most current research.

2. Definitions

Hypoglycemia is defined as a state in which there are neuroglycopenic symptoms concurrent with a low blood glucose level. The definition of "low blood glucose" can differ significantly across the major medical associations. While the American Diabetes Association (ADA) defines low blood glucose as glucose levels less than or equal to 70 mg/dL (3.9 mM) (ADA, 2005), the European Medicines Agency (EMA) defines the condition as glucose levels under 54 mg/dL (3.0 mM) (EMA, 2010). The ADA definition of "low blood glucose" will be used for the purposes of this article.

It should be noted that despite this baseline threshold, the symptoms of hypoglycemia present at different levels in different patients. For example, in patients averaging blood glucose levels above 200 mg/dL, neurogenic symptoms associated with hypoglycemia can appear when the blood glucose falls to what should be a normal level, near or below 100 mg/dL. This not only presents a significant difficulty in preventing hypoglycemic symptoms, but the glucose situation of each patient must be considered individually as well.

2.1 Artifactual hypoglycemia

In determining whether a patient is experiencing hypoglycemia, it is essential to recognize the situations that can frequently result in false-positives. Artifactual hypoglycemia can be the product of a number of factors, including some that are a result of the methodology employed. These include the absence of an antiglycolytic agent in the blood collection tube,

delayed blood processing, and imperfect glucose monitoring machines, which are often accurate only to within +/- 40 mg/dL. In this last example, a patient meeting both the EMA and the ADA criteria for hypoglycemia may actually be in the normal blood glucose range.
Patient health factors that affect the true detection of hypoglycemia are typically those that result in an abnormal consumption of blood glucose by circulating cells. In patients with leukemia, elevated levels of glycolysis in leukocytes result in significantly decreased levels of blood glucose from the time blood is drawn to the time blood is monitored (Spiller, 2011). The effect is similar in patients suffering from erythrocytosis and polycythemia vera.

3. Symptoms of hypoglycemia

The symptoms of hypoglycemia can be divided into two distinct categories: neuroglycopenic and neurogenic. In both types of diabetes, neuroglycopenic and neurogenic hypoglycemic symptoms can appear with a large change in blood glucose levels without achieving actual numerical hypoglycemia.

3.1 Neuroglycopenic symptoms

The neuroglycopenic symptoms of hypoglycemia include (Ben-Ami et al., 2009; Warren, 2005):

- Behavioral changes, including irritability and nightmares
- Cognitive impairments, including confusion and difficulty concentrating
- Psychomotor abnormalities, including dizziness, weakness, and poor coordination
- Seizure
- Coma

3.2 Neurogenic symptoms

The neurogenic symptoms of hypoglycemia include (Warren, 2005):

- Adrenergic tremor
- Palpitations and anxiety
- Colinergic sweating
- Hunger
- Paresthesias or neurological symptoms, such as numbness in the mouth and tongue

4. Causes of hypoglycemia in diabetic patients

In patients with either type I or type II diabetes, the root cause of factual hypoglycemia is always hyperinsulinemia. However, the etiology of hyperinsulinemia varies depending on the type of treatment strategy in place. For type I diabetes, hypoglycemia is always due to excessive insulin dosage. In type II diabetes, it results from the use of insulin or sulfonureas. The combination of a GLP-1 agent and a sulfonurea is a potent mixture and may cause hypoglycemia.
The risk of hypoglycemia in patients with type II diabetes beginning insulin treatment is fairly low, and is comparable to patient populations being treated with sulfonureas alone. However with time the incidence increases remarkably. For type II diabetics, the incidence increases from 5% for patients on insulin for less than two years to 24% for type II patients taking insulin for more than five years (Heller, 2010). In type I diabetics, the incidence of

hypoglycemia increases from 22% in patients with the condition for less than 5 years to 44% in patients who have had diabetes for more than 15 years.

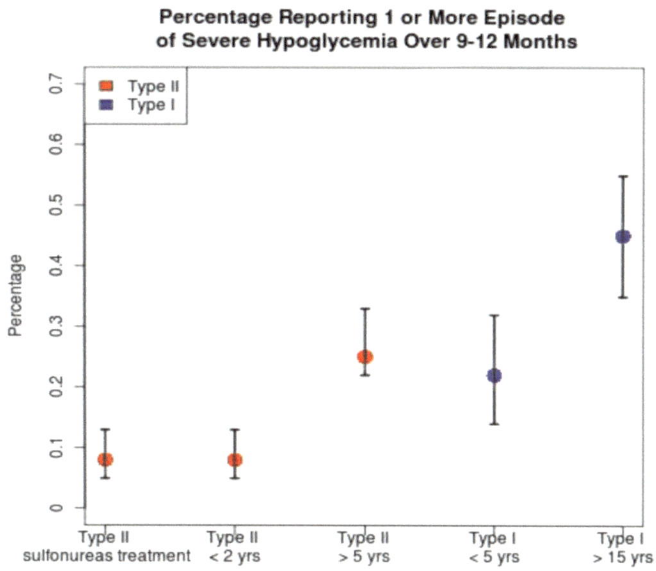

Fig. 1. Incidence of hypoglycemia increases with the duration of illness. (adapted from Heller, 2010).

The increase of hypoglycemia likely results from impaired counter-regulatory hormone release (Bolli, 1983; Matyka, 1997). Within five years of the onset of type I diabetes, expression of the hypoglycemia-protective hormone glucagon is less responsive to instances of hypoglycemia by 66%. This imbalance is partially mitigated by normal epinephrine levels during this time. However, by fifteen years of the disease, type I diabetics typically present with glucagon levels decreased by 80% of baseline and epinephrine levels reduced by 66% (Heller, 2010). This situation presents a significant difficultly for the patient's counter-regulatory hormones to correct. Type II diabetics also develop the same hormonal deficiencies, which are proportional to the duration of the disease.

In both type I and type II diabetes patients, the situation is enhanced by physiological unawareness of hypoglycemia. Hypoglycemic unawareness occurs in 17% of patients who have had type I diabetes (Heller, 2010). The causes are:

- Having diabetes for many years with decreased counter-regulatory hormones
- Autonomic neuropathy
- Frequent low blood sugar with desensitization to hypoglycemia
- Stress or depression
- Poor self-care
- Alcohol consumption
- A previous low blood sugar in the last 24 to 48 hours
- Beta blockers

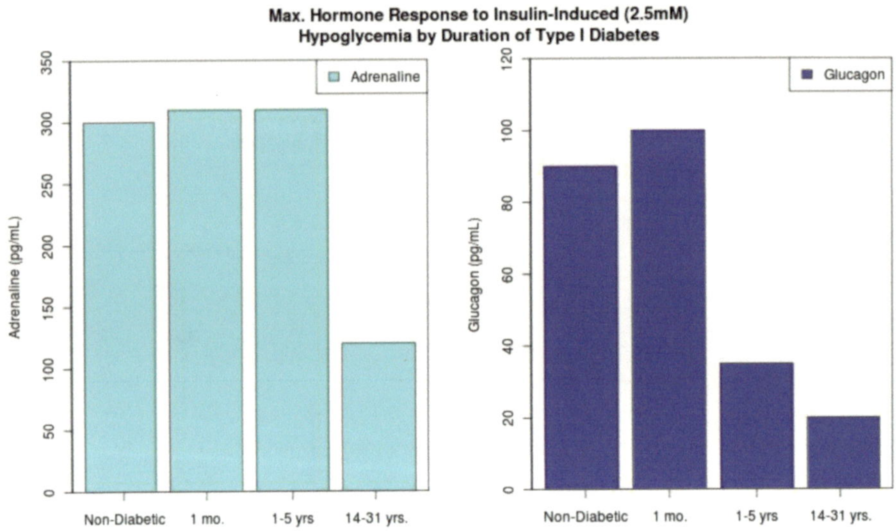

Fig. 2. Progressive decrease in endocrine counter-regulation depending on duration of Type I diabetes. (adapted from Heller, 2010).

4.1 Normal physiological response to of hypoglycemia

As the brain cannot synthesize glucose or store substantial amounts as glycogen in neurons, it requires a continuous supply of glucose from the circulation to function. Hypoglycemia therefore causes brain dysfunction. The normal physiologic response to hypoglycemia appears in stages. Epinephrine release begins at 63 mg/dL (Cryer, 2007). Secondary symptoms of tremor, palpitations and sweating begin at 58 mg/dL. Cognitive dysfunction presents consistently at 54 mg/dL. Confusion and disorientation appear at 45 mg/dL. At 18 mg/dL, coma and seizure result. Prolonged blood glucose levels less than 18 mg/dL result in brain damage.

4.2 Impaired physiological responsiveness

In diabetics exhibiting impaired physiological responsiveness to hypoglycemia and hypoglycemic unawareness, the levels of blood glucose corresponding to the stages of cognitive dysfunction are unchanged. However, the release of epinephrine occurs at 50-52 mg/dL, which is lower by 10 mg/dL than the typical release point observed in normal patients. It should be noted that epinephrine release does not occur until *after* cognitive dysfunction appears. Thus, the warning symptoms of tremor, palpitations and sweating actually follow cognitive dysfunction instead of preceding it. This type of brain desensitization to hypoglycemia is caused by acclimation to frequent episodes of hypoglycemia. The brain becomes accustomed to the low glucose levels and does not signal for epinephrine to be released during such times. Because of neuroglycopenia, the patient with an impaired epinephrine response cannot reliably treat his or her own condition. In these cases, the only hopes for the patient to combat the episode of hypoglycemia are natural insulin degradation, delayed epinephrine and glucagon release, or intervention by a third party.

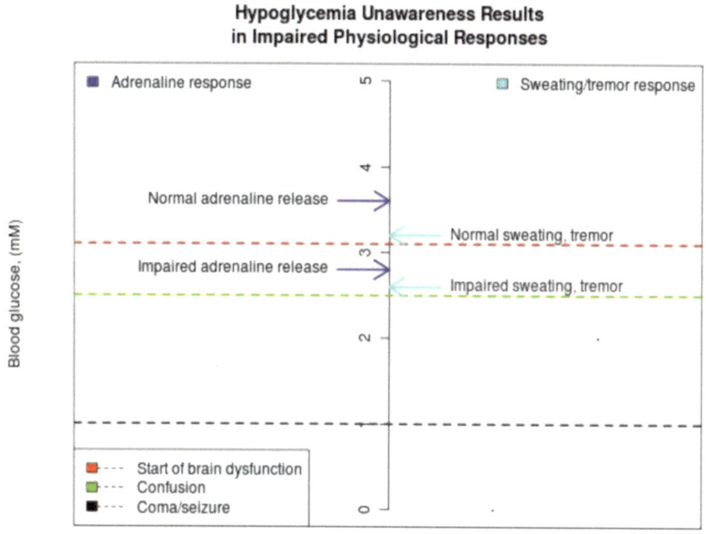

Fig. 3. Impaired physiological responses due to hypoglycemia unawareness (adapted from Cryer, 2007). Note: 1 mM = 18 mg/dL

The reason for this reduced responsiveness is the brain's adaptation to frequent episodes of hypoglycemia. In patients experiencing frequent bouts of hypoglycemia, glucose transporters in the neurons of the brain increase in number, permitting the brain to receive a more steady supply of glucose. As a result, the blood hypoglycemic threshold for the brain to signal epinephrine release becomes lower. This creates a state of hypoglycemic unawareness, as the brain has adapted to hypoglycemia. The patient can then develop perilously low glucose levels without realizing it.

Since repeated hypoglycemia is common in people with diabetes who strive to keep their glucose levels under tight control near a pre-defined 'normal' level, the incidence of hypoglycemic unawareness is higher in this population. The more intensive the treatment protocol, the greater the incidence of hypoglycemia and hypoglycemia unawareness. This situation is abetted by the rigidity of the patient's diabetes control, as many patients will ignore and attempt to tolerate their hypoglycemic episodes to meet the specifications of their physician. This population is at serious risk of becoming accustomed to hypoglycemia, and unfortunately, these patients run a risk of developing a major hypoglycemic reaction and the associated medical consequences. To successfully monitor this situation, the physician must realize that some patients experience difficulty in loosening their tight blood glucose control, and these patients should be warned repeatedly about the dangers of hypoglycemic episodes and its consequences.

In addition, stress, depression, poor self-care, alcohol or drug use or any situation that renders the patient less attentive or aware of his or her bodily sensations can contribute to hypoglycemic unawareness. In particular, depression, which is found in approximately 30% of diabetics, needs to be addressed (ADA, 2005; Piette et al., 2004). It is very difficult for patients suffering from clinical depression to control their diabetes. As a physician, one must be alert for classic depressive symptoms in their diabetic patients, principally fatigue. It takes energy and effort to care for diabetes, and if the patient is depressed, he or she will experience great difficulty in performing simple self-care. Many of these patients lack the energy to monitor their diabetes, the self-motivation to adhere to a diet, and the focus to coordinate to two. This frequently leads to hypoglycemic reactions.

Beta blockers can also contribute to the incidence of hypoglycemia. These drugs decrease the beta adrenergic symptoms, such as palpitations and tremor, that are associated with the onset of hypoglycemia. On occasion, these medications may prevent the patient from recognizing the adrenergic warning symptoms, resulting in hypoglycemic unawareness. Beta blockers also prevent epinephrine from increasing the release of glucose from the liver.

5. Prevalence of hypoglycemia

The prevalence of hypoglycemia is profound and worrisome, especially considering the lack of attention given to the condition. In one study in which patients self-reported hypoglycemic events, 50% of patients with type II diabetes on insulin and 30% of patients taking sulfonureas without insulin reported such an event (Cryer, 2003). It has been shown that 62% of type I diabetics exhibit asymptomatic hypoglycemia, as do 46% of type II diabetics. There is also evidence that type I diabetics can expect to experience a major hypoglycemic event at least once per year, while type II diabetics can anticipate a similar event once every 2.5 years. As the prevalence of type II diabetes is far greater than type I diabetes, the absolute number of hypoglycemic events in type II diabetes is significantly higher than in type I diabetics, but the incidence per capita is lower.

5.1 Determinants of hypoglycemic events

Several determinants can be used to predict an increased risk of symptomatic hypoglycemia. These include:

- Advanced age
- Irregular meal schedule
- Regularity of exercise
- Hemoglobin A1c $\geq$ 7%
- Having diabetes > 8 years
- Duration of insulin therapy
- Renal impairment
- Diabetic neuropathy
- Previous history of hypoglycemia
- Anticoagulant therapy
- Concurrent medication of five or more prescription drugs hospitalization within the last 12 months

The state of the patient's health is therefore a indicator of the incidence of significant hypoglycemia. The more fragile the patient, the more likely he or she is to experience a severe hypoglycemic event.

6. Hypoglycemia and increased mortality

There are two potential causative reasons for increased mortality in patients with hypoglycemia. The main one is cardiovascular. Diabetics have a higher incidence of cardiovascular disease than the general population, including coronary artery disease, cardiac hypertrophy, and cardiac autonomic neuropathy (Johnston, 2011). This is because with hypoglycemia, there is an increase adrenergic load causing a faster heart rate with subsequent cardiac ischemia and possibly myocardial infarction. Hypoglycemia also causes a increased QT interval on the electrocardiogram. The QT interval is increased more in those with diabetic autonomic neuropathy. It is well documented that an increased QT interval can lead to ventricular fibrillation and sudden death (Lee, 2004).

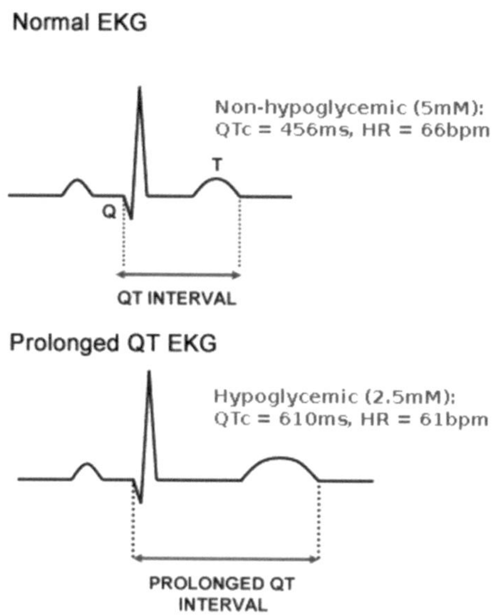

Fig. 4. QT interval prolongation during hypoglycemia (adapted from Heller 2010).

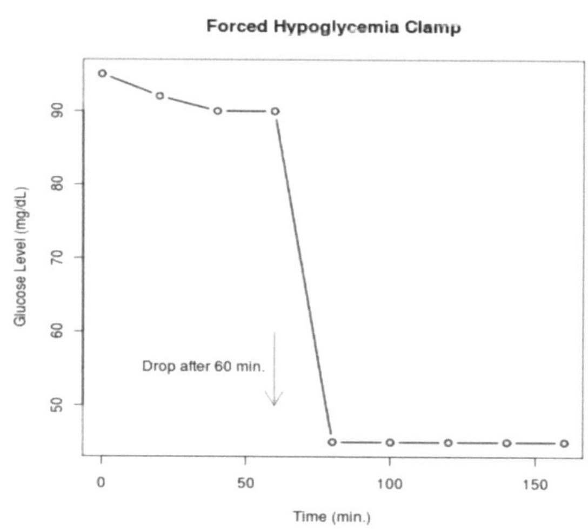

Fig. 5. Drop in glucose after 60 minutes with a insulin-glucose clamp. Glucose lowered with insulin from 95 mg/dL to 45 mg/dL (adapted from Lee, 2004). Please refer to Figure 6 to connect the drop in blood glucose with prolonged QTc interval.

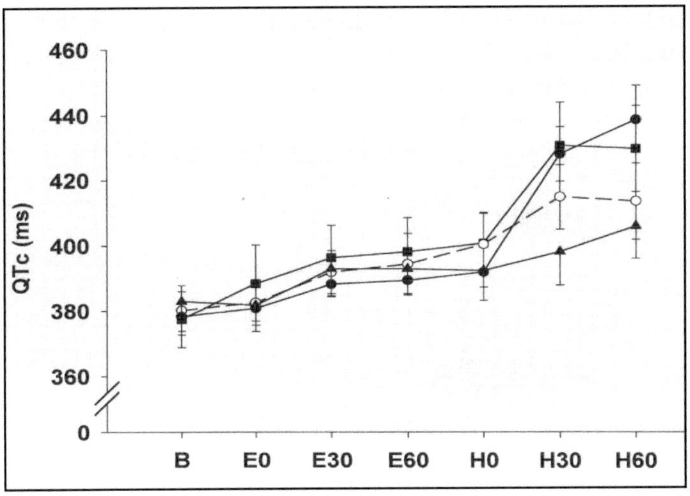

Fig. 6. The effect of noted hypoglycemia on QTc interval in ms. Mean ± SE QTc at baseline (B) after 0, 30, and 60 min of euglycemia (E0, E30, and E60, respectively) and hypoglycemia (H0, H30, and H60, respectively) (adapted from Lee, 2004).

6.1 Hypoglycemia and the brain

As glucose is necessary for the brain's metabolic function, frequent *severe* hypoglycemia results in an increased risk of brain cell death, and has been linked to an increased incidence of dementia (Bruce, 2009).

However, the Fremantle study presents a strong counter argument to this hypothesis, finding that elderly patients with hypoglycemia do not have persistent adverse neurological effects (Fremantle Diabetes Study, 2009). It should be noted that elderly patients with dementia are highly susceptible to hypoglycemia. This group hypothesized that the well recognized brain damage associated with repeated severe hypoglycemia is more likely in incidences in which symptom recognition and the ability to self-correct or seek assistance are impaired, for example in patients with cognitive impairment or dementia. Hypoglycemia may be the cause of death in type I and type II diabetics and is found in those who have severe secondary complications of diabetes, such as end stage renal failure or severe autonomic neuropathy.

However, hypoglycemia is a part of life for many diabetics. Some patients may be hypoglycemic, with blood glucose less than 50 mg/dL, up to 10% of the time (Cryer, 2007). As previously noted, type I diabetics can statistically expect to experience at least one major hypoglycemic reaction per year. Thankfully, death is rare in these instances. In primate studies, it takes 5-6 hours of hypoglycemia (blood glucose less than 20 mg/dL with an average of 13 mg/dL) to produce brain damage and brain death (Cryer, 2007). Thus, it is extremely difficult to cause brain death by isolated instances of hypoglycemia in diabetics who have good hormonal protective mechanisms and who do not have major complications. Brain dysfunction caused by temporal hypoglycemia, a condition that many clinicians treat daily, is usually reversed quickly with the reintroduction of glucose. Fully 70% of major hypoglycemic reactions which necessitate professional assistance are treated in outpatient facilities. In fact, a small benefit of recurrent moderate hypoglycemia is that the increase in neuronal glucose uptake transporters may actually ameliorate brain damage and cognitive dysfunction induced by severe instances of hypoglycemia, as the brain is able to obtain more glucose than would be expected in a naïve patient.

7. Recent hypoglycemia trial results (ACCORD, ADVANCE, VADT, NICE-SUGAR)

Hypoglycemia was found to be a major health issue for diabetics in four recent large-scale studies: the Action to Control Cardiovascular Risk in Diabetes Trial (ACCORD), the Action in Diabetes and Vascular Disease: Controlled Evaluation (ADVANCE), VA Diabetes Trial (VADT) and the Normoglycaemia in Intensive Care Evaluation and Survival Using Glucose Algorithm Regulation Trial (NICE-SUGAR). (NICE-SUGAR Study, 2009).

Each of the ACCORD, ADVANCE and VADT studies examined intensively treated diabetics as outpatients, and compared this population with standard treatments, with the major endpoints looking at CV death, non-fatal myocardial infarctions and strokes. Other macrovascular events were looked at in the ADVANCE and VADT.

Study Designs: **ACCORD, ADVANCE, VADT**

	ACCORD	ADVANCE	VADT
Major Endpoints	CV death -or- Non-fatal MI/stroke	CV death -or- Non-fatal MI/stroke -or- macrovacs event	CV death -or- Non-fatal MI/stroke -or- macrovacs event
Study	RCT	RCT	RCT
Design	Glucose intensive vs. standard arm, 2x2 BP control, +/- fenofibrate vs. placebo	Glucose intensive vs. standard arm, 2x2, +indamine vs. placebo	Glucose intensive vs. standard arm, 2x1, all BP and lipid Rx

Fig. 7. Comparison of the ACCORD, ADVANCE, and VADT studies.

7.1 The ACCORD study

In the landmark ACCORD study which revealed surprising results to the medical community, an increase in mortality in the intensively treated diabetes group was observed as compared to the standard therapy group. So adverse was the intensively treated regimen that the study was halted two years early.

The study's authors attributed increased mortality to weight gain, hypoglycemia and possibly specific medications. However, it is reasonable to assume that hypoglycemia was a major contributing factor. In the ACCORD study, the incidence of severe hypoglycemia was significantly higher in the intensively treated group. Over 15% of patients had severe hypoglycemia as compared to 5% in the standard treatment group. Increased mortality stemmed from cardiac issues such as cardiac arrhythmias, cardiovascular changes from hyperadrenalism (e.g. heart rate), vascular constriction with its attendant angina, myocardial ischemia and even myocardial infarction, or increased thrombotic tendency with decreased thrombolysis. Regardless of the absolute cause of increased mortality among intensively treated patients, it is clear that intensive treatment, with its extra time, cost, dedication, and more frequent episodes of hypoglycemia and anxiety, did not benefit long-term diabetic patients.

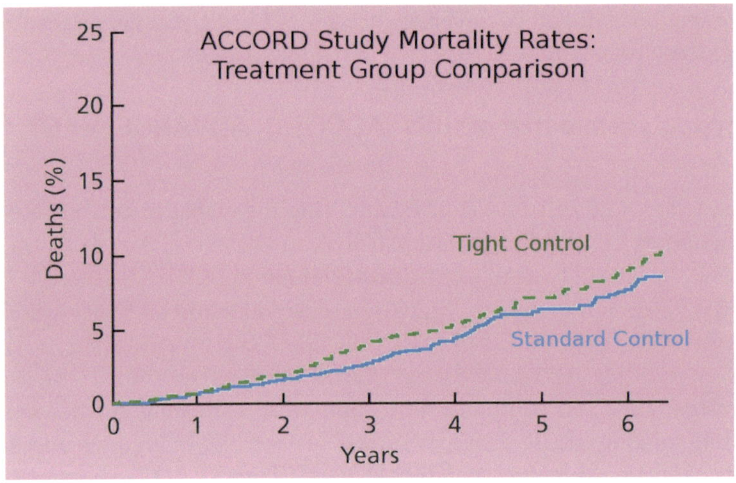

Fig. 8. Mortality rates among treatment regimens in the ACCORD study (adapted from ACCORD Study Group, 2011).

7.2 The ADVANCE study

In the ADVANCE study, gliclizide was used in the intensively treated group of type II diabetes patients and compared with standard therapy in over 11,000 patients. Though severe hypoglycemia was infrequent in both arms of the study, nearly twice the proportion of patients in the intensively treated group reported episodes of hypoglycemia (2.7% vs. 1.5%). The intensity of diabetes control was an independent predictor of microvascular and macrovascular events. There is also a significant correlation between severe hypoglycemia and all-cause mortality. This is true of both non-cardiovascular and cardiovascular mortality. From the results of the ADVANCE study, it can be concluded that hypoglycemia is at least a key marker if not the cause of clinical outcomes.

7.3 The VADT study

From the VADT trial, it appears that there can be harm from intense glucose control. This study examined the benefit of tight control in type II diabetics and developed the conclusions that tight control did not lower the risk of cardiovascular events, and that while tight control may be beneficial during the first ten years of diabetes treatment, it may be harmful to elderly patients.

7.4 The NICE-SUGAR trial

The NICE-SUGAR trial examined 6,108 patients in the intensive-care unit (NICE-SUGAR Study, 2009). There were two comparable groups who were treated differently, the intensively treated group (goal glucose 81-108 mg/dl) and the conventional therapy group (goal glucose glucose < 180 mg/dL). A total of 829 patients (27.5%) in the intensive-control group and 751 (24.9%) in the conventional-control group died during the study. In the trial there was a significant increase in severe hypoglycemic events observed in the intensively treated group as compared to the conventional therapy group, and an increase in mortality without any clear evidence of health outcome benefit. Indeed, mortality increased in the intensively treated group across all subgroups, including surgical patients. In critically ill patients, an association was revealed between even mild or moderate hypoglycemia and mortality. The more severe the hypoglycemia, the greater the risk of death. Again, with the added expense, increased work load on hospital staff and patients, and increased hypoglycemia, it can be concluded that there is no benefit in intensely treating diabetes in enfeebled populations, such as those in the intensive-care unit. Intensive treatment may very well be harmful.

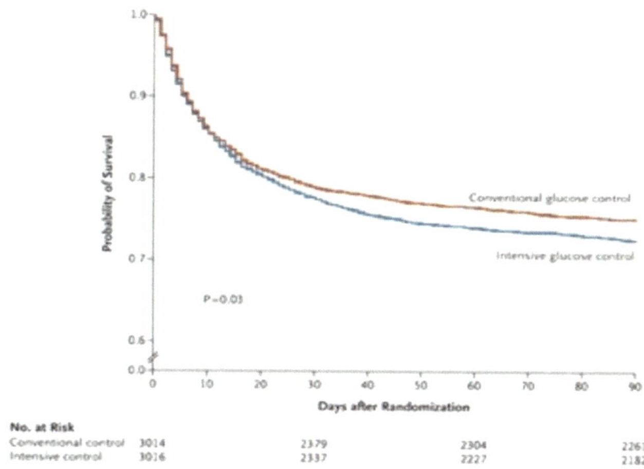

Fig. 9. Comparison of survival rates in the NICE-SUGAR study (adapted from NICE-SUGAR Study Investigators, 2009).

8. Hypoglycemia, anxiety and diabetes control

A non-trivial aspect of treating a diabetic patient with a history of hypoglycemic incidents is the potential resistance of the patient to an aggressive diabetes management plan. It has been shown that more than 54% of patients with diabetes are anxious about hypoglycemia most of or all of the time (Álvarez et al., 2008; Zhang, 2010). Diabetic patients with episodes of hypoglycemia reported significantly higher rates of shakiness, sweating, excessive fatigue, drowsiness, inability to concentrate, dizziness, hunger, asthenia and headache. These patients tend to allow their average glucose level to become higher, and are resistant to suggestions as to how to improve their diabetes control.

In treating patients clinically, it is clear that the worry of developing hypoglycemia stops many patients from achieving diabetes management goals. The more episodes of hypoglycemia, the lesser the compliance.

9. Hypoglycemia and health care costs

Hypoglycemia increases a patient's overall health costs significantly. In a cohort of 2,664 patients evaluated with a health-care claims database, the average annual health-care expenditure for diabetic patients with hypoglycemia was $3,169 versus $1,812 for diabetics who do not have hypoglycemia (Zhang, 2010). The average usage of short term disability in diabetic patients with hypoglycemia is approximately twice that of patients who do not have hypoglycemia (19.5 days annually vs. 11 days annually). In Sweden, a study assessed the burden of hypoglycemia in a 309 patient diabetic population over 35 years of age (Lundkvist et al., 2005). The results showed that 37% of patients reported symptoms of hypoglycemia during the preceding month. These patients were more affected by their diabetes, reported lower general health, and were more anxious about hypoglycemia than those without hypoglycemia. In this study, the direct and indirect costs of hypoglycemia per patient were estimated to be an additional $27 per month (in Sweden).

10. Hypoglycemia prevention

One antecedent hypoglycemic reaction decreases the epinephrine and symptoms score significantly for at least twenty-four hours. This blunted epinephrine response and hypoglycemic unawareness allows for increased incidences of hypoglycemia. Thus, hypoglycemia begets hypoglycemia, making it imperative for a patient to be particularly vigilant following a hypoglycemic reaction. This is especially important for two days following a hypoglycemic reaction. This entails more blood glucose monitoring and relaxing the blood glucose goal.

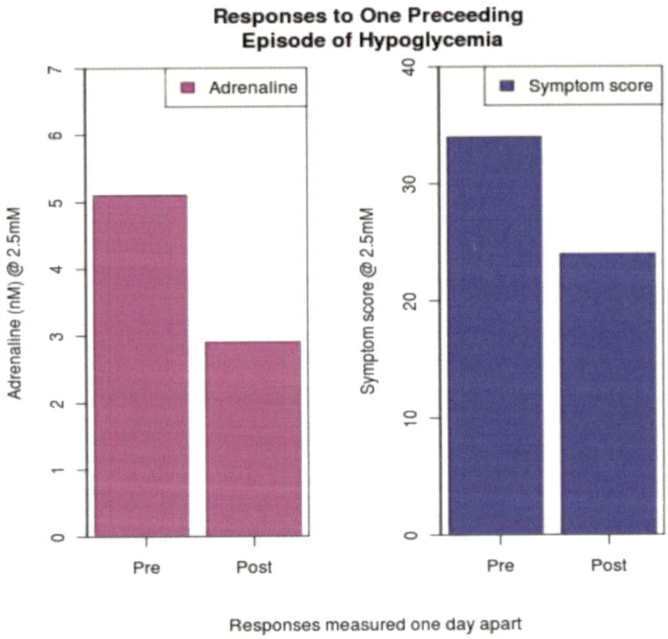

Fig. 10. Epinephrine and symptoms score, pre- and post-hypoglycemia (adapted from Heller, 2010).

For those with hypoglycemic unawareness, the pre-meal glucose level should be no lower than 140 mg/dL. The art of diabetic control comes into play, as the patient must be keenly aware of early signs of hypoglycemia. If hypoglycemia is anticipated, the patient must check his or her blood glucose levels using finger-sticks more often and he or she must try to identify patterns in a monitoring diary to predict potential causes of this insulin side effect. The insulin dose must do be adjusted with consideration of activity and lifestyle.

Without patient understanding and cooperation, there is little the physician can do to prevent hypoglycemia. Even raising the average glucose goal to very high levels will not suffice without the additional effort of more monitoring on the part of the patient. Training programs exist to help those with hypoglycemic unawareness (blood glucose awareness training, BGAT), and these have been shown to help patients significantly (Cox, 2001).

There is a novel approach of giving an *alpha glucosidase inhibitor* of the enteric enzyme which slows carbohydrate breakdown and thus prolongs absorption of carbohydrates in order to make glucose available for longer periods. This has been shown to decrease hypoglycemia.

Continuous glucose monitors are a new tool that enhances a patient's ability to achieve this. Currently, several continuous glucose monitoring devices are available (Guardian Real-time, Dexcom Seven Plus, Abbott Freestyle Navigator).

These devices all measure interstitial glucose levels, and though this metric lags whole blood glucose levels by at least 15 minutes, this provides the patient with relatively up-to-date information. It should be noted that these devices are designed to be supplemental to finger-stick glucose monitoring (Chico et al., 2003). They are designed to alert the patient if blood glucose levels fall past a pre-set level. These devices are particularly beneficial for patients who have frequent hypoglycemia and/or hypoglycemia unawareness (Beck, 2011). It can also identify dangerously low overnight blood glucose levels, as patients do not monitor their glucose level during this time. The STAR trial has shown that using these machines allows a 1% decrease in hemoglobin A1c levels without an increase in hypoglycemia.

10.1 Risks associated with elderly populations

In elderly diabetic patients who are experiencing episodes of hypoglycemia, the intensity of diabetes treatment should be reduced. A looser blood glucose range is more tolerable than hypoglycemic events, as this population is particularly vulnerable to accidents stemming from low blood sugar. A single hypoglycemic reaction could mean a fall, a broken hip, and a 50% six month mortality rate corresponding to elderly patients post-fracture.

In addition, elderly populations show a decrease in the counter-regulatory hormonal responses to hypoglycemia, and also a decrease in the symptomatic responses to hypoglycemia. Decreased cognition, renal impairment or polypharmacy are contributing causes. Hypoglycemia should be carefully monitored, as presenting features may be atypical and easily misinterpreted, resulting in delayed treatment. It should be noted that simply raising the hemoglobin A1c target level may not be adequate to prevent hypoglycemia in those with poor glucose control (Munshi, 2011).

10.2 Prevention in elderly populations

More frequent glucose monitoring is perhaps the best method for preventing hypoglycemia. With this approach, the elderly patient will be more quickly able to respond to dangerously decreasing blood glucose levels.

As recommended by the by the American Academy of Clinical Endocrinologists, elderly patients should avoid medications that cause hypoglycemia, such as sulfonureas. While these medications have excellent uses in other populations, they are more likely to be hazardous to elderly patients.

11. Treatment of hypoglycemia

During symptoms, whenever possible, a patient's blood glucose level should be checked. If the patient is found to be hypoglycemic, eating or drinking a sugary food is rapidly beneficial. The meal does not have to be large, but should provide a good deal of sugar. Examples are 2-3 glucose tablets, glucose gel, ½ cup fruit juice or soft drink, 1 tablespoon table sugar, or 4-6 pieces of hard candy. Following ingestion, the patient's glucose level should be checked within 20 minutes to make sure that glucose is rising. If blood glucose remains low (under 70 mg/dL), more sugar should be ingested. For patients with a history of hypoglycemia, a snack or drink containing sugar should be available at all times to take as soon as symptoms appear.

If a patient is found to exhibit hypoglycemia during sleep, decreasing the evening insulin and/or ingesting a complex carbohydrate or protein prior to bedtime should be recommended.

In situations where a hypoglycemic diabetic is non-cooperative or non-responsive, injectable glucagon may be given. The typical dose in a glucagon kit is 1 mg, which is sufficient to dose a 200 lb person. A full dose is usually not needed for someone weighing less than 150 pounds, such as a child. Side effects include nausea with an excess dosage, and for most patients a half dosage should be sufficient. If glucose hasn't risen in ten to fifteen minutes after the injection, the other half dose can always be given. This approach works rapidly, usually within 15-20 minutes, by causing a large egress of glucose from the liver.

A classic method for treatment of hypoglycemia is 1 ampule of intravenous 50% dextrose. The dosage for D50W is one half of the ampule, with verification of IV patency after the half of the ampule is given, and a recheck of blood glucose levels before administering the other half. 50% dextrose is heavily necrotic due to its hyperosmolarity, and should only be given through a patent IV line. Any infiltration can cause massive tissue necrosis.

12. Conclusion

As shown in the United Kingdom Prospective Diabetes Study (UKPDS) (UK Hypoglycaemia Study Group, 2007), patients with type II diabetes who tightly control their glucose levels during the first decade after diagnosis (hemoglobin A1c average of 7% vs 7.9%) exhibited a reduced risk of heart attack and death in subsequent years. This engenders within many patients a comfort with tight glucose control. However, patients who attempt tight control for longer durations of diabetes have significantly increased incidences of hypoglycemia, which increases morbidity and mortality. This is evident in both an outpatient or an inpatient setting. In general, patients with more complications from diabetes, older patients, more frequent episodes of hypoglycemia, and longer durations of diabetes lead to more severe instances of hypoglycemia. There are many possible pathological pathways for hypoglycemia to cause sudden death. Less intensive glucose goals to avoid the possibility of hypoglycemia are imperative to consider in the treatment of diabetics.

13. References

ACCORD Study Group. Long-Term Effects of Intensive Glucose Lowering on Cardiovascular Outcomes. N Engl J Med 2011; 364:818-828

American Diabetes Association. Defining and reporting hypoglycemia in diabetes. *Diabetes Care*. 2005; 28(5): 1245-1249.

Álvarez, Guisasola F., Tofé, Povedano S., Krishnarajah, G., Lyu, R., Marvos, P., Yin, D. Hypoglycaemic symptoms, treatment satisfaction, adherence and their associations with glycaemic goal in patients with type 2 diabetes mellitus: findings from the Real-Life Effectiveness and Care Patterns of Diabetes Management (RECAP-DM) Study. *Diabetes Obes Metab*. 2008; 10(suppl 1): 25-32.

Beck, R. Juvenile Diabetes Research Foundation continous glucose monitoring study group: Factors predictive of severe hypoglycemia in type 1 diabetes. *Diabetes Care*. 2011; 10: 1111.

Ben-Ami, H., Nagachandran, P., Mendelson, A.and Edoute, Y. Drug-induced hypoglycemic coma in 102 diabetic patients. Arch. Intern. Med. 1999. 159:281–284.

Bolli, G. Abnormal glucose counter-regulation in insulin-dependent diabetes mellitus: Interaction of anti-insulin antibodies and impaired glucagon and epinephrine secretion. *Diabetes*. 1983. Vol. 32, No. 2: 134-141.

Bruce, D.G. Severe hypoglycaemia and cognitive impairment in older patients with diabetes: the Fremantle Diabetes Study. *Diabetologia*. 2009; 52: 1808-1815.

Chan, S.P., Ji, L.N., Nitiyanant, W., Baik, S.H., Sheu, W.H.H. Hypoglycemic symptoms in patients with type 2 diabetes in Asia-Pacific Real-life effectiveness and Care Patterns of Diabetes Management: the RECAP-DM study. *Diabetes Res. Clin. Pract.* 2010; 89(2): e30-e32.

Chico, A., Vidal-Ríos, P., Subirà, M., Novials, A. The continuous glucose monitoring system is useful for detecting unrecognized hypoglycemias in patients with type 1 and type 2 diabetes but is not better than frequent capillary glucose measurements for improving metabolic control. *Diabetes Care*. 2003. 26(4): 1153-1157.

Canadian Diabetes Association. Clinical Practice Guidelines Expert Committee. Hypoglycemia. *Can J Diabetes*. 2008. 32(suppl 1): S62-S64.

Cox, D. Blood Glucose Awareness Training (BGAT-2): Long-term benefits. *Diabetes Care*. 2001. Vol. 24, No. 4: 637-642

Cryer, P.E. Mechanisms of sympathoadrenal failure and hypoglycemia in diabetes. *J. Clin. Invest*. 2006. 116(6): 1470-1473.

Cryer, P.E. Hypoglycemia, functional brain failure, and brain death. *J. Clin. Invest*.2007. 117(4): 868-870.

Cryer, P.E., Davis, S.N., Shamoon, H. Hypoglycemia in diabetes. *Diabetes Care*.2003. 26(6): 1902-1912.

Davis, T. Determinants of severe hypoglycemia complicating type 2 diabetes: The Fremantle Diabetes Study. *Journal of Clinical Endocrinology and Metabolism*. 2009.

Donnelly, L.A. Frequency and predictors of hypoglycaemia in Type 1 and insulin-treated Type 2 diabetes: a population-based study. *Diabet. Med.* 2005. ;22(6): 749-755.

European Medicines Agency. Note for guidance on clinical investigation of medicinal products in the treatment of diabetes mellitus. Published May 30,2002. http://www.ema.europa.eu/docs/en_GB/document_library/Scientific_guideline/2009/09/WC500003262.pdf. Accessed September 7, 2010.

Heller, Simon. Hypoglycemia in Type II diabetes Module 1 and 2. *Ourceatus.org*. 2010.

Johnston, S. Evidence linking hypoglycemic events to an increased risk of acute cardiovascular events in patients with type 2 diabetes. *Diabetes Care*. 2011. 10-15.

Lee, S. Influence of Autonomic Neuropathy on QTc Interval Lengthening During Hypoglycemia in Type 1 Diabetes. *Diabetes.* 2004. Vol. 53, No. 6: 535-1542.

Lundkvist, J., Berne, C., Bolinder, B., Jönsson, L. The economic and quality of life impact of hypoglycemia. *Eur. J. Health Econom.* 2005. 6(3): 197-202.

Matyka, K., Evans, M., Lomas, J., Cranston, I., MacDonald, I., Amiel, S.A. Altered hierarchy of protective responses against severe hypoglycemia in normal aging in healthy men. *Diabetes Care.* 1997. 20(2): 135-141.

McCrimmon, R., Sherwin, R. Hypoglycemia in Type 1 Diabetes. *Diabetes.* 2010. 59(10): 2333-2339.

Meneilly, G.S., Cheung, E., Tuokko, H. Altered responses to hypoglycemia of healthy elderly people. *J. Clin. Endocrinol. Metab.* 1994. 78(6): 1341-1348.

Munshi, M. Frequent Hypoglycemia Among Elderly Patients With Poor Glycemic Control. *Arch. Intern. Med.* 2011. 171(4): 363-364.

NICE-SUGAR Study Investigators. Intensive versus Conventional Glucose Control in Critically Ill Patients. *N. Engl. J. Med.* 2009. 360: 1283-1297.

Piette, J.D., Richardson, C., Valenstein, M. Addressing the Needs of Patients With Multiple Chronic Illnesses: The Case of Diabetes and Depression. *The American Journal of Managed Care.* 2004. 10:152-162.

Rossetti, P. Prevention of hypoglycemia while achieving good glycemic control in type 1 diabetes: the role of insulin analogs. *Diabetes Care.* 2008. *31: S113-20.*

Spiller, H.A. Unintentional Therapeutic Errors Involving Insulin in the Ambulatory Setting Reported to Poison Centers. *The Annals of Pharmacotherapy.* 2011. 45(1): 1-6.

UK Hypoglycaemia Study Group. *Diabetolgia.* 2007. 50: 1140-1147.

Warren, R.E., Hypoglycaemia and cognitive function. *Diabetes Obes. Metab.* 2005. 7: 493-503.

Yale, J.F., Begg, I., Gerstein, H. Canadian Diabetes Association clinical practice guidelines for the prevention and management of hypoglycemia in diabetes. *Can. J. Diabetes.* 2001. 26(1): 22-35.

Zhang, Y. The Burden of hypoglycemia in type 2 diabetes: A systemic review of patient and economic perspectives. *JCOM Journal.* 2010. Vol 17, No. 12: 547-557.